D0853691

Thyroid Disorders and Diseases

Guest Editor

KENNETH D. BURMAN, MD

MEDICAL CLINICS
OF NORTH AMERICA

www.medical.theclinics.com

March 2012 • Volume 96 • Number 2

SAUNDERS an imprint of ELSEVIER, Inc.

W.B. SAUNDERS COMPANY
A Division of Elsevier Inc.

1600 John F. Kennedy Boulevard ● Suite 1800 ● Philadelphia, Pennsylvania 19103-2899

http://www.theclinics.com

MEDICAL CLINICS OF NORTH AMERICA Volume 96, Number 2
March 2012 ISSN 0025-7125, ISBN-13: 978-1-4557-3891-5

Editor: Rachel Glover
Developmental Editor: Teia Stone

© **2012 Elsevier Inc. All rights reserved.**

This journal and the individual contributions contained in it are protected under copyright by Elsevier, and the following terms and conditions apply to their use:

Photocopying
Single photocopies of single articles may be made for personal use as allowed by national copyright laws. Permission of the Publisher and payment of a fee is required for all other photocopying, including multiple or systematic copying, copying for advertising or promotional purposes, resale, and all forms of document delivery. Special rates are available for educational institutions that wish to make photocopies for non-profit educational classroom use. For information on how to seek permission visit www.elsevier.com/permissions or call: (+44) 1865 843830 (UK)/(+1) 215 239 3804 (USA).

Derivative Works
Subscribers may reproduce tables of contents or prepare lists of articles including abstracts for internal circulation within their institutions. Permission of the Publisher is required for resale or distribution outside the institution. Permission of the Publisher is required for all other derivative works, including compilations and translations (please consult www.elsevier.com/permissions).

Electronic Storage or Usage
Permission of the Publisher is required to store or use electronically any material contained in this journal, including any article or part of an article (please consult www.elsevier.com/permissions). Except as outlined above, no part of this publication may be reproduced, stored in a retrieval system or transmitted in any form or by any means, electronic, mechanical, photocopying, recording or otherwise, without prior written permission of the Publisher.

Notice
No responsibility is assumed by the Publisher for any injury and/or damage to persons or property as a matter of products liability, negligence or otherwise, or from any use or operation of any methods, products, instructions or ideas contained in the material herein. Because of rapid advances in the medical sciences, in particular, independent verification of diagnoses and drug dosages should be made.

Although all advertising material is expected to conform to ethical (medical) standards, inclusion in this publication does not constitute a guarantee or endorsement of the quality or value of such product or of the claims made of it by its manufacturer.

Medical Clinics of North America (ISSN 0025-7125) is published bimonthly by Elsevier Inc., 360 Park Avenue South, New York, NY 10010-1710. Months of issue are January, March, May, July, September, and November. Periodicals postage paid at New York, NY, and additional mailing offices. Subscription prices are USD 232 per year for US individuals, USD 424 per year for US institutions, USD 117 per year for US students, USD 295 per year for Canadian individuals, USD 551 per year for Canadian institutions, USD 184 per year for Canadian students, USD 358 per year for international individuals, USD 551 per year for international institutions and USD 184 per year for international students. To receive student/resident rate, orders must be accompanied by name of affiliated institution, date of term, and the *signature* of program/residency coordinator on institution letterhead. Orders will be billed at individual rate until proof of status is received. Foreign air speed delivery is included in all *Clinics* subscription prices. All prices are subject to change without notice. **POSTMASTER:** Send address changes to *Medical Clinics of North America*, Elsevier Health Sciences Division, Subscription Customer Service, 3251 Riverport Lane, Maryland Heights, MO 63043. **Customer Service: Telephone: 1-800-654-2452** (U.S. and Canada); **1-314-447-8871** (outside U.S. and Canada). **Fax: 1-314-447-8029.** E-mail: journalscustomerservice-usa@elsevier.com (for print support); journalsonlinesupport-usa@elsevier.com (for online support).

Reprints. For copies of 100 or more of articles in this publication, please contact the Commercial Reprints Department, Elsevier Inc., 360 Park Avenue South, New York, NY 10010-1710. Tel.: 212-633-3812; Fax: 212-462-1935; E-mail: reprints@elsevier.com.

Medical Clinics of North America is also published in Spanish by McGraw-Hill Interamericana Editores S. A., P.O. Box 5-237, 06500 Mexico, D.F., Mexico.

Medical Clinics of North America is covered in *MEDLINE/PubMed (Index Medicus), Current Contents, ASCA, Excerpta Medica, Science Citation Index, and ISI/BIOMED.*

Printed in the United States of America.

GOAL STATEMENT

The goal of *Medical Clinics of North America* is to keep practicing physicians up to date with current clinical practice by providing timely articles reviewing the state of the art in patient care.

ACCREDITATION

The *Medical Clinics of North America* is planned and implemented in accordance with the Essential Areas and Policies of the Accreditation Council for Continuing Medical Education (ACCME) through the joint sponsorship of the University of Virginia School of Medicine and Elsevier. The University of Virginia School of Medicine is accredited by the ACCME to provide continuing medical education for physicians.

The University of Virginia School of Medicine designates this enduring material activity for a maximum of 15 *AMA PRA Category 1 Credit*(s)™ for each issue, 90 credits per year. Physicians should only claim credit commensurate with the extent of their participation in the activity.

The American Medical Association has determined that physicians not licensed in the US who participate in this CME enduring material activity are eligible for a maximum of 15 *AMA PRA Category 1 Credit*(s)™ for each issue, 90 credits per year.

Credit can be earned by reading the text material, taking the CME examination online at http://www.theclinics.com/home/cme, and completing the evaluation. After taking the test, you will be required to review any and all incorrect answers. Following completion of the test and evaluation, your credit will be awarded and you may print your certificate.

FACULTY DISCLOSURE/CONFLICT OF INTEREST

The University of Virginia School of Medicine, as an ACCME accredited provider, endorses and strives to comply with the Accreditation Council for Continuing Medical Education (ACCME) Standards of Commercial Support, Commonwealth of Virginia statutes, University of Virginia policies and procedures, and associated federal and private regulations and guidelines on the need for disclosure and monitoring of proprietary and financial interests that may affect the scientific integrity and balance of content delivered in continuing medical education activities under our auspices.

The University of Virginia School of Medicine requires that all CME activities accredited through this institution be developed independently and be scientifically rigorous, balanced and objective in the presentation/discussion of its content, theories and practices.

All authors/editors participating in an accredited CME activity are expected to disclose to the readers relevant financial relationships with commercial entities occurring within the past 12 months (such as grants or research support, employee, consultant, stock holder, member of speakers bureau, etc.). The University of Virginia School of Medicine will employ appropriate mechanisms to resolve potential conflicts of interest to maintain the standards of fair and balanced education to the reader. Questions about specific strategies can be directed to the Office of Continuing Medical Education, University of Virginia School of Medicine, Charlottesville, Virginia.

The faculty and staff of the University of Virginia Office of Continuing Medical Education have no financial affiliations to disclose.

The authors/editors listed below have identified no professional or financial affiliations for themselves or their spouse/partner:
Jaime P. Almandoz, MD, BCh; Rebecca S. Bahn, MD; Gabriela Brenta, MD; Rosalinda Y. Camargo, MD, PhD; Maria Grazia Castagna, MD, Sara Danzi, PhD; Leonidas H. Duntas, MD; James A. Garrity, MD; Hossein Gharib, MD, MACP, MACE; Rachel Glover, (Acquisitions Editor); Megan R. Haymart, MD; Steven P. Hodak, MD; Jacqueline Jonklaas, MD, PhD; Irwin Klein, MD; Joanna Klubo-Gwiezdzinska, MD, PhD; Priya Kundra, MD; Geraldo Medeiros-Neto, MD, MACP; Furio Pacini, MD; Maria Papaleontiou, MD; Geanina Popoveniuc, MD; Mary H. Samuels, MD; Stuart C. Siegel, MD; Marius N. Stan, MD; Nikolaos Stathatos, MD; Shannon D. Sullivan, MD, PhD; Eduardo K. Tomimori, MD, PhD; Andrew Wolf, MD (Test Author); and Cynthia F. Yazbeck, MD.

The authors/editors listed below identified the following professional or financial affiliations for themselves or their spouse/partner:
Kenneth D. Burman, MD (Guest Editor) is an industry funded research/investigator for Pfizer and Eisai; is an author for UpToDate and Medscape; is on the Advisory Board for the FDA, Endocrine Committee; is the Deputy Editor, Journal of Clinical Endocrinology & Metabolism; is on the Editorial Board, Medullary Thyroid Cancer Committee, for the American Thyroid Association.
Leonard Wartofsky, MD, MPH, MACP is a consultant for Asurogen.

Disclosure of Discussion of Non-FDA Approved Uses for Pharmaceutical Products and/or Medical Devices.

The University of Virginia School of Medicine, as an ACCME provider, requires that all faculty presenters identify and disclose any off-label uses for pharmaceutical and medical device products. The University of Virginia School of Medicine recommends that each physician fully review all the available data on new products or procedures prior to clinical use.

TO ENROLL

To enroll in the Medical Clinics of North America Continuing Medical Education program, call customer service at 1-800-654-2452 or visit us online at http://www.theclinics.com/home/cme. The CME program is available to subscribers for an additional fee of USD 228.

VISIT US ONLINE!
Access your subscription at:
www.theclinics.com

Contributors

GUEST EDITOR

KENNETH D. BURMAN, MD
Director, Endocrine Section, Washington Hospital Center, Washington, DC

AUTHORS

JAIME P. ALMANDOZ, MB, BCh
Fellow, Division of Endocrinology, Diabetes, Metabolism and Nutrition; Mayo School of Graduate Medical Education, College of Medicine, Mayo Clinic, Rochester, Minnesota

REBECCA S. BAHN, MD
Professor of Medicine, Division of Endocrinology, Metabolism and Nutrition, Mayo Clinic, Rochester, Minnesota

GABRIELA BRENTA, MD
Department of Endocrinology, Dr César Milstein Hospital, Buenos Aires, Argentina

KENNETH D. BURMAN, MD
Director, Endocrine Section, Washington Hospital Center, Washington, DC

ROSALINDA Y. CAMARGO, MD, PhD
Assistant Professor of Medicine, Thyroid Unit, Division of Endocrinology, University of São Paulo Medical School, São Paulo, Brazil

MARIA GRAZIA CASTAGNA, MD
Section of Endocrinology and Metabolism, University of Siena, Siena, Italy

SARA DANZI, PhD
Assistant Professor, Department of Biological Sciences and Geology, Queensborough Community College, Bayside, New York

LEONIDAS H. DUNTAS, MD
Professor of Endocrinology, Endocrine Unit, Evgenidion Hospital, University of Athens, Athens, Greece

JAMES A. GARRITY, MD
Consultant in Ophthalmology, Professor of Ophthalmology, Department of Ophthalmology, Mayo Clinic School of Medicine, Mayo Clinic, Rochester, Minnesota

HOSSEIN GHARIB, MD, MACP, MACE
Consultant, Division of Endocrinology, Diabetes, Metabolism, and Nutrition, Mayo Clinic, Rochester, Minnesota

MEGAN R. HAYMART, MD
Assistant Professor of Medicine, Division of Metabolism, Endocrinology and Diabetes, and Hematology/Oncology, Department of Medicine, University of Michigan Health System, Ann Arbor, Michigan

STEVEN P. HODAK, MD
Clinical Associate Professor of Medicine, Medical Director, Centre for Diabetes and Endocrinology, Division of Endocrinology and Metabolism, Department of Medicine, University of Pittsburgh School of Medicine, Pittsburgh, Pennsylvania

JACQUELINE JONKLAAS, MD, PhD
Associate Professor, Division of Endocrinology, Georgetown University Medical Center, Washington, DC

IRWIN KLEIN, MD
Private Practice, Great Neck, New York

JOANNA KLUBO-GWIEZDZINSKA, MD, PhD
Division of Endocrinology, Department of Medicine, Washington Hospital Center, Washington, DC; Department of Endocrinology and Diabetology, Collegium Medicum in Bydgoszcz, Nicolaus Copernicus University in Torun, Bydgoszcz, Poland

PRIYA KUNDRA, MD
Endocrine Section, Washington Hospital Center; Assistant Clinical Professor of Medicine, Georgetown University Hospital, Washington, DC

GERALDO MEDEIROS-NETO, MD, MACP
Senior Professor of Endocrinology, Division of Endocrinology, Department of Medicine, University of Sao Paulo Medical School, Sao Paulo, Brazil

FURIO PACINI, MD
Section of Endocrinology and Metabolism, Department of Internal Medicine, Endocrinology and Metabolism and Biochemistry, University of Siena, Siena, Italy

MARIA PAPALEONTIOU, MD
Fellow, Division of Metabolism, Endocrinology and Diabetes, Department of Medicine, University of Michigan Health System, Ann Arbor, Michigan

GEANINA POPOVENIUC, MD
Endocrine Fellow, Division of Endocrinology, Georgetown University Medical Center; Section of Endocrinology, Washington Hospital Center, Washington, DC

MARY H. SAMUELS, MD
Professor of Medicine, Division of Endocrinology, Diabetes and Clinical Nutrition, Oregon Health and Science University, Portland, Oregon

STUART C. SEIGEL, MD
Fellow, Division of Endocrinology and Metabolism, Department of Medicine, University of Pittsburgh School of Medicine, Pittsburgh, Pennsylvania

MARIUS N. STAN, MD
Consultant in Endocrinology, Division of Endocrinology, Metabolism and Nutrition, Assistant Professor of Medicine, Mayo Clinic School of Medicine, Mayo Clinic, Rochester, Minnesota

NIKOLAOS STATHATOS, MD
Thyroid Unit, Department of Medicine, Massachusetts General Hospital, Harvard Medical School, Boston, Massachusetts

SHANNON D. SULLIVAN, MD, PhD
Assistant Professor of Medicine, Georgetown University School of Medicine; Staff Physician, Department of Endocrinology, Washington Hospital Center, Washington, DC

EDUARDO K. TOMIMORI, MD, PhD
Assistant Professor, Section of Ultrasonography at the Hospital das Clínicas, University of São Paulo Medical School, São Paulo, Brazil

LEONARD WARTOFSKY, MD, MPH, MACP
Professor of Medicine, Department of Medicine, Washington Hospital Center, Washington, DC

CYNTHIA F. YAZBECK, MD
Fellow, Division of Endocrinology and Metabolism, University of Pittsburgh Medical Center, Pittsburgh, Pennsylvania

Contents

The thyroid gland produces thyroid hormone, which has clinically important actions practically in every system in the human body. Detailed knowledge of the physiology of the thyroid gland is critical for the proper management of thyroid disorders. The molecular biology of thyroid function is being studied in great detail. Clinically important molecules, such as the thyroid-stimulating hormone receptor and the sodium/iodide symporter, have been identified and well characterized. Such discoveries have significantly improved our understanding of thyroid physiology. As a result, new diagnostic and therapeutic approaches for the management of thyroid disorders are now available or in development.

Hyperthyroidism describes the sustained increase in thyroid hormone biosynthesis and secretion by a thyroid gland with increased metabolism. Although the use of radioiodine scanning serves as a useful surrogate that may help characterize the cause of thyrotoxicosis, it only indirectly addresses the underlying physiologic mechanism driving the increase in serum thyroid hormones. In this article, thyrotoxic states are divided into increased or decreased thyroid metabolic function. In addition to the diagnosis, clinical presentation, and treatment of the various causes of hyperthyroidism, a section on functional imaging and appropriate laboratory testing is included.

Hypothyroidism is the result of inadequate production of thyroid hormone or inadequate action of thyroid hormone in target tissues. Primary hypothyroidism is the principal manifestation of hypothyroidism, but other causes include central deficiency of thyrotropin-releasing hormone or thyroid-stimulating hormone (TSH), or consumptive hypothyroidism from excessive inactivation of thyroid hormone. Subclinical hypothyroidism is present when there is elevated TSH but a normal free thyroxine level. Treatment involves oral administration of exogenous synthetic thyroid hormone. This review presents an update on the etiology and types of hypothyroidism, including subclinical disease; drugs and thyroid function; and diagnosis and treatment of hypothyroidism.

Subacute, silent, and postpartum thyroiditis are temporary forms of thyroid dysfunction caused by thyroid gland inflammation. They classically present with a triphasic course: a brief period of thyrotoxicosis due to release of preformed thyroid hormone that lasts for 1 to 3 months, followed by a more prolonged hypothyroid phase lasting up to 6 months, and eventual return to a euthyroid state. However, the types and degree of thyroid dysfunction are variable in these disorders, and individual patients may present with mild or more severe cases of thyrotoxicosis alone, hypothyroidism alone, or both types of thyroid dysfunction.

Thyroid disorders are common in women during pregnancy. If left untreated, both hypothyroidism and hyperthyroidism are associated with adverse effects on pregnancy and fetal outcomes. It is important to correctly identify these disorders and treat them appropriately to prevent pregnancy-related complications. Levothyroxine is the indicated treatment for hypothyroidism, and thionamides are the treatment of choice for hyperthyroidism; thyroidectomy may be indicated in select cases. When thyroid cancer is diagnosed during pregnancy, a decision must be made regarding performing thyroidectomy during the pregnancy or postponing surgical resection until the postpartum period. Radioactive iodine is absolutely contraindicated during pregnancy and lactation.

Thyroid hormone has profound effects on the heart and cardiovascular system. This article describes the cellular mechanisms by which thyroid hormone acts at the level of the cardiac myocyte and the vascular smooth muscle cell to alter phenotype and physiology. Because it is well established that thyroid hormone, specifically T_3, acts on almost every cell and organ in the body, studies on the regulation of thyroid hormone transport into cardiac and vascular tissue have added clinical significance. The characteristic changes in cardiovascular hemodynamics and metabolism that accompany thyroid disease states can then be best understood at the cellular level.

Thyroid hormones regulate cholesterol and lipoprotein metabolism, whereas thyroid disorders, including overt and subclinical hypothyroidism, considerably alter lipid profile and promote cardiovascular disease. Good evidence shows that high thyroid-stimulating hormone (TSH) is associated with a nonfavorable lipid profile, although TSH has no cutoff threshold for its association with lipids. Thyromimetics represent a new class of hypolipidemic drugs: their imminent application in patients with severe dyslipidemias, combined or not with statins, will improve the lipid profile, potentially accelerate energy expenditure and, as a consequence, vitally lessen the risk of cardiovascular disease.

> The main causes of simple diffuse goiter (SDG) and multinodular goiter (MNG) are iodine deficiency, increase in serum thyroid-stimulating hormone (TSH) level, natural goitrogens, smoking, chronic malnutrition, and lack of selenium, iron, and zinc. Increasing evidence suggests that heredity is equally important. Treatment of SDG and MNG still focuses on L-thyroxine-suppressive therapy surgery. Radioiodine alone or preceded by recombinant human TSH stimulation is widely used in Europe and other countries. Each of these therapeutic options has advantages and disadvantages, with acute and long-term side effects.

> Thyroid cancer is the most common endocrine malignancy, although representing fewer than 1% of all human tumors. Differentiated thyroid carcinoma (DTC) includes the papillary and follicular histotypes and their variants, accounting for more than 90% of all thyroid cancers. Given the changing presentation of DTC in the last years, the aim of DTC management is to ensure the most effective but least invasive treatment, and adequate follow-up for a disease that nowadays is mostly cured just with surgery and is rarely fatal. This review addresses the multiple steps of current management, based on previous assumptions.

> This review presents current knowledge about the thyroid emergencies known as myxedema coma and thyrotoxic storm. Understanding the pathogenesis of these conditions, appropriate recognition of the clinical signs and symptoms, and their prompt and accurate diagnosis and treatment are crucial in optimizing survival.

Preface

Thyroid Disorders and Diseases

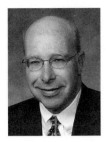

Kenneth D. Burman, MD
Guest Editor

Thyroid disorders and diseases are common and thyroid cancer is increasing at an alarming rate. It seems particularly propitious to have an issue of *Medical Clinics of North America* devoted to these general topics at the present time. Indeed, we are extremely fortunate to have contributions from a group of internationally respected authorities who review recent developments and put them into a practical clinical perspective. Important, clinically relevant topics such as thyroid hormone pathophysiology, evaluation and treatment of hyperthyroidism and hypothyroidism, and approach to thyroid emergencies are discussed. There are many newer aspects of thyroid pathophysiology and thyroid diseases that are being explored. For example, the normal TSH reference range in elderly patients is now considered different from younger individuals; thus, decisions with regard to which patients should be treated for hypothyroidism are now more complex. The application of modern technology, such as the use of molecular diagnostic techniques, sonographic elastography, and surgical approaches to patients with thyroid nodules and cancer, has already modified clinical practice. The variable and important effects of thyroid hormone excess and deficiency on cardiac function and lipid metabolism are also discussed. The pathophysiology, assessment, and treatment of Graves' ophthalmopathy, a particularly difficult disorder to treat, are reviewed. Diagnostic evaluation and management approach to patients with thyroid nodules, thyroid cancer, goiters, and thyroiditis are also discussed with practical, clinical advance given. Thyroid function in pregnancy is reviewed with clinical discussion regarding the expected changes in thyroid hormone metabolism during pregnancy. There are new recommendations regarding the approach to hypothyroid pregnant women who require additional levothyroxine therapy during gestation. There is an increasing movement toward developing evidence-based clinical guidelines. Recent guidelines regarding thyroid nodules and thyroid cancer, as well as thyroid physiology and perturbations in disease during pregnancy, are also highlighted.

Med Clin N Am 96 (2012) xiii–xiv
doi:10.1016/j.mcna.2012.02.004
0025-7125/12/$ – see front matter © 2012 Elsevier Inc. All rights reserved.

Chekhov said "Knowledge is of no value unless you put it into practice." We hope this issue will help you understand important and common thyroid disorders and diseases and that this knowledge will be applied in both clinical and research spheres to help humankind.

I am indebted to each of the authors, who eagerly discussed their topics in a detailed and clinically relevant manner. The editor is also indebted to Ms Forcina and Ms Glover from Elsevier, without whose assistance this edition could not have been accomplished.

Kenneth D. Burman, MD
Endocrine Section
Washington Hospital Center
110 Irving Street, NW, Room 2A-72
Washington, DC 20010-2975, USA

E-mail address:
Kenneth.D.Burman@Medstar.net

Thyroid Physiology

Nikolaos Stathatos, MD

KEYWORDS

- Thyroid physiology • Thyroxine • Triiodothyronine • Deiodinase
- Nuclear receptors

The thyroid gland is a butterfly-shaped organ located anteriorly to the trachea at the level of the second and third tracheal rings. It was so named by Thomas Wharton in 1656, not because of its shape (*thyreos* in Greek means "shield"), but because of its similarity in shape to the nearby thyroid cartilage of the larynx.[1]

Three major components play a role in regulating the production of thyroid hormones: First is the thyroid gland itself with its functional unit, the thyroid follicle; this is the location of synthesis and release into the circulation of thyroid hormone. The other 2 components are the hypothalamus and the pituitary gland.

THYROID EMBRYOLOGY

Embryologically, the thyroid gland is the earliest endocrine structure to appear during human development.[2] It originates from the embryonic endoderm. The earliest morphologic evidence for the thyroid gland is the thyroid enlage (or thyroid placode), a thickening of the endodermal layer in an area overarching the aortic arch.[3] The appearance is evident at about embryonic day 22 in humans. With the development of modern techniques in molecular biology, there is now evidence that the development of the thyroid enlage is not the first step in the development of the primitive thyroid follicular cells. The expression of transcription factors (such as the NK2 homeobox [Nkx2]-1 and paired box [Pax]-8) that are critical for the development of the thyroid gland has been documented 12 to 24 hours before thickening occurs. It is obvious that a complex, but recently more clearly elucidated sequence of embryonic events needs to take place for the normal development of the thyroid gland.[3] A defect in any of these events can lead to number of developmental thyroid anomalies that range from complete or partial agenesis of the thyroid gland[4] resulting in congenital hypothyroidism, to syndromes of reduced sensitivity to thyroid hormone.[5]

The primitive thyroid gland continues to expand ventrally while remaining attached to the pharyngeal floor by a stalk, called thyroglossal duct. As the gland expands laterally to form the 2 lobes, the lumen of the thyroglossal duct disappears, and in most cases the duct itself is no longer present at the end of this process. Occasionally,

The author has nothing to disclose.
Department of Medicine, Thyroid Unit, Massachusetts General Hospital, Harvard Medical School, 15 Parkman Street, WACC 730S, Boston, MA 02114, USA
E-mail address: nstathatos@partners.org

Med Clin N Am 96 (2012) 165–173
doi:10.1016/j.mcna.2012.01.007
0025-7125/12/$ – see front matter © 2012 Elsevier Inc. All rights reserved.

however, a significant remnant is not only detectable after birth or during adult life,[6] but significant abnormality can originate there, including thyroid malignancies.[7] Remnants of thyroid tissue or, occasionally, the only thyroid tissue in the body can be detected as distantly from the normal adult anatomic position of the thyroid gland as the base of the tongue, the embryonic origin of the gland.[8]

Thyroid hormone is first detected in the human fetal circulation at about 11 to 13 weeks of gestation. The responsiveness of the different developing tissues to thyroid hormones seems to be tightly regulated, as evidenced by a sufficient amount of thyroid hormone being critical for the proper development of specific cellular functions in embryonic neural cells[9] as well as the expression of different deiodinases at different time points, usually before specific developmental points. There is evidence, for example, that the development of specific parts of the brain is preceded by the increased expression of deiodinases in those regions that allows conversion of thyroxine (T_4) to the more active triiodothyronine (T_3). This step seems to be a critical and necessary one for the proper development of these regions of the brain. A large body of literature is now available, including guidelines from the major medical organizations (eg, the American Thyroid Association and the Endocrine Society), indicating the importance of proper management of thyroid dysfunction during pregnancy.[10]

A developmentally separate part of the thyroid gland is a group of cells that are present in between the thyroid follicles, called parafollicular cells (also called C-cells). Parafollicular cells are the main source of the hormone calcitonin, but their embryologic origin is different. These cells originate in the embryonic ectoderm and migrate into the thyroid gland during the development of the gland itself.

HYPOTHALAMIC-PITUITARY-THYROID AXIS

One of the most important regulators of thyroid function is the thyroid-stimulating hormone (TSH). TSH is a peptide hormone produced in the anterior pituitary gland, itself under the influence of both thyrotropin-releasing hormone (TRH), produced in the hypothalamus, and thyroid hormone (negative feedback, **Fig. 1**). TSH is very sensitive to small changes in levels of serum thyroid hormone (**Fig. 2**). This feedback system requires the regulatory action of the hypothalamus with the production of TRH. Thyroid hormone has a direct inhibitory effect on TRH production. By contrast, low levels of thyroid hormone lead to increased TRH synthesis in the hypothalamus, which is released into the portal circulation of the hypothalamic-pituitary system. TRH in turn stimulates TSH production in the pituitary gland, resulting in an improved level of serum thyroid hormone (through TSH stimulation of the thyroid gland) and restoration of the axis. TSH measurement in serum is now thought to be the most sensitive test available to clinicians for the diagnosis of most states of thyroid dysfunction, such as hypothyroidism or hyperthyroidism (exemptions include pituitary or hypothalamic disorders).[11]

Damage to the pituitary gland or the hypothalamus can lead to what is known as secondary hypothyroidism, which represents rare but challenging forms of hypothyroidism.[12] On rare occasions pituitary tumors can secrete TSH in excess, leading to secondary hyperthyroidism.[13]

PHYSIOLOGY OF THE THYROCYTE

The functional unit of the thyroid gland is the thyroid follicle (**Fig. 3**). This follicle is a cystic structure the wall, made up of a single layer of specialized epithelial cells often referred to as thyrocytes or follicular cells. The content of the follicle is termed colloid.

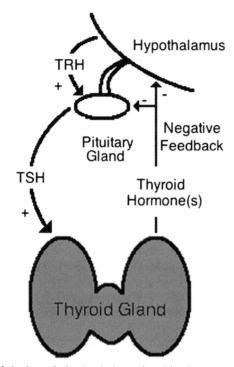

Fig. 1. Regulation of the hypothalamic-pituitary-thyroid axis.

It is largely made up of thyroglobulin (Tg), a large glycoprotein (∼660 kDa) that serves as the main storage form of thyroid hormone.

TSH exerts its effects on thyrocytes through its specific receptor known as the TSH receptor (TSHR),[14] located on the basolateral thyrocyte membrane. TSHR is a 7-trans-membrane G-coupled receptor protein. Its structure and role in thyroid pathology has been extensively studied. Antibodies against this receptor are central in the development of Graves disease, the most common form of hyperthyroidism.[15] The intracellular effects of activation of this receptor are mainly mediated by the stimulation of adenylyl

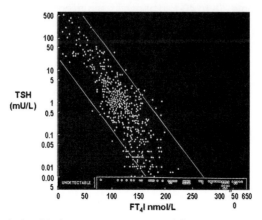

Fig. 2. Log-linear relationship between serum TSH and free T_4.

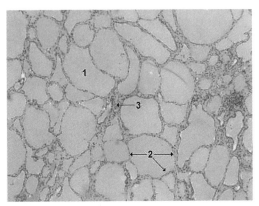

Fig. 3. Thyroid histology. (1) Thyroid follicle. (2) Follicular cells. (3) Parafollicular (C-) cells.

cyclase and the resulting increase in concentrations of intracellular cyclic adenosine monophosphate (cAMP).[16] TSH has a stimulatory effect on thyrocytes that results in increased iodine uptake and increased production of thyroid hormone. It also has a trophic effect on the thyroid gland. These actions have very important physiologic, pathophysiologic, diagnostic, and therapeutic implications. In cases of prolonged hypothyroidism, chronic exposure of the thyroid gland to increased levels of TSH results in the formation of an enlarged gland, also known as a goiter. Stimulating thyroid cells with TSH (endogenous or synthetic) is a critical and necessary step for both the diagnostic and therapeutic use of radioactive iodine in cases of thyroid cancer.

There are 2 main types of thyroid hormone: thyroxine (also called T_4 because it carries 4 iodine atoms) and triiodothyronine (also called T_3 because it carries 3 iodine atoms) (**Fig. 4**). Under normal circumstances, about 90% of the thyroid output is in the form of T_4 and about 10% is T_3. As evidenced by the amount of iodine in each molecule of thyroid hormone, this element is central and critical for the function of the thyroid gland. Thyrocytes concentrate iodine against a concentration gradient to be able to synthesize thyroid hormone. A complex molecular mechanism is in place for this synthesis (see **Fig. 4**) involving an active, energy-consuming process, with the sodium/iodide symporter (NIS) playing a key role.[17] The NIS is a transporter protein located at the basolateral membrane (**Fig. 5**). It has the ability to concentrate iodine in the thyrocytes some 20- to 40-fold above its serum concentration. This transporter has been studied intensively because it is a critical factor in many pathologic states,

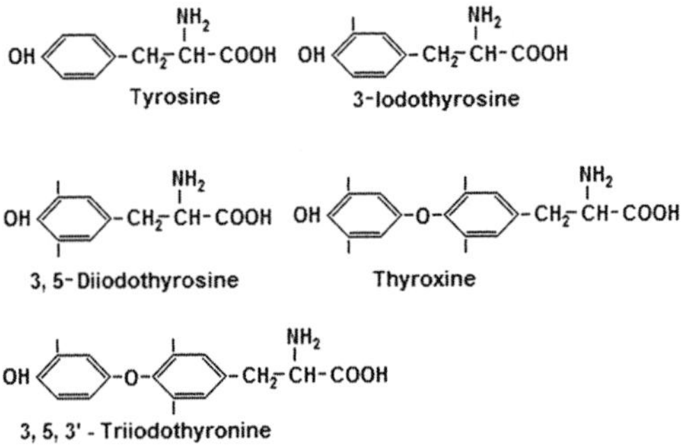

Tyrosine

3-Iodothyrosine

3, 5-Diiodothyrosine

Thyroxine

3, 5, 3' - Triiodothyronine

Fig. 4. Iodotyrosine compounds including T_3 and T_4.

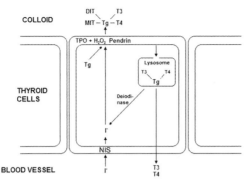

Fig. 5. Organification of iodine. DIT, diiodothyronine; MIT, monoiodothyronine; NIS, sodium/iodide symporter; Tg, thyroglobulin; TPO, thyroid peroxidase.

including thyroid cancer. Loss of expression in thyroid cancer cells leads to decreased iodine uptake in malignant thyrocytes, resulting in a reduced efficacy of radioactive iodine as both a diagnostic and therapeutic tool. Medications that may induce redifferentiation and reexpression of NIS have been investigated (lithium, rosiglitazone[18]) or are currently under investigation (eg, BRAF inhibitors).

Once in the thyrocytes, iodine is organified into tyrosine residues present in Tg. This process takes place at the apical membrane of these cells facing the colloid (see **Fig. 5**). The thyroid peroxidase (TPO) enzyme is a key player in this process, together with hydrogen peroxide.[19] TPO is a selenoprotein (a protein with selenium incorporated into its tertiary structure). The regulation of the activity of this enzyme is quite complex, iodine being a very important factor. Exposure to excess amounts of iodine is known to block TPO activity, a phenomenon known as the Wolff-Chaikoff effect.[20] Clinically this can lead to hypothyroidism. However, over time thyrocytes can eventually overcome this blockade, and this can lead to increased production of thyroid hormone. This phenomenon is known as the escape from the Wolff-Chaikoff effect.[21] These events are characteristically seen in thyrocytes that are replete of iodine. By contrast, when a thyrocyte deplete in iodine is exposed to iodine, it increases production of thyroid hormone significantly, often leading to biochemical and clinical hyperthyroidism. This process is known as the Jod-Basedaw effect.[22] The mechanism for this phenomenon is unclear, but it is thought to be caused either by rapid iodination of poorly iodinated Tg or by the fueling of a subclinical autonomous functioning thyroid tissue, as in a "hot" nodule or in Graves disease.[23]

TPO also seems to be a target in the autoimmune processes such as Hashimoto thyroiditis. Detection of antibodies against TPO is diagnostic of thyroid autoimmunity, usually Hashimoto thyroiditis,[24] although they are detectable in the majority of patients with Graves disease as well.[25]

Another protein closely involved in the organification of iodine together with TPO is pendrin (see **Fig. 5**).[26] A rare genetic disorder called Pendred syndrome includes the clinical findings of sensorineural deafness and a goiter attributable to partial iodine organification defect.[27]

Tg, as already mentioned, is a large glycoprotein that represents the main storage form of thyroid hormone. When thyrocytes are stimulated by TSH, Tg is endocytosed and cleaved to release T_4 and/or (T_3). Tg is critical for the normal function of the thyroid gland and its measurement is a very important clinical tool, mainly in the management of thyroid cancer. It is one of the more immunogenic thyroid-related proteins, and antibodies against Tg have been reported even in approximately 20% of people with no apparent thyroid pathology.

PERIPHERAL ACTIONS OF THYROID HORMONES

Thyroid hormones circulate in blood mainly bound to carrier proteins (less than 1% is circulating in a free unbound form). It is the small free amount of thyroid hormone that is thought to be metabolically active at the tissue level. More than 95% of the serum thyroid hormones are bound to 3 carrier proteins: thyroid-binding globulin (TBG), transthyretin, and albumin.[28] Thyroid hormone has also been shown to be bound to lipoproteins[29] and thyroid hormone autoantibodies of the immunoglobulin G class.[30] These carrier proteins function on one hand as an extrathyroidal depot of thyroid hormone, containing hormone that can be immediately available to peripheral tissues as needed, while on the other hand protecting them from exposure to excess amounts of thyroid hormone. The role of these carrier proteins is best illustrated in those unusual situations whereby genetic mutations lead to altered amounts and/or structures of these proteins and the resulting clinical and biochemical picture of the patients carrying these mutations. One such example is a condition known as familial dysalbuminemic hyperthyroxinemia, the result of mutations of the albumin gene, which leads to a 60-fold increase in the affinity of albumin for thyroxine.[31] Biochemically this results in an elevated level of serum thyroxine, a normal TSH, and a state of clinical euthyroidism.

Passive diffusion had been postulated to be the main mode whereby thyroid hormone(s) enter target cells. However, transporting proteins that seem to be critical in this process have now been identified. Members of this group include the monocarboxylate transporter 8 (MCT8), MCT10, and the organic anion transporting polypeptide 1C1 (OATP1C1).[32] Differential tissue expression has been documented, with OATP1C1, for example, being predominantly expressed in brain capillaries. OATP1C1 has a higher affinity for T_4 than for other iodinated compounds.[33] The clinical relevance of transporting proteins is again demonstrated in cases of genetic mutations. For example, mutations of the gene encoding MCT8 result in a clinical phenotype of severe psychomotor retardation and elevated levels of serum T_3.[34]

T_4 is often referred to as the prohormone, indicating that conversion to the active T_3 is required for biological activity. This conversion is catalyzed by a group of selenoproteins called diodinases. Three different isoforms have been described: D1, D2, and D3. Tissue-specific expression and different functions have been described for each of these.

Type 1 deiodinase (D1) has been shown to catalyze the conversion of T_3 to both the active triiodothyronine and its inactive counterpart, reverse T_3 (rT_3).[35] However, it seems to have an increased affinity for rT_3. As a result, it has been described a scavenger enzyme with a role of deiodinizing inactive iodothyronines, clearing them from the circulation, and recycling of iodine. A more recently noted function of D1 is in the biosynthesis of thyronamines, a class of endogenous compounds that appears to antagonize actions of thyroid hormone.[36] Although their exact role in thyroid physiology remains largely unknown, a promising therapeutic potential has already been described for thyronamines, as they represent the only endogenous compounds able to induce hypothermia as a prophylactic or for acute treatment of stroke.[37]

Type 2 deiodinase (D2) is the main thyroid hormone activator, converting the prohormone T_4 to the active T_3.[38] Furthermore, D2 regulates intracellular T_3 actions by regulating the availability of its nuclear receptors (thyroid receptors α and β). D2, together with D3, is the most important regulator of serum T_3 levels.

Type 3 deiodinase (D3) catalyzes the conversion of T_4 to the biologically inactive rT_3 and T_3 to 3,3′-diiodothyronine, which is also inactive. D3 likely represents the physiologic inactivator of thyroid hormones.[39] Rare cases of consumptive hypothyroidism have been described whereby D3 is overexpressed in hemangiomas. The result is a state of hypothyroidism caused by excessive degradation of T_3 and T_4.[40]

Thyroid hormones exert their actions mainly by binding and activating specific nuclear receptors. These receptors are transcriptionally active proteins that cause expression of thyroid hormone–responsive genes. The actions of thyroid hormones through these receptors are called genomic.

There are 2 major subtypes of thyroid receptors (TR): TRα and TRβ. However, there are several isoforms (TRα1, TRα2, TRβ1, TRβ2). Each isoform seems to have a tissue-specific function. For example, T_3-mediated cardiovascular effects are mediated by the TRα1 isoform,[41,42] whereas those on plasma cholesterol are mediated by TRβ1.[43] Recently, not only has manipulation of specific isoforms been shown to be clinically possible, but pharmacologic agents such as sobetirome or eprotirome, selective TRβ1 agonists, are currently entered in clinical trials for the management of hypercholesterolemia.[44]

More recently, nongenomic actions of thyroid hormone have been described that are mediated through either nonnuclear actions of these receptors[45–47] or novel cell-surface receptors.[48,49]

REFERENCES

1. Werner SC, Ingbar SH, Braverman LE, et al. Werner & Ingbar's the thyroid: a fundamental and clinical text. 8th edition. Philadelphia: Lippincott Williams & Wilkins; 2000.

2. Sgalitzer KE. Contribution to the study of the morphogenesis of the thyroid gland. J Anat 1941;75(Pt 4):389–405.

3. De Felice M, Di Lauro R. Minireview: intrinsic and extrinsic factors in thyroid gland development: an update. Endocrinology 2011;152(8):2948–56.

4. Topaloglu AK. Athyreosis, dysgenesis, and dyshormonogenesis in congenital hypothyroidism. Pediatr Endocrinol Rev 2006;3(Suppl 3):498–502.

5. Refetoff S, Dumitrescu AM. Syndromes of reduced sensitivity to thyroid hormone: genetic defects in hormone receptors, cell transporters and deiodination. Best Pract Res Clin Endocrinol Metab 2007;21(2):277–305.

6. Organ GM, Organ CH Jr. Thyroid gland and surgery of the thyroglossal duct: exercise in applied embryology. World J Surg 2000;24(8):886–90.

7. Klubo-Gwiezdzinska J, Manes RP, Chia SH, et al. Clinical review: ectopic cervical thyroid carcinoma—review of the literature with illustrative case series. J Clin Endocrinol Metab 2011;96(9):2684–91.

8. Toso A, Colombani F, Averono G, et al. Lingual thyroid causing dysphagia and dyspnoea. Case reports and review of the literature. Acta Otorhinolaryngol Ital 2009;29(4):213–7.

9. Oppenheimer JH, Schwartz HL. Molecular basis of thyroid hormone-dependent brain development. Endocr Rev 1997;18(4):462–75.

10. Haddow JE. The new American Thyroid Association Guidelines for thyroid disease during pregnancy and postpartum: a blueprint for improving prenatal care. Thyroid 2011;21(10):1047–8.

11. Spencer CA, LoPresti JS, Patel A, et al. Applications of a new chemiluminometric thyrotropin assay to subnormal measurement. J Clin Endocrinol Metab 1990; 70(2):453–60.

12. Yamada M, Mori M. Mechanisms related to the pathophysiology and management of central hypothyroidism. Nat Clin Pract Endocrinol Metab 2008;4(12):683–94.
13. Losa M, Fortunato M, Molteni L, et al. Thyrotropin-secreting pituitary adenomas: biological and molecular features, diagnosis and therapy. Minerva Endocrinol 2008;33(4):329–40.
14. Davies TF, Yin X, Latif R. The genetics of the thyroid stimulating hormone receptor: history and relevance. Thyroid 2010;20(7):727–36.
15. Smith BR, Sanders J, Furmaniak J. TSH receptor antibodies. Thyroid 2007; 17(10):923–38.
16. Kleinau G, Krause G. Thyrotropin and homologous glycoprotein hormone receptors: structural and functional aspects of extracellular signaling mechanisms. Endocr Rev 2009;30(2):133–51.
17. Hingorani M, Spitzweg C, Vassaux G, et al. The biology of the sodium iodide symporter and its potential for targeted gene delivery. Curr Cancer Drug Targets 2010;10(2):242–67.
18. O'Neill CJ, Oucharek J, Learoyd D, et al. Standard and emerging therapies for metastatic differentiated thyroid cancer. Oncologist 2010;15(2):146–56.
19. Mansourian AR. Metabolic pathways of tetraidothyronine and triiodothyronine production by thyroid gland: a review of articles. Pak J Biol Sci 2011;14(1):1–12.
20. Markou K, Georgopoulos N, Kyriazopoulou V, et al. Iodine-induced hypothyroidism. Thyroid 2001;11(5):501–10.
21. Eng PH, Cardona GR, Fang SL, et al. Escape from the acute Wolff-Chaikoff effect is associated with a decrease in thyroid sodium/iodide symporter messenger ribonucleic acid and protein. Endocrinology 1999;140(8):3404–10.
22. Woeber KA. Iodine and thyroid disease. Med Clin North Am 1991;75(1):169–78.
23. Ermans AM, Camus M. Modifications of thyroid function induced by chronic administration of iodide in the presence of "autonomous" thyroid tissue. Acta Endocrinol 1972;70(3):463–75.
24. Dayan CM, Daniels GH. Chronic autoimmune thyroiditis. N Engl J Med 1996; 335(2):99–107.
25. Chardes T, Chapal N, Bresson D, et al. The human anti-thyroid peroxidase autoantibody repertoire in Graves' and Hashimoto's autoimmune thyroid diseases. Immunogenetics 2002;54(3):141–57.
26. Scott DA, Wang R, Kreman TM, et al. The Pendred syndrome gene encodes a chloride-iodide transport protein. Nat Genet 1999;21(4):440–3.
27. Bizhanova A, Kopp P. Genetics and phenomics of Pendred syndrome. Mol Cell Endocrinol 2010;322(1-2):83–90.
28. Schussler GC. The thyroxine-binding proteins. Thyroid 2000;10(2):141–9.
29. Benvenga S, Gregg RE, Robbins J. Binding of thyroid hormones to human plasma lipoproteins. J Clin Endocrinol Metab 1988;67(1):6–16.
30. Benvenga S, Trimarchi F, Robbins J. Circulating thyroid hormone autoantibodies. J Endocrinol Invest 1987;10(6):605–19.
31. Pannain S, Feldman M, Eiholzer U, et al. Familial dysalbuminemic hyperthyroxinemia in a Swiss family caused by a mutant albumin (R218P) shows an apparent discrepancy between serum concentration and affinity for thyroxine. J Clin Endocrinol Metab 2000;85(8):2786–92.
32. Heuer H, Visser TJ. Minireview: pathophysiological importance of thyroid hormone transporters. Endocrinology 2009;150(3):1078–83.
33. Tohyama K, Kusuhara H, Sugiyama Y. Involvement of multispecific organic anion transporter, Oatp14 (Slc21a14), in the transport of thyroxine across the blood-brain barrier. Endocrinology 2004;145(9):4384–91.

34. Brockmann K, Dumitrescu AM, Best TT, et al. X-linked paroxysmal dyskinesia and severe global retardation caused by defective MCT8 gene. J Neurol 2005;252(6):663–6.
35. Maia AL, Goemann IM, Meyer EL, et al. Deiodinases: the balance of thyroid hormone: type 1 iodothyronine deiodinase in human physiology and disease. J Endocrinol 2011;209(3):283–97.
36. Piehl S, Hoefig CS, Scanlan TS, et al. Thyronamines—past, present, and future. Endocr Rev 2011;32(1):64–80.
37. Doyle KP, Suchland KL, Ciesielski TM, et al. Novel thyroxine derivatives, thyronamine and 3-iodothyronamine, induce transient hypothermia and marked neuroprotection against stroke injury. Stroke 2007;38(9):2569–76.
38. Williams GR, Bassett JH. Deiodinases: the balance of thyroid hormone: local control of thyroid hormone action: role of type 2 deiodinase. J Endocrinol 2011;209(3):261–72.
39. Dentice M, Salvatore D. Deiodinases: the balance of thyroid hormone: local impact of thyroid hormone inactivation. J Endocrinol 2011;209(3):273–82.
40. Jassam N, Visser TJ, Brisco T, et al. Consumptive hypothyroidism: a case report and review of the literature. Ann Clin Biochem 2011;48(Pt 2):186–9.
41. Johansson C, Vennstrom B, Thoren P. Evidence that decreased heart rate in thyroid hormone receptor-alpha1-deficient mice is an intrinsic defect. Am J Physiol 1998;275(2 Pt 2):R640–6.
42. Gloss B, Trost S, Bluhm W, et al. Cardiac ion channel expression and contractile function in mice with deletion of thyroid hormone receptor alpha or beta. Endocrinology 2001;142(2):544–50.
43. Gullberg H, Rudling M, Forrest D, et al. Thyroid hormone receptor beta-deficient mice show complete loss of the normal cholesterol 7alpha-hydroxylase (CYP7A) response to thyroid hormone but display enhanced resistance to dietary cholesterol. Mol Endocrinol 2000;14(11):1739–49.
44. Ladenson PW. Thyroid hormone analogues: ready for prime time. Thyroid 2011;21(2):101–2.
45. Hiroi Y, Kim HH, Ying H, et al. Rapid nongenomic actions of thyroid hormone. Proc Natl Acad Sci U S A 2006;103(38):14104–9.
46. Lei J, Nowbar S, Mariash CN, et al. Thyroid hormone stimulates Na-K-ATPase activity and its plasma membrane insertion in rat alveolar epithelial cells. Am J Physiol Lung Cell Mol Physiol 2003;285(3):L762–72.
47. Moeller LC, Cao X, Dumitrescu AM, et al. Thyroid hormone mediated changes in gene expression can be initiated by cytosolic action of the thyroid hormone receptor beta through the phosphatidylinositol 3-kinase pathway. Nucl Recept Signal 2006;4:e020.
48. Bergh JJ, Lin HY, Lansing L, et al. Integrin alphaVbeta3 contains a cell surface receptor site for thyroid hormone that is linked to activation of mitogen-activated protein kinase and induction of angiogenesis. Endocrinology 2005;146(7):2864–71.
49. Davis PJ, Davis FB, Cody V. Membrane receptors mediating thyroid hormone action. Trends Endocrinol Metab 2005;16(9):429–35.

Thyrotoxicosis

Stuart C. Seigel, MD, Steven P. Hodak, MD*

KEYWORDS
- Hyperthyroidism • Thyroid metabolic function • Thyrotoxicosis

Thyrotoxicosis describes a clinical syndrome that results from high concentrations of free thyroxine, free triiodothyronine, or both. However, the term hyperthyroidism is more specific and is used to describe the sustained increase in thyroid hormone biosynthesis and secretion by a thyroid gland with increased metabolism.[1] The causes of thyrotoxicosis have traditionally been arranged according to their pattern of radio-iodine uptake. Although the use of radioiodine scanning serves as a useful surrogate that may help characterize the cause of thyrotoxicosis, it only indirectly addresses the underlying physiologic mechanism driving the increase in serum thyroid hormones. We prefer to characterize the causes of thyrotoxicosis based on underlying thyroid metabolism as opposed to its imaging characteristics. In this article, thyrotoxic states are therefore divided into 2 main categories: increased or decreased thyroid metabolic function. In addition to the diagnosis, clinical presentation, and treatment of the various causes of hyperthyroidism, a section on functional imaging and appropriate laboratory testing is included. These sections are integral to establishing the foundation required to understand this article.

EPIDEMIOLOGY

Several large studies conducted in varying populations have contributed to the understanding of the prevalence of thyrotoxicosis (**Table 1**).

Generally, the prevalence of thyrotoxicosis is more common in women and populations with iodine deficiency.[2–4] Subclinical hyperthyroidism (SH), a condition associated with thyroid autonomy, is more common in areas of iodine deficiency.[2,4,5]

CLINICAL PRESENTATION

Disease-specific signs and symptoms of thyrotoxicosis are discussed throughout this article. These signs and symptoms are summarized in **Table 2**.[6]

Division of Endocrinology and Metabolism, Department of Medicine, University of Pittsburgh School of Medicine, 3601 Fifth Avenue, Suite 587, Pittsburgh, PA 15213, USA
* Corresponding author.
E-mail address: sph12@pitt.edu

Med Clin N Am 96 (2012) 175–201
doi:10.1016/j.mcna.2012.01.016
0025-7125/12/$ – see front matter © 2012 Elsevier Inc. All rights reserved.

medical.theclinics.com

Table 1
Epidemiology of thyroid disease

Study	Study Population	Prevalence of Thyrotoxicosis
Iodine-Sufficient Population		
Wickham survey[2]	Mixed urban and rural community aged 18 years and older in northeast England	1.9%–2.7% of women had thyrotoxicosis <0.16%–0.23% of men had thyrotoxicosis
NHANES III[3]	US civilian noninstitutionalized population aged 12 years and older	1.2% or the equivalent of 2,610,097 people had thyrotoxicosis
Iodine-Deficient Population		
Pescopagano survey[4]	Population of all ages located in Pescopagano, Italy, a southern Italian village	2.9% of adults had thyrotoxicosis of which only 0.9% was toxic diffuse goiter whereas 2.0% was toxic nodular goiter.
Subclinical hyperthyroidism (SH)		
NHANES III[3]	US civilian noninstitutionalized population	0.7% of the population have SH
Colorado Thyroid Disease Prevalence Study[5]	Participants in a statewide health fair in Colorado, 1995 aged 18 years and older	2.1% of individuals had SH More common in women than in men
Wickham survey[2]	Mixed urban and rural community in northeast England	Prevalence of SH was 0.6%
Pescopagano survey[4]	Population of all ages located in Pescopagano, Italy, a southern Italian village	Prevalence of SH was 6.4%

FUNCTIONAL THYROID IMAGING

There are multiple imaging modalities that can be used to help determine the cause of a thyrotoxic state. In this section the usefulness of radioiodine, technetium 99m (Tc 99m) pertechnetate, and ultrasonography is discussed. Although they are all helpful

Table 2
Clinical symptoms and signs of thyrotoxicosis

Symptoms of Thyrotoxicosis in Order of Decreasing Frequency	Clinical Signs of Thyrotoxicosis
Weight loss (most common)	Atrial fibrillation[a]
Heat intolerance	Tremor
Tremor	Palpable goiter[b]
Palpitations	Thyroid eye disease in Graves disease
Anxiety	
Increased frequency of bowel movement	
Neck enlargement	
Shortness of breath	
Weight gain	

[a] More common in elderly patients.
[b] Less common in elderly patients.
Data from Boelaert K, Torlinska B, Holder RL, et al. Older subjects with hyperthyroidism present with a paucity of symptoms and signs: a large cross-sectional study. J Clin Endocrinol Metab 2010;95(6):2715–26.

in the diagnosis of thyrotoxicosis, they each have specific benefits and limitations. An appreciation of these factors can help the clinician choose the most appropriate test in any given clinical context.

Radionuclide Imaging

Radionuclide imaging of the thyroid continues to be an important diagnostic tool in the investigation of hyperthyroidism. Of the many different radioactive compounds, Tc 99m and iodine 123 (I 123) are the most commonly used agents for imaging the thyroid.[7] These tracers undergo trapping by the sodium iodide symporter in the thyroid.

In contrast to Tc 99m, I 123 undergoes organification and is incorporated into thyroid hormones, allowing for the determination of true uptake, which may be more reflective of thyroid physiology.[7,8] I 123 has a relatively short half-life of 13 hours and emits only photons and is therefore preferred for diagnostic testing. After administration, uptake measurements are made 4 to 24 hours later.[7,9] The fractional uptake of radioactive iodine in the thyroid gland reflects the function of the sodium iodide symporter, the rate of internal iodine binding, and the rate of release of iodine from the thyroid. As noted by McDougall,[8] uptake within the first hour reflects iodine trapping, whereas uptake during hours 6 to 8 reflects uptake, oxidation, and organification. Measurements after this period reflect the balance of organification and radioiodine release from the thyroid. Standard protocols generally include a fractional uptake at 4 to 6 hours, followed by a repeat assessment at 12 to 24 hours. Early uptake at 4 to 6 hours is most helpful when the thyroid gland or nodule has markedly increased metabolism. In such cases, 24-hour uptake may be deceptively low because of increased iodine turnover. Otherwise, 24-hour uptake, which is a better integrative reflection of thyroid metabolism, is preferred.[9]

Thyroid imaging with Tc 99m represents an appealing alternative to I 123 scanning in some clinical settings. Unlike I 123, Tc 99m requires only 5 minutes to establish an estimate of thyroid activity.[7,9] Because of its shorter image-acquisition time, Tc 99m is often considered more patient friendly and may be the radionuclide of choice for patients who are unable to lie flat with their neck extended for long periods.[9] However, because Tc 99m is trapped but not organified by thyroid tissue, hypofunctioning or cold nodules may be misidentified as hyperfunctioning or hot nodules and vice versa.[9] Nonetheless, Tc 99m remains an effective agent for radionuclide imaging when it is necessary to distinguish diffuse increased uptake associated with Graves disease from the diffuse low uptake associated with thyroiditis. In such cases, Tc 99m scanning represents a quick and effective alternative to I 123 scanning. However, when thyroid nodules are present and the functional disposition of the nodules is in question, I 123 scanning remains the best mode of evaluation.

In patients with thyrotoxicosis, a radioactive iodine uptake should be performed when the clinical presentation is not clearly diagnostic of Graves disease or when thyroid nodularity is present.[10]

The pattern of radionuclide uptake enables the clinician to rapidly narrow the differential diagnosis of thyrotoxicosis. Diseases caused by increased thyroid gland metabolism such as Graves, toxic multinodular goiter (TMNG), and toxic adenoma (TA) typically show increased uptake because of either the increased activation of the thyroid-stimulating hormone (TSH) receptor via stimulating autoantibodies as in Graves disease or the autonomous function of nodules inherent to TMNG and TA. Disease states caused by decreased thyroid gland metabolism such as subacute (painful) or lymphocytic (silent, painless, or postpartum) thyroiditis show very low radionuclide uptake. T4 and T3 released during the inflammatory destruction of thyroid follicles suppress TSH, leading to decreases in thyroid metabolism, iodine trapping, and organification.[11] However, as TSH production increases during the recovery phase of thyroiditis, suppression of thyroid metabolism is reversed. If a radionuclide scan is performed during this phase of acute thyroiditis, it often shows increased uptake. If the clinician does not realize that the patient is going through the recovery phase, the pattern of diffusely increased uptake can be mistaken for the pattern associated with Graves disease, leading to erroneous diagnosis. This problem can be avoided by ensuring that TSH is suppressed at the time the radionuclide scan is performed.[7,9]

Ultrasonography

Thyroid ultrasonography can be used to differentiate between thyrotoxic states caused by increased and decreased thyroid gland metabolism. Increased blood flow and systolic velocity both in the thyroid arteries and the thyroid parenchyma may be used to clarify the cause of thyrotoxicosis. Kurita and colleagues[12] showed that a total blood flow area of 8% (calculated as thyroid blood flow area/thyroid area) measured using color Doppler ultrasonography has a sensitivity and specificity of 84% and 90%, respectively, for distinguishing Graves disease and destructive thyroiditis. Ota and colleagues[13] found that a thyroid blood flow of greater than 4% (measured quantitatively using power Doppler ultrasonography) differentiated Graves disease from thyrotoxicosis caused by thyroiditis. However, Doppler ultrasonography is operator dependent, and results may vary based on Doppler gain settings and the type of ultrasonographic equipment used. In addition, a standardized approach for assessing the cause of thyrotoxicosis with Doppler ultrasonography has not been codified, limiting widespread acceptance of this approach.[14] Nonetheless, this method has been shown in multiple publications to be reliable and is most useful when radioactive iodine scanning is contraindicated, such as during pregnancy and breast feeding, or not possible because of recent iodine exposure.[10]

LABORATORY TESTING

The most sensitive and specific assay for assessment of suspected thyrotoxicosis is TSH.[15] TSH is reported on a log-linear scale such that very small changes in free T4 are expressed as larger changes in TSH. This situation explains why TSH is considerably more sensitive than direct thyroid hormone measurements in detecting thyroid hormone excess. If hyperthyroidism is strongly suggested, the presence of an increased serum free T4 in conjunction with a suppressed TSH at the time of initial evaluation improves diagnostic accuracy because it confirms that the suppression of TSH is a result of thyrotoxicosis and not another cause.[10]

Typically, overt thyrotoxicosis presents with suppression of TSH and increases in either T4 or T3 or both. However, in milder thyrotoxicosis, TSH may be suppressed because of T3 toxicosis and present with normal levels of T4 and an isolated increase of T3. Such a pattern can occur during early stages of Graves disease, TMNG, or an autonomously functioning thyroid nodule.[10,16] For that reason, we recommend assessment of T3 in addition to T4 whenever a clinical suspicion of thyrotoxicosis exists.

The ratio of T3 to T4 may help distinguish whether thyrotoxicosis is caused by increased or decreased thyroid gland metabolism. Patients with hyperthyroidism related to Graves disease or TMNG have an increased serum ratio of total T3 to total T4. This finding is secondary to the production of thyroglobulin, with a higher T3 content and the increased thyroidal deiodination of T4 to T3 because of an accelerated and disordered thyroid metabolism.[17] Usually patients with Graves disease or TMNG have a T3/T4 ratio greater than 20, whereas patients with thyroiditis have a ratio less than 20.[18]

Thyroid receptor antibodies are not routinely required and are rarely needed to establish the cause of a thyrotoxic state. However, they do have some clinical usefulness. If thyrotoxicosis develops during pregnancy when radionuclide thyroid scanning is contraindicated, the measurement of thyroid receptor antibodies may prove useful for distinguishing Graves disease from gestational thyrotoxicosis. Because maternal TSH receptor antibodies also cross the placenta, they can stimulate the neonatal thyroid gland, resulting in fetal goiter or hyperthyroidism.[19] Therefore, mothers with a history of Graves disease, even if already adequately treated with radioiodine or a thyroidectomy, should have thyroid receptor antibody levels measured at 22 to 26 weeks of gestation to determine whether closer neonatal monitoring is needed.[10] Thyroid receptor antibodies may be helpful in establishing the diagnosis of Graves disease in the approximately 10% of patients who present without overt biochemical thyrotoxicosis but nonetheless have Graves ophthalmopathy.[20]

Two major types of assays are used to measure thyroid receptor antibodies. Radioreceptor assays measure the inhibition of binding of labeled TSH to TSH receptors in the presence of the patient's serum or serum IgG fraction. Antibodies measured by this assay are termed TSH receptor binding inhibitory antibodies (TBIIs).[20] TBIIs are found in 95% of untreated patients with Graves thyrotoxicosis, 50% of patients with Graves thyrotoxicosis who are in remission after cessation of thionamide therapy, and 15% of patients with chronic autoimmune thyroiditis.[21] In vitro bioassays measure the ability of the patient's serum or serum IgG fraction to increase the levels of cyclic adenosine monophosphate (cAMP) production in cultured cells. Antibodies measured by this assay are called thyroid receptor-stimulating antibodies or thyroid-stimulating immunoglobulins (TSIs). These antibodies are both more sensitive and since they are positive in 94% of patients with untreated Graves' disease, 91% of patients who relapse after a course of antithyroid medications, and only 10% of patients with chronic autoimmune thyroiditis.[22,23]

THYROTOXICOSIS CAUSED BY INCREASED THYROID GLAND METABOLISM
Graves Disease

Graves disease is the most common cause of hyperthyroidism. It is 5 to 10 times more common in women and the peak age of onset is between 40 and 60 years of age.[24,25] The typical symptoms of hyperthyroidism are present in most patients with Graves disease. Signs more specific to Graves disease include ophthalmopathy and, although rare, localized pretibial myxedema and clubbing of the digits known as thyroid acropachy.[25] Older patients when compared with younger patients are more likely to present with weight loss or depression than tachycardia and tremor.[26] This condition is sometimes termed apathetic hyperthyroidism. In addition, atrial fibrillation is a common presenting symptom in patients more than 50 years of age.[25]

Graves disease is primarily caused by circulating IgG antibodies against the TSH receptor.[24,25] These antibodies cause release of thyroid hormone and thyroglobulin, stimulation of iodine uptake, protein synthesis, and thyroid cell growth. Davies[27] noted that although most patients with Graves disease have both B-cell and T-cell lymphocytes directed against thyroglobulin, thyroid peroxidase, and the TSH receptor, it is primarily the TSH receptor antibodies that are responsible for the manifestations of this disease. Other antibodies are only secondarily involved.

Ophthalmopathy is a potentially sight-threatening disease that occurs in patients with Graves disease and has an annual incidence of 16 women and 3 men per 100,000.[28] Cigarette smokers are more likely to develop severe and treatment refractory ophthalmopathy.[28] Smoking therefore represents one of the most potent modifiable risk factor for Graves ophthalmopathy. Almost 50% of patients with Graves disease report symptoms of Graves ophthalmopathy, which include the sensation of dry and gritty eyes, photophobia, excessive tearing, double vision, and a sense of pressure behind the eyes.[28] Of patients with Graves ophthalmopathy, 3% to 5% have severe disease, with intense pain, inflammation, corneal ulceration or infection, and optic neuropathy secondary to optic nerve compression.[28,29] Enzmann and colleagues[30] showed that in patients without clinical ophthalmopathy, an orbital computed tomography (CT) scan still showed orbital muscle enlargement in up to 40% of patients. Up to 13% of patients with severe ophthalmopathy have pretibial myxedema, and 25% of patients with pretibial myxedema have thyroid acropathy.

Laboratory evaluation typically shows an undetectable TSH, an increased free T4 with an increased T3/T4 ratio. Evidence of thyroid enlargement and thyroid bruit with concomitant ophthalmopathy strongly suggests Graves disease and often obviates radionuclide scanning and thyroid antibody testing. However, a radioactive iodine uptake and scan may be useful when the diagnosis is in question.[10] Radionuclide testing usually shows diffuse increased homogeneous uptake. If a radioactive uptake and scan are contraindicated, as is the case during pregnancy or lactation, or are not feasible because of recent iodine exposure, measurement of Graves disease-associated antibodies such as TSI or TBII may be useful if Graves disease is suspected. As discussed previously, color Doppler ultrasonography may show increased thyroidal blood flow, which can be used to make the diagnosis of Graves disease as well.[10,12,13]

There are multiple options for the treatment of Graves disease. In patients with symptomatic thyrotoxicosis, a resting heart rate more than 90 beats per minute, or coexistent cardiovascular disease, a β-adrenergic antagonist should be started.[10] Adrenergic signs and symptoms such as tremor, tachycardia, systolic hypertension, nervousness, and anxiety also rapidly respond to β-adrenergic blockade.[31] For definitive therapy, patients with overt Graves hyperthyroidism should be treated with antithyroid medication (antithyroid drugs [ATDs]), I 131 ablation, or thyroidectomy.[10]

In contrast to European physicians, who favor ATDs and thyroidectomy as the therapies of choice, US physicians have been shown to prefer radioactive iodine ablation.[32,33] Radioactive iodine ablation is generally well tolerated and is associated with a relapse rate of about 21%.[25] About 80% to 90% of patients with Graves disease who undergo radioiodine ablation develop hypothyroidism.[34] Complications may include short-term worsening of hyperthyroidism and rarely include thyroid storm. Pretreatment and posttreatment with ATDs may thus be beneficial.[10] In addition, studies have shown an increased risk of worsening Graves ophthalmopathy in patients treated with radioactive iodine therapy. This situation is believed to be caused by an increase in thyrotropin receptor antibody (TRAb) levels as a response to greater antigen exposure as the thyroid gland is destroyed after treatment.[35–37]

In contrast to radioactive iodine therapy, thyroidectomy results in a relapse rate of only 5%.[25] Concern about possible adverse surgical outcomes has contributed to the decreased preference for thyroidectomy as the definitive treatment of Graves disease among physicians in the United States. However, high-volume surgeons have been shown to have very low complication rates of permanent hypocalcemia and recurrent laryngeal nerve injury. In addition, recent studies have shown a statistically significant association between increasing surgical experience and improved patient outcomes.[33,38,39]

The goal of antithyroid medication is to induce a euthyroid state by decreasing the production of thyroid hormones. Although spontaneous remission after ATDs is possible, Graves disease recurs in approximately 40% of patients.[25] ATDs are generally well tolerated; however, mild adverse side effects, including an abnormal sense of taste, pruritis, arthralgias, and urticaria, may occur in 1% to 5% of cases.[40] Agranulocytosis, a rare but dangerous complication, occurs with an incidence of 0.2% to 0.5% in patients taking methimazole or propylthiouracil (PTU), and often presents with a fever or sore throat.[41] In addition, both methimazole and PTU may cause hepatotoxicity, a serious side effect, which is reported in 0.1% to 0.2% of treated patients.[42] PTU-related hepatotoxicity usually takes the form of an allergic hepatitis associated with markedly increased aminotransferase levels and submassive or massive hepatic necrosis on liver biopsy.[42] The hepatic abnormalities associated with methimazole therapy are typical of a cholestatic process, with biopsy specimens showing preserved hepatocellular architecture along with intracanalicular cholestasis and mild periportal inflammation.[42] Antineutrophil cytoplasmic antibody-positive vasculitis has also been reported to be associated with ATD therapy.[42]

Given that ATDs, radioactive iodine ablation, and thyroidectomy have been shown to be effective and relatively safe, it is important to consider the logistics, benefits, expected speed of recovery, drawbacks, potential side effects, and cost before committing to a specific treatment modality (**Table 3**).[10] The physician can make a recommendation based on clinical judgment, taking into account the patient's personal values and preferences.

Toxic Adenoma

A solitary thyroid nodule that autonomously secretes a supranormal amount of T4 or T3 is termed a TA. Autonomous nodules typically cause suppression of TSH, resulting in metabolic suppression of the surrounding gland. This situation produces an archetypal radionuclide scan pattern, showing a focal area of increased uptake with marked photopenia of the surrounding thyroid. As opposed to Graves disease, which is mediated by an activating antibody, TAs are believed to result from a somatic mutation that intrinsically activates the cAMP cascade, causing increased growth and function of the follicular cells.[43]

There is an increased prevalence of autonomously functioning nodules in areas of iodine deficiency. In these regions, TAs can account for up to 10% of cases of thyrotoxicosis.[44] In areas of sufficient iodine supply, thyroid autonomy is rare. In the United States, Hamburger,[45] a clinical thyroidologist, showed that TAs represented 1% of his referral base of 39,487 patients. He also found that in addition to being more prevalent in women, solitary adenomas greater than 3.0 cm were more likely to be found in older patients and had a significantly higher likelihood of being toxic. Patients with TAs may present with signs and symptoms of overt thyrotoxicosis or SH or may be symptomatically euthyroid.[44]

The diagnosis of a TA is made using a combination of laboratory data and imaging. In addition to TSH, it is important to check levels of T3 as well as T4, because an increased incidence of predominant T3 hypersecretion is reported with solitary thyroid adenomas.[46] Once evidence of hyperthyroidism has been established, the next step is to order an uptake scan, which often confirms the diagnosis with the typical pattern of uptake noted earlier. This uptake pattern can be associated with overt or even subclinical thyrotoxicosis.[7] TAs occasionally undergo spontaneous infarction and involution. However, most TAs require definitive management with either I,131 radioactive ablation or thyroidectomy. Surgical resection has a risk of less than 1% for treatment failure, but a 2.3% risk of developing persistent hypothyroidism.[10] On the other hand, patients who undergo I 131 ablation have a 6% to 18% risk of persistent hyperthyroidism and a 5% risk of recurrent hyperthyroidism.[10]

Table 3
Factors that may play a role in determining the treatment of Graves disease

Modality	Favorable Factors	Contraindications
Radioactive iodine ablation	Women planning a future pregnancy in 4–6 mo Individual with high surgical risk Patients with history of external beam radiation to the neck or previous neck surgeries Contraindication to ATDs Lack of access to a high-volume thyroid surgeon	Pregnancy Lactation Coexisting thyroid cancer Suspicion of thyroid cancer Women planning a pregnancy in 4–6 months Inability to comply with radiation safety
ATDs	Patients with a high likelihood of remission (women, mild disease, small goiters, and negative or low titers of TRAb) High surgical risk or elderly patients with low life expectancy Patients with history of external beam radiation to the neck or previous neck surgeries Lack of access to a high-volume thyroid surgeon Patients with moderate to severe GO	Previous known major adverse drug reactions to ATDs
Thyroidectomy	Large goiters or symptomatic compression Low uptake of radioiodine Documented or suspected thyroid malignancy Coexisting hypoparathyroidism requiring surgery Women planning a pregnancy in <4–6 mo Patients with moderate to severe GO	Substantial comorbidity, cardiopulmonary disease, or end-stage cancer Pregnancy (relative contraindication)

Abbreviations: ATDs, antithyroid drugs; GO, Graves ophthalmopathy.
Data from Bahn RS, Burch HB, Cooper DS, et al. Hyperthyroidism and other causes of thyrotoxicosis: management guidelines of the American Thyroid Association and American Association of Clinical Endocrinologists. Endocr Pract 2011;17(3):456–520.

Toxic Multinodular Goiter

TMNGs show multiple autonomously functioning nodules that cause subclinical or overt hyperthyroidism. Like TAs, many studies have shown that the development of TMNG is also strongly correlated with iodine deficiency.[4,47,48] TMNG accounts for up to 50% of cases of thyrotoxicosis in iodine-deficient areas. In contrast, in regions of iodine sufficiency, TMNG accounts for only 3% to 10% of thyrotoxicosis.[44] Smoking, female sex, and having an enlarged thyroid gland are all risk factors for the development of TMNG.[49]

The pathophysiology of TMNG involves a multistep process, as theorized by Krohn and colleagues.[49] The first step consists of the development of thyroid hyperplasia from iodine deficiency, nutritional goitrogens, or autoimmunity. Increased proliferation and an increased rate of mutation then occur through several proposed mechanisms. When mutations include the TSH receptor and Gs-α signaling proteins, clones with constitutive activation of the cAMP cascade then arise. Such constitutively activated clones are then believed to further proliferate under the influence of growth factors, forming small clonal populations of autonomously functional tissue. These small lesions eventually expand to become clinically relevant autonomously functioning thyroid nodules.

Patients with TMNG may present with signs and symptoms of subclinical or overt hyperthyroidism. The diagnosis can be made based on a combination of laboratory, clinical, and imaging data similar to that described for TAs. However, the pattern of radionuclide scanning shows multiple nodules with increased uptake. Physical examination may reveal a heterogeneously enlarged thyroid. Nodules may also be palpable; however, even nodules greater than 1.5 cm elude detection by palpation in up to 60% of cases.[50] A radionuclide uptake and scan typically show areas of both increased and decreased activity scattered throughout the gland, reflecting the presence of hyperfunctioning nodules distributed within suppressed extranodular thyroid tissue.[9]

As with toxic solitary nodules, multiple toxic nodules also rarely involute and resolve spontaneously. Up to 95% of affected patients require definitive management with thyroidectomy or radioactive iodine ablation.[51] In patients undergoing I 131 radioiodine ablation, euthyroidism is achieved in 50% to 60% by 3 months and 80% by 6 months. Retreatment is required in approximately 20% of cases.[10] Surgical treatment with near-total or total thyroidectomy results in euthyroidism within days after surgery. In contrast to radioactive I 131 therapy, which can result in hypothyroidism, requiring exogenous replacement in 3% of patients at 1 year and 64% at 24 years, total thyroidectomy results in hypothyroidism nearly 100% of the time.[10]

Iodine-induced Hyperthyroidism

Iodine-induced hyperthyroidism (IIH) is typically a transient form of hyperthyroidism that occurs after iodine exposure in patients with several underlying thyroid conditions (**Box 1**). IIH is most commonly found in iodine-deficient areas and in elderly patients with long-standing nodular goiter.[52] In 1 endemic goiter area, the incidence of IIH was estimated to be up to 2%.[53] In contrast, within the iodine-sufficient United States, the prevalence of goiter is about 3% and the incidence of iodide-induced thyrotoxicosis is low.[52] Increased release of thyroid hormone by autonomous thyroid tissue after iodide repletion (**Box 2**) is believed to explain IIH.[54] Normally, excess iodine administration does not lead to increased thyroid hormone synthesis and release because of the Wolff-Chaikoff effect, which describes the inhibitory effect of iodine excess on thyroid iodide organification. In patients with underlying thyroid autonomy,

---

Box 1
Conditions in which iodine supplementation may lead to IIH

Endemic iodide-deficiency goiter

Euthyroid patients with Graves disease especially after ATD therapy

Patients with multinodular goiters who reside in areas of iodine repletion or deficiency

Nontoxic nodular goiter

Nontoxic diffuse goiter

Nodular functional autonomy

Data from Roti E, Vagenakis AG. Effect of excess iodide: clinical aspects. In: Braverman LE, Utiger RD, editors. Werner's and Ingbar's the thyroid. 9th edition. Philadelphia: Lippincott Williams & Wilkins; 2005. p. 290–300.

Box 2
Iodine-rich products

Iodine-containing vitamins

Kelp

Kombu, an edible kelp

Iodinated contrast agents

Amiodarone

---

there is an escape from this protective effect, known as the Jod-Basedow phenomenon.

In IIH, serum thyroid hormone levels are increased with a suppressed TSH. Radionuclide scanning typically shows uniformly diminished activity secondary to the competitive inhibition of radioiodine tracer uptake by the excess iodine.[9] β-Adrenergic antagonists alone or in combination with methimazole should be used to treat IIH, which typically resolves within 1 to 18 months.[10] Thyroidectomy may also be considered in patients who are allergic or resistant to ATDs.

Hyperemesis Gravidarum

Hyperemesis gravidarum (HG), a condition that is defined by persistent vomiting, marked ketonuria, and a weight loss greater than 5% during pregnancy, also causes abnormal thyroid function tests and hyperthyroidism.[55] The thyrotropic action of human chorionic gonadotropin (HCG), which is typically increased in HG, leads to an increase in T4 and suppression of TSH in 60% of affected women.[56–60] True hyperthyroidism, unrelated to HG, occurs infrequently during pregnancy, with a prevalence of about 0.1% to 0.4%. Graves disease accounts for 85% of these cases and should be excluded when primary thyrotoxicosis is considered.[19] The presence of a goiter, ophthalmopathy, severe tachycardia, or significantly increased TSH receptor or thyroid peroxidase antibodies (TPOAbs) may help distinguish patients with Graves disease clinically from those with HG.[61] HG usually spontaneously resolves by 20 weeks' gestation and pregnancy outcomes are generally excellent.[19,61] Unless symptoms are severe, treatment of HG with ATDs is rarely necessary. Affected patients with HG and thyrotoxicosis should be followed closely because of the associated anorexia, vomiting, and weight loss. Repeat thyroid function tests at intervals of 3 to 4 weeks are recommended.[10]

Gestational Trophoblastic Disease

Some forms of gestational trophoblastic disease (GTD) may present with significantly increased levels of circulating β-hCG. However, these patients rarely experience symptomatic hyperthyroidism. Walkington and colleagues[62] showed that among 196 patients with choriocarcinoma treated with chemotherapy in Sheffield, England, 14 (7%) were found to have biochemical hyperthyroidism, but only 4 were symptomatic. Lockwood and colleagues[63] found that women with hCG concentrations of greater than >400,000 IU/L, consistently had TSH suppression; however, few of these women showed signs and symptoms of hyperthyroidism.

Treatment of hyperthyroidism in patients with molar pregnancies should be directed toward the cause of the increased HCG levels. Extirpation of the tumor results in rapid resolution of the thyrotoxic state.[62,64] In symptomatically thyrotoxic patients with GTD, in addition to treating the primary tumor, treatment with ATDs may also be helpful.[10]

Although exceptionally rare, it has been shown that patients with molar pregnancy can develop thyroid storm, which requires appropriately intensive management.[64]

Testicular Germ Cell Tumors

There have been multiple case reports of thyrotoxicosis in patients with testicular cancer.[65,66] Most patients with hyperthyroidism from testicular germ cell tumors have metastatic choriocarcinoma.[67] The positive correlation between HCG and T4 levels suggests that HCG is also the cause of hyperthyroidism in these patients.[68]

Of patients with metastatic nonseminomatous germ cell tumors, 3.5% have hyperthyroidism and HCG levels greater than 50,000 IU/L. In addition, 50% of patients with HCG levels greater than 50,000 IU/L have hyperthyroidism.[66]

Recognition of thyrotoxic symptoms in patients with metastatic testicular germ cell tumors can be difficult because they may overlap with those of metastatic disease.[66] Therefore, screening thyroid function tests should be obtained in patients with HCG levels more than 50,000.[66]

Treatment of these patients with chemotherapy results in rapid decline in HCG and FT4; however, an initial rapid surge in HCG may occur and can rarely result in thyroid storm.[66] Treatment of hyperthyroidism may include a thionamide and a β-adrenergic antagonist if necessary in addition to treatment of the primary tumor.[10,66]

TSH-secreting Pituitary Adenoma

TSH-secreting pituitary adenoma (TSHoma) is a rare disease and accounts for less than 2% of all pituitary tumors, with an incidence of 1 case per million.[69] The number of recorded cases has tripled in the last decade as a result of the improved sensitivity of the immunometric assays for TSH. Although the tumor can occur at any age, most patients are diagnosed between the third and sixth decade of life.[70] These tumors are almost always benign; however, transformation into pituitary carcinoma has been reported.[71]

TSHoma presents with increased levels of circulating thyroid hormones in the presence of an unsuppressed TSH. When this pattern of thyroid function tests is present, the differential diagnosis includes TSHoma and pituitary resistance to thyroid hormone (PRTH), which is discussed later. Because most TSH-secreting tumors are macroadenomas, sellar imaging is important for confirming the diagnosis. The use of a molar α subunit/TSH ratio is also helpful when TSHoma is suspected. It is calculated by dividing the α subunit value (expressed as μg/L) by the TSH value (expressed as mU/L) and multiplying by 10. A normal ratio should be less than 1. This calculation is most helpful for assessment of TSH macroadenomas because it is increased in greater than 80% of cases. The calculation is less reliable in the uncommon setting of TSH macroadenomas, in which it is reported to be normal in 60% of cases. In addition, the ratio may be falsely increased in some normal patients, and may be substantially higher in normal postmenopausal women. This ratio should therefore be interpreted with appropriate caution.[72,73]

The diagnosis of TSHoma is often delayed. It is not infrequently confused with Graves disease because of the presence of a goiter, which often occurs as a result of chronic stimulation of the thyroid by the autonomous production of TSH. Inappropriate thyroidectomies and radioiodine ablations have been reported in such patients, who are often incorrectly diagnosed until they present with headaches and visual field deficits related to the mass effect of the tumor.[74] The initial treatment of choice is surgical revision of the tumor. If surgery fails or is not possible, somatostatin analogues and stereotactic radiation therapy can be considered. For thyrotoxic symptoms, ATDs and β-adrenergic blockers are helpful.[75]

Pituitary Resistance to Thyroid Hormone

PRTH is defined as an imbalance between hypothalamic-pituitary and peripheral response to thyroid hormone.[76] The mechanism underlying PRTH involves genetic mutations in one of 2 isoforms of the thyroid hormone receptor β subunits (TR-β1 or 2). Normal regulation of thyroid hormone secretion requires appropriate function of both peripheral thyroid hormone receptors (which contain TR- β1) as well as hypothalamic and pituitary thyroid hormone receptors (which contain TR-β2). Mutations affecting TR-β2 disproportionately more than TR-β1 lead to the development of PRTH.[77]

Patients with this condition may present with typical thyrotoxic signs and symptoms such as palpitations and tachycardia. On physical examination, a goiter is the most common finding.[78]

Similar to TSHoma, PRTH presents with increased levels of thyroxine and triiodothyronine in the presence of a detectable TSH. In contrast to TSHoma, PRTH typically presents with a normal α-glycoprotein subunit level/TSH molar ratio. In addition, a negative pituitary magnetic resonance imaging scan in a patient with thyrotoxicosis, increased T3 and T4 levels, and an inappropriately normal TSH is supportive of the diagnosis of PRTH.[75]

Treatment with 3,5,3′-triiodothyroacetic acid (a T3 analogue) and dextrothyroxine (a T4 analogue) have been used in patients with PRTH and have been reported to decrease peripheral hormone levels and TSH.[79] Bromocriptine, a dopamine agonist, blocks TSH secretion and can be used alone or in combination with thyroid hormone analogues. PTU, because it preferentially blocks type 1 deiodinase but not type 2, should reduce the intracellular content of T3 in the peripheral tissues but not in the pituitary thyrotrophic cells, which may restore the balance between peripheral and pituitary resistance in patients with PRTH.[76] Thyroidectomy can also be used in patients refractory to medical therapy.[80]

THYROTOXICOSIS CAUSED BY DECREASED THYROID GLAND METABOLISM
Postpartum Thyroiditis

Differing methodologies, study populations, and screening protocols have contributed to the varying prevalence of postpartum thyroiditis (PPT) reported in the literature. A large meta-analysis found that the pooled prevalence of PPT for the general population is 8.1%, whereas the prevalence across the world ranges from 4.4% to 9.3%.[81]

PPT is an autoimmune disease that develops during the period of immunologic rebound that can occur at any time during the first year after delivery. It has been shown that women who develop PPT are more likely to have specific alterations in T cells, an HLA-DR5 cell surface receptor, and increased titers of antimicrosomal autoantibodies and TPOAbs, implicating an autoimmune process.[81–83] Women with positive TPOAbs or a history of type 1 diabetes are respectively 5.7 times and 3 to 4 times more likely to develop PPT.[81]

PPT presents during the first postpartum year as transient hyperthyroidism, transient hypothyroidism, or transient hyperthyroidism followed by transient hypothyroidism. Most women recover to euthyroidism; however, 38% to 54% develop persistent hypothyroidism.[84,85] Recently, Stuckey and colleagues showed that a low urinary iodine concentration (UIC) at 6 months post partum was predictive of long-term hypothyroidism 12 years later. The investigators proposed that the low UIC was reflective of a more destructive thyroiditis, resulting in a greater depletion of intrathyroidal iodine stores and a greater TSH-driven retention of iodine in the hypothyroid phase.

Most affected patients present with a hypothyroid phase. However, 32% of women have an antecedent hyperthyroid phase, with 93% of the hyperthyroid episodes occurring at 6 months post partum.[85] Although most thyrotoxic patients develop symptoms, about one-third of patients are asymptomatic.[86] The thyrotoxicosis typically resolves in 2 to 3 months if left untreated. The TSH is usually low, and free T4 levels are increased or normal. Most often, TPOAbs are positive, whereas TSI and TBII are negative.

The development of postpartum Graves disease is less common than PPT, but it is necessary to distinguish between the 2 because management differs. Women with Graves disease typically have a more pronounced goiter and thyroid bruit. Ophthalmopathy when present is strongly suggestive of Graves disease, as is a marked increase in the T3/T4 ratio. An I 123 or technetium scan may be necessary to make the distinction between Graves disease and PPT. Both of these agents are excreted in breast milk, which contraindicates active nursing if a scan is performed. However, both agents have a short half-life, of 15 hours to 3 days and up to 36 hours for Tc 99m and I 123, respectively. Breast feeding should be discontinued for an appropriate period after treatment with one of these agents. Nursing can safely resume thereafter. β-Adrenergic blockers are also excreted in breast milk but may still be used to reduce the hyperadrenergic symptoms during the thyrotoxic phase of thyroiditis. If β-blockade is required for a nursing mother, the lowest dose possible should be used to minimize exposure to the nursing infant.[10] Although all β-blockers are excreted in breast milk, some have more favorable pharmacokinetics making use during pregnancy when medically necessary. Water-soluble β-adrenergic blockers with low protein binding such as atenolol, sotalol, and acebutalol are excreted in high levels in breast milk and should be avoided.[87] Because of their more favorable pharmacokinetics, we recommend use of the nonselective β-adrenergic antagonist propranolol or the β-1–selective agent metoprolol when symptomatic treatment is necessary. For propranolol, the maximum dose ingested by the infant is reported to be 0.1% of the maternal dose.[88] Metoprolol is rapidly cleared by infants with normal liver function.[10,88] Cessation of nursing should not be necessary when either of these medications is used at low to moderate doses.

Silent Painless Thyroiditis

Painless thyroiditis, also known as silent lymphocytic thyroiditis, is an uncommon cause of thyrotoxicosis, representing about 1% of all cases.[89] PPT and silent thyroiditis are similar and differ only because of the former's temporal relation to pregnancy. This disease is characterized pathologically by a focal or diffuse infiltrate of lymphocytes and is difficult to distinguish from chronic lymphocytic thyroiditis on biopsy specimens.[90]

Silent thyroiditis is an autoimmune disease manifested by positive anti-TPO antibodies in most patients, but the cause remains unclear. The search for viral antibodies in patients with silent thyroiditis has been unrevealing, but a case showing a familial pattern of silent thyroiditis suggests that genetic and environmental factors may play a role.[91,92] Medications such as lithium, sunitinib, interferon α, and interleukin 2 (IL-2) have also been reported to cause silent thyroiditis.[93–95]

Patients follow a clinical course similar to PPT, with a thyrotoxic phase lasting from 2 to 9 weeks followed by a short interval of euthyroidism and then a hypothyroid phase lasting about 4 to 16 weeks.[90] A return to normal thyroid function occurs in approximately 80% of patients.[89] However, even if normal thyroid function recovers, continued screening is recommended because long-term studies have shown that up to 50% of patients develop permanent hypothyroidism after an episode of silent thyroiditis.[96] It is possible to have repeated episodes of silent thyroiditis because there have been case reports of patients having up to 9 recurrences.[97]

Treatment of the thyrotoxic phase of silent thyroiditis involves β-adrenergic antagonists. Because new hormone synthesis is already suppressed in these patients, ATDs are not useful. Although not commonly required, corticosteroids have been used to improve symptoms and shorten the time course of the disease.[10] Thyroid replacement may be necessary during the hypothyroid phase, but should be reduced or stopped after 3 to 6 months to assess for recovery of normal thyroid function.

Subacute Thyroiditis

Subacute thyroiditis (SAT), also known as de Quervain thyroiditis or granulomatous thyroiditis, is a self-limited inflammatory disorder associated with thyroid tenderness and pain as well as abnormal thyroid function. The incidence of SAT has been reported to be 4.9 cases per 100,000 per year.[98] It occurs in up to 5% of patients with symptomatic thyroid disease and presents more often in women who are 40 to 50 years old.[89,98] SAT often follows an upper respiratory infection (URI), tends to be seasonal and geographic, and has been associated with infections by adenovirus, Coxsackie, Epstein-Barr, and influenza viruses. For these reasons a viral cause seems plausible; however, studies suggest that genetics may play a role as well.[99]

Clinically, as shown in a study of 94 individuals with SAT, patients often present with moderate to severe spontaneous thyroid pain and a history of an antecedent URI. In addition, they may have dysphagia, arthralgia, myalgia, tremor, sweating, and weight loss. On physical examination, the patient may be febrile and have a palpable goiter, with either diffuse or unilateral tenderness on palpation. In most patients, an initial thyrotoxic phase resolves after several weeks and hypothyroidism subsequently develops, with a course similar to that of postpartum and silent thyroiditis.[89] Fatourechi and colleagues[98] showed that although early transient hypothyroidism is common, only 15% of patients with SAT develop persistent permanent hypothyroidism. SAT has been shown to recur in 4% of patients.

A markedly increased erythrocyte sedimentation rate (ESR) is a hallmark of painful SAT. One study found that 86% of patients with untreated SAT had an increased C-reactive protein (CRP) level.[100] Free T4 levels are usually increased with ratios of T4/T3 of less than 20, whereas TSH is low or undetectable.[89] Serum thyroid antibodies are typically normal; however, they can be transiently increased during the acute phase, reflecting the release of antigen during inflammation as opposed to an autoimmune event.[99] Radioiodine uptake is low and thyroid ultrasonography shows decreased color-flow Doppler.

The initial treatment in these patients should include a β-blocker and a nonsteroidal antiinflammatory drug (NSAID) for pain relief. For patients who fail to respond to NSAID therapy, corticosteroids can be considered. Although corticosteroid therapy does result in symptomatic improvement, it does not prevent early-onset and late-onset hypothyroidism. Levothyroxine replacement therapy can be used in patients with symptoms of hypothyroidism; however, it should be withdrawn in 3 to 6 months to assess for recovery of normal thyroid function.[10]

Suppurative Thyroiditis

Acute suppurative thyroiditis (AST) is effectively an abscess within the thyroid. It is a rare but life-threatening endocrine emergency and is also a cause of thyrotoxicosis.[101–103] The rarity of this disease is related to the encapsulation, rich blood supply, extensive lymphatic drainage, and other various protective mechanisms inherent to the thyroid gland.[89] Patients have been reported to develop AST by direct inoculation through intravenous drug use, interventional procedures, esophageal rupture, or neck trauma or indirectly by hematogenous or lymphatic spread of infection. In addition, anatomic variants such as a pyriform sinus fistula, thyroid nodule, or thyroid cancer may predispose patients to AST.[104] Immunosuppressed, elderly, and debilitated patients are at a higher risk of acquiring AST.[89]

AST is most commonly caused by gram-positive and gram-negative aerobes; however, fungal, parasitic, mycobacterial, and opportunistic infections have also been reported.[105–109]

Patients can present with anterior neck pain, swelling, fever, dysphagia, dysphonia, and thyroid mass on palpation in addition to the other signs and symptoms of thyrotoxicosis.

Most patients with AST have normal thyroid function. However, thyrotoxicosis can develop secondary to the release of thyroxine and triiodothyronine from inflammatory destruction of thyroid follicles. Because both SAT and AST can be associated with acute thyroid pain and tenderness, thyrotoxicosis, an increased white blood cell count, and a low radioactive iodine uptake, thyroid imaging and fine-needle aspiration (FNA) may be necessary to distinguish between the two.[104]

Initial laboratory studies should include thyroid function tests, complete blood count, comprehensive metabolic panel, blood cultures, and human immunodeficiency virus screen. A CT scan with contrast of the neck and chest provides a detailed anatomic assessment of the soft tissue for enhancement and determines whether there is an abscess and the degree to which it may have extended into the retropharyngeal space or mediastinum.[110] In addition, CT may locate an anatomic abnormality contributing to the development of the infection.[111] Although ultrasonographic examination is useful and may be able to identify a fluid collection in the thyroid, it is less comprehensive in the evaluation of extrathyroidal involvement. If a fluid collection is seen on imaging, an ultrasound-guided FNA biopsy may be both diagnostic and therapeutic.

Treatment involves effective antibiotic therapy and elimination of formed abscesses. Anatomic abnormalities such as a pyriform sinus fistula, the most common source of infection in children, often require surgical resection or nonsurgical obliteration to prevent recurrent infection.[104] In patients with thyrotoxicosis, treatment with β-adrenergic blockers is effective. Similar to other forms of destructive thyroiditis, there is no role for ATDs.[10]

Radiation Thyroiditis

Radiation thyroiditis, a side effect of radioactive iodine therapy, is a painful inflammation of the thyroid and occurs in 1% of patients undergoing treatment. It can result in thyrotoxicosis as a result of the destruction-mediated release of thyroid hormone.[34] Treatment usually consists of NSAIDs, and β-blockers; however, steroids should be considered in patients with refractory pain. External beam radiation can also have effects on the thyroid, as shown by Nishiyama and colleagues,[112] who prospectively assessed acute reactions of the thyroid to external neck irradiation. These investigators followed thyroid function tests among 22 individuals who underwent radiation therapy with a treatment field that included the thyroid. Patients showed both mild biochemical thyrotoxic and hypothyroid phases; however, clinical symptoms did not occur. Increases in total T4, free T4, and total T3 trended upwards during radiotherapy but did not reach significance. At 6 months, which was the duration of the study, the TSH level was significantly higher than the initial baseline levels, whereas the free t4 was significantly lower. The investigators believed the small changes in thyroid function were a direct effect of radiation exposure, probably caused by mild thyroid inflammation.

Thyrotoxicosis Factitia

Thyrotoxicosis as a result of the exogenous administration of thyroid hormone is most often iatrogenic, occurring frequently in patients taking thyroid replacement for various reasons.[113] In addition, there have been reports of thyroid hormone abuse for the purpose of weight loss and energy enhancement.[114,115]

Distinguishing thyrotoxicosis factitia from painless sporadic thyroiditis may be difficult and requires a high degree of clinical suspicion. Both diseases may present with increased levels of thyroid hormones, a suppressed TSH, and a low radioactive iodine uptake. A serum thyroglobulin may be helpful because it is typically undetectable in thyrotoxicosis factitia and increased in thyroiditis.[116,117]

SPECIAL CASES
Struma Ovarii

Struma ovarii is an ovarian tumor, typically associated with a teratoma, that contains differentiated and potentially functional thyroid epithelium. Thyrotoxicosis is an unusual manifestation occurring in only 8% of patients with struma ovarii and is most commonly caused by autonomous function of the thyroid epithelium of the tumor.[10] Patients with Graves disease have rarely been reported to have persistent or recurrent hyperthyroidism caused by the action of the TRAb on the ectopic thyroid tissue.[118]

Laboratory evaluation reveals a suppressed TSH, an increased thyroglobulin level, and T3 level may be increased.[119] Radioactive iodine uptake is decreased at the thyroid; however, a whole-body radioactive iodine scan usually shows positive uptake in the pelvis.[120]

Surgical resection is the initial treatment of choice because of the risk of developing carcinoma. In cases of malignant struma ovarii, total thyroidectomy usually follows resection of the tumor to facilitate the subsequent use of ablative radioactive iodine therapy. Preoperative treatment with β-adrenergic blocking agents and ATDs may be necessary to establish euthyroidism before surgery.[10]

Metastatic Functioning Differentiated Thyroid Cancer

Thyrotoxicosis caused by metastatic thyroid cancer is rare. Most reported cases are caused by follicular carcinoma with functioning metastases in the lungs and bones at presentation. Papillary thyroid carcinoma has been reported in only 5 cases.[121]

Establishing the diagnosis of metastatic thyrotoxicosis requires the exclusion of a hyperfunctioning thyroid gland, evidence of radioactive iodine uptake in the metastatic lesions, and failure of the thyrotoxicosis to resolve after thyroidectomy.[122]

In most reported cases, hyperthyroidism was already established at the time the thyroid cancer was discovered. In the remainder of the cases, hyperthyroidism occurred after the diagnosis of thyroid carcinoma.[122]

The symptoms of hyperthyroidism in these patients can range from those of mild thyroxicosis to overt thyroid storm, which is reported occasionally.[113,123]

Treatment of these patients includes local debulking with surgery, interventional vascular procedures to disrupt tumor blood supply, and radioactive iodine with the addition of ATDs as needed. Thyrotoxicosis has been reported after thyrotropin injections used for imaging and iodine ablation and should therefore be used with appropriate caution in these patients.[10]

Subclinical Hyperthyroidism

SH is defined as a suppressed TSH, generally to less than 0.3 mIU/L, with a normal level of T4 and T3. In light of recent studies evaluating the long-term consequences of this disease, establishing the diagnosis and instituting treatment may be beneficial in certain patients.

Differing TSH cutoff values have contributed to the variably reported prevalence of SH reported in the literature. The NHANES III (National Health and Nutrition Examination Survey III) study, which represents the US civilian noninstitutionalized population, defined SH using a TSH cutoff value of 0.1 mU/L, and found the overall prevalence of SH to be 0.7%.[3] The Colorado thyroid disease prevalence study, which involved participants in a statewide health fair aged 18 years and older, used a TSH cutoff value of 0.3 mU/L and found the overall prevalence of SH to be 2.1%.[5] Generally, men and women more than 65 years of age have the highest prevalence of SH.[48]

To establish the diagnosis of SH, other causes of a low TSH level should be excluded. They may include pituitary or hypothalamic disease, euthyroid sick syndrome, certain medications, such as dobutamine, dopamine, or steroids, and excessive thyroid hormone ingestion. In addition, excess endogenous thyroid hormone production by Graves disease or a nodular goiter must be ruled out.[124]

There are multiple potential consequences of prolonged SH, which have led to the consideration of treatment. It has been shown that SH is an independent risk factor for atrial fibrillation.[125–127] The TEARS study (Thyroid Epidemiology, Audit, and Research Study) showed that patients with endogenous SH have an increased risk of cardiovascular disease and dysrhythmias.[128] The cardiovascular health study showed that patients with SH had no increased risk of developing heart failure. However, a more recent study showed that exogenous SH was associated with decreased myocardial strain on an echocardiogram, implying impaired cardiac function.[129,130] Some studies have shown an association between SH and dementia, whereas others have not.[131,132] An increased risk of hip fracture in men with SH has also been reported.[133]

SH is generally asymptomatic and typically discovered incidentally. Few patients with SH (about 0.5% to 0.7%) develop overt hyperthyroidism, whereas most continue to have SH. About one-third of patients with SH become euthyroid.[134]

Establishing the diagnosis of SH should include a thorough medical history, a repeat TSH test over a 3-month to 6-month period to establish that the abnormal thyroid function tests are not transient, and thyroid ultrasonography to evaluate for nodular thyroid disease. If nodules are noted on ultrasonography, then a radionuclide scan to evaluate for a TMNG or a TA should be obtained.

Once the diagnosis of SH is established, treatment is based on age, TSH level, symptoms, and comorbidities. If the TSH level is persistently less than 0.1 mU/L, treatment should be considered in all patients older than 65 years, postmenopausal women not on estrogens or bisphosphonates, patients with osteoporosis, cardiac risk factors or heart disease, and individuals with symptoms of thyrotoxicosis. If the TSH level is persistently less than normal, but greater than 0.1 mU/L, then treatment should be considered in individuals older than 65 year and in patients with cardiac disease or symptoms of thyrotoxicosis. The treatment should be based on the cause of the thyroid dysfunction and follow the same principles, as described throughout this article, for the various causes of overt hyperthyroidism.[10]

Amiodarone-induced Thyrotoxicosis

Amiodarone is an iodine-rich antiarrhythmic drug used for the treatment of cardiac arrhythmias. The iodine in amiodarone accounts for one-third of its total mass. This measurement is clinically significant because each 200-mg dose of amiodarone results in 6 mg of free iodine in the blood circulation. This dose is 20 to 40 times higher than the daily iodine intake in the United States.[135]

There are 2 types of amiodarone-induced thyrotoxicosis (AIT). Type 1 AIT is a form of IIH caused by the high iodine content of amiodarone. It occurs most commonly in patients with underlying hypermetabolic thyroid disease such as latent Graves disease or MNG.[135] These patients are often unable to regulate hormone synthesis in the setting of such a high iodine load. Type 2 AIT is a drug-induced destructive thyroiditis resulting from the direct toxicity of amiodarone and its metabolite, desethylamiodarone, to thyroid follicles.[136] The thyrotoxicosis in these patients is related to the release of thyroid hormone into the bloodstream from damaged thyroid follicular epithelium.

The reported prevalence of AIT varies based on regional iodine sufficiency. A recent study conducted in the Netherlands, which is a relatively iodine-deficient country, reported a 14% prevalence of thyroid dysfunction among 303 patients taking amiodarone, who were followed for 3 years. Among the patients with thyroid dysfunction, 8% developed AIT and the remaining 6% developed amiodarone-induced hypothyroidism.[137] An inverse correlation between dietary iodine intake and prevalence of AIT is reported in a study by Martino and colleagues[138] showing that hyperthyroidism was a more frequent complication of amiodarone therapy in the relatively iodine-deficient region of western Tuscany, but hypothyroidism was more frequent in Worcester, MA, where iodine intake is sufficient.

Clinically, the presentation of AIT is similar for both type 1 and 2. The onset of symptoms can develop early or after many years of amiodarone treatment. Because of the tissue storage and slow release of the drug and its metabolite, the effect of amiodarone can persist for a long time even after drug withdrawal. The classic symptoms of thyrotoxicosis may be absent because of the β-adrenergic–blocking properties of amiodarone and its impairment of T4 to T3 conversion. Patients may present with worsening of the underlying arrhythmia that initially led to the use of amiodarone. Ophthalmopathy is typically absent unless the patient has underlying undiagnosed Graves disease.[139]

Distinguishing the type of AIT is crucial because it determines the therapeutic approach. Imaging can often help differentiate between the 2 types of AIT. Thyroid ultrasonography may show a diffuse or nodular goiter, which suggests type 1 AIT. Color-flow Doppler sonography (CFDS) shows an absence of vascularity in patients with type 2 AIT and increased vascularity and blood flow velocity in patients with type 1.[140] Radioactive iodine uptake is usually very low in type 2 AIT, similar to other types of thyroiditis. Literature suggests that in type 1 AIT, RAI uptake may be normal or even increased.[141] However, in our experience we find iodine uptake is low in all forms of AIT, likely due to the systemic iodine intoxication resulting from the high iodine content of amiodarone. A Tc 99m thyroid scan has also been suggested as a useful tool.[141] Laboratory evaluation with IL-6 and CRP has been shown to have limited usefulness because of the considerable overlap that exists between affected patients and controls. Similarly, although a greater frequency of positive thyroid antibodies, particularly TRAb, is reported in patients with type 1 AIT, patients with type 2 AIT also have positive antibodies in 8% of cases.[141,142] This overlap reduces the clinical usefulness of this means of assessment.

Treatment depends on the type of AIT that is present. Type 1 AIT is treated with ATDs, because these drugs directly inhibit the increased thyroid metabolism responsible for the increased production of thyroid hormone. Because these patients often have iodine-replete thyroid glands, conferring resistance to the inhibitory action of thionamides, higher drug dosages (40 mg daily) and longer treatment periods (3–6 months) are necessary.[10] Potassium perchlorate 250 mg to 500 mg twice a day has also been used to improve the response to thionamides by decreasing thyroid iodine uptake and increasing thyroidal iodine discharge.[141] However, potassium perchlorate has been rarely associated with potentially fatal blood dyscrasias and is available in the United States only through compounding pharmacies that prepare the medication from reagent-grade chemical stock.[143] Our experience is that in many cases of type I AIT, perchlorate is an indispensable treatment adjunct.

Type 2 AIT, an inflammatory thyroiditis, is treated with corticosteroids and typically resolves in a few weeks. These patients should be treated with 40 mg prednisone once daily for 2 to 4 weeks followed by a gradual taper over 2 to 3 months.[10]

Occasionally, patients may not respond to single modality therapy caused by a mix of type 1 and type 2 AIT. These patients may require combined antithyroid and antiinflammatory medications.[10] The decision to stop amiodarone in the setting of thyrotoxicosis is controversial and should be made on an individual basis.

Hashitoxicosis

Hashimoto thyroiditis is the most common cause of hypothyroidism and goiter in the United States.[89] Patients may present with symptoms of hypothyroidism, goiter, or both.[144] Increased TPOAbs and thyroglobulin antibodies are present in 90% and 20% to 50% of patients, respectively.[89] Rarely, patients with Hashimoto thyroiditis may present with hashitoxicosis or the presence of biochemical hyperthyroidism. One study[145] performed in children found that of 69 total patients with autoimmune thyroiditis, 11.5% developed hashitoxicosis. All of these patients had spontaneous resolution of the thyrotoxicosis, with subsequent development of euthyroidism or hypothyroidism confirming the diagnosis. The duration of hyperthyroidism in these patients ranged from 31 to 168 days.

It is important to differentiate Graves disease from hashitoxicosis. CFDS may be helpful because it typically shows significantly increased vascularity in Graves disease and normal to only slightly increased vascularity in hashitoxicosis; however, the vascularity can be variable.[146] In addition, in Hashimoto thyroiditis, ultrasonographic examination usually shows a heterogeneous thyroid parenchyma with innumerable scattered small hypoechoic nodules separated by echogenic septa.[146] The presence of increased TPO and thyroglobulin antibodies with a negative TSI is also suggestive of hashitoxicosis.

Medication-induced Thyrotoxicosis

When evaluating a patient for hyperthyroidism, the differential diagnosis should include drug-induced thyroid dysfunction. This next section discusses some of the medications that have been reported to be a cause of thyrotoxicosis.

Drugs that contain iodine can cause IIH. As discussed earlier, patients with underlying thyroid autonomy or who live in iodine-deficient areas are at the highest risk of developing IIH. Some of the medications that contain clinically significant amounts of iodine include radiocontrast dyes, amiodarone, and topical povidone-iodine.[147] Ioxaglic acid, a component of intravenous contrast, has been associated with severe thyrotoxicosis, presenting with fever and marked neck tenderness.[148] Lithium, which is metabolized in the thyroid in a manner similar to iodine, has been reported to cause hyperthyroidism, with an incidence rate of 2.7 cases per 1000 person-years. It has been postulated that lithium may have a direct toxic effect on the thyroid gland because intrathyroidal lithium concentrations are higher than in the blood.[95] Sunitinib, a tyrosine kinase inhibitor, has also been associated with the development of destructive thyroiditis. The mechanism is not believed to be immune mediated but remains unclear.[94] One study found that the combination of IL-2 and IFN-α-2a led to thyroid dysfunction in 4 of 8 patients. These patients developed a self-limited autoimmune thyroiditis, with a hyperthyroid phase of 2 weeks followed by a hypothyroid phase lasting up to 24 weeks.[93] Recently, epoprostenol, a prostacyclin analogue used in the treatment of pulmonary arterial hypertension, has been found to be associated with seronegative hyperthyroidism. Chadha and colleagues[149] found that 6.7% of patients being treated with epoprostenol developed TSI-negative thyrotoxicosis with large goiters and increased uptake on thyroid scan. The investigators believe that epoprostenol can stimulate the thyroid tissue, induce growth of the thyroid gland, and lead to the development of hyperthyroidism.

SUMMARY

Thyrotoxicosis is a clinical syndrome resulting from increased levels of thyroid hormones caused by either increased or decreased thyroid metabolic function. Clinical symptoms, laboratory data, and radiologic imaging are often needed to make an accurate diagnosis. Because appropriate treatment is dependent on the pathophysiologic process behind the thyrotoxic state, establishing the proper diagnosis is of utmost importance.

REFERENCES

1. Braverman LE, Utiger RD. Introduction to thyrotoxicosis. In: Braverman LE, Utiger RD, editors. Werner's and Ingbar's the thyroid. 9th edition. Philadelphia: Lippincott Williams & Wilkins; 2005. p. 453–4.
2. Tunbridge WM, Evered DC, Hall R, et al. The spectrum of thyroid disease in a community: the Whickham survey. Clin Endocrinol 1977;7(6):481–93.
3. Hollowell JG, Staehling NW, Flanders WD, et al. Serum TSH, T(4), and thyroid antibodies in the United States population (1988 to 1994): National Health and Nutrition Examination Survey (NHANES III). J Clin Endocrinol Metab 2002; 87(2):489–99.
4. Aghini-Lombardi F, Antonangeli L, Martino E, et al. The spectrum of thyroid disorders in an iodine-deficient community: the Pescopagano survey. J Clin Endocrinol Metab 1999;84(2):561–6.
5. Canaris GJ, Manowitz NR, Mayor G, et al. The Colorado thyroid disease prevalence study. Arch Intern Med 2000;160(4):526–34.
6. Boelaert K, Torlinska B, Holder RL, et al. Older subjects with hyperthyroidism present with a paucity of symptoms and signs: a large cross-sectional study. J Clin Endocrinol Metab 2010;95(6):2715–26.
7. Smith JR, Oates E. Radionuclide imaging of the thyroid gland: patterns, pearls, and pitfalls. Clin Nucl Med 2004;29(3):181–93.
8. Mcdougall R. In vivo radionuclide test and imaging. In: Braverman LE, Utiger RD, editors. Werner's and Ingbar's the thyroid. 9th edition. Philadelphia: Lippincott Williams & Wilkins; 2005. p. 310–28.
9. Intenzo CM, dePapp AE, Jabbour S, et al. Scintigraphic manifestations of thyrotoxicosis. Radiographics 2003;23(4):857–69.
10. Bahn RS, Burch HB, Cooper DS, et al. Hyperthyroidism and other causes of thyrotoxicosis: management guidelines of the American Thyroid Association and American Association of Clinical Endocrinologists. Endocr Pract 2011; 17(3):456–520.
11. Intenzo CM, Capuzzi DM, Jabbour S, et al. Scintigraphic features of autoimmune thyroiditis. Radiographics 2001;21(4):957–64.

12. Kurita S, Sakurai M, Kita Y, et al. Measurement of thyroid blood flow area is useful for diagnosing the cause of thyrotoxicosis. Thyroid 2005;15(11):1249–52.

13. Ota H, Amino N, Morita S, et al. Quantitative measurement of thyroid blood flow for differentiation of painless thyroiditis from Graves' disease. Clin Endocrinol 2007;67(1):41–5.

14. Bogazzi F, Vitti P. Could improved ultrasound and power Doppler replace thyroidal radioiodine uptake to assess thyroid disease? Nat Clin Pract Endocrinol Metab 2008;4(2):70–1.

15. de los Santos ET, Starich GH, Mazzaferri EL. Sensitivity, specificity, and cost-effectiveness of the sensitive thyrotropin assay in the diagnosis of thyroid disease in ambulatory patients. Arch Intern Med 1989;149(3):526–32.

16. Woeber KA. Triiodothyronine production in Graves' hyperthyroidism. Thyroid 2006;16(7):687–90.

17. Laurberg P, Vestergaard H, Nielsen S, et al. Sources of circulating 3,5,3'-triiodothyronine in hyperthyroidism estimated after blocking of type 1 and type 2 iodothyronine deiodinases. J Clin Endocrinol Metab 2007;92(6):2149–56.

18. Shigemasa C, Abe K, Taniguchi S, et al. Lower serum free thyroxine (T4) levels in painless thyroiditis compared with Graves' disease despite similar serum total T4 levels. J Clin Endocrinol Metab 1987;65(2):359–63.

19. LeBeau SO, Mandel SJ. Thyroid disorders during pregnancy. Endocrinol Metab Clin North Am 2006;35(1):117–36, vii.

20. Marcocci C, Marino M. Thyroid directed antibodies. In: Braverman LE, Utiger RD, editors. Werner's and Ingbar's the thyroid. 9th edition. Philadelphia: Lippincott Williams & Wilkins; 2005. p. 361–71.

21. Costagliola S, Morgenthaler NG, Hoermann R, et al. Second generation assay for thyrotropin receptor antibodies has superior diagnostic sensitivity for Graves' disease. J Clin Endocrinol Metab 1999;84(1):90–7.

22. Morgenthaler NG, Pampel I, Aust G, et al. Application of a bioassay with CHO cells for the routine detection of stimulating and blocking autoantibodies to the TSH-receptor. Horm Metab Res 1998;30(3):162–8.

23. Vitti P, Elisei R, Tonacchera M, et al. Detection of thyroid-stimulating antibody using Chinese hamster ovary cells transfected with cloned human thyrotropin receptor. J Clin Endocrinol Metab 1993;76(2):499–503.

24. Cooper DS. Hyperthyroidism. Lancet 2003;362(9382):459–68.

25. Brent GA. Clinical practice. Graves' disease. N Engl J Med 2008;358(24): 2594–605.

26. Nordyke RA, Gilbert FI Jr, Harada AS. Graves' disease. Influence of age on clinical findings. Arch Intern Med 1988;148(3):626–31.

27. Davies TF. The pathogenesis of Graves' disease. In: Braverman LE, Utiger RD, editors. Werner's and Ingbar's the thyroid. 9th edition. Philadelphia: Lippincott Williams & Wilkins; 2005. p. 458–70.

28. Bahn RS. Graves' ophthalmopathy. N Engl J Med 2010;362(8):726–38.

29. Wiersinga WM, Bartalena L. Epidemiology and prevention of Graves' ophthalmopathy. Thyroid 2002;12(10):855–60.

30. Enzmann DR, Donaldson SS, Kriss JP. Appearance of Graves' disease on orbital computed tomography. J Comput Assist Tomogr 1979;3(6):815–9.

31. Klein I, Becker DV, Levey GS. Treatment of hyperthyroid disease. Ann Intern Med 1994;121(4):281–8.

32. Wartofsky L, Glinoer D, Solomon B, et al. Differences and similarities in the diagnosis and treatment of Graves' disease in Europe, Japan, and the United States. Thyroid 1991;1(2):129–35.

33. Roher HD, Goretzki PE, Hellmann P, et al. Complications in thyroid surgery. Incidence and therapy. Chirurg 1999;70(9):999–1010 [in German].
34. Ross DS. Radioiodine therapy for hyperthyroidism. N Engl J Med 2011;364(6): 542–50.
35. Bartalena L, Marcocci C, Bogazzi F, et al. Relation between therapy for hyperthyroidism and the course of Graves' ophthalmopathy. N Engl J Med 1998;338(2):73–8.
36. Tallstedt L, Lundell G, Torring O, et al. Occurrence of ophthalmopathy after treatment for Graves' hyperthyroidism. The Thyroid Study Group. N Engl J Med 1992;326(26):1733–8.
37. Laurberg P, Wallin G, Tallstedt L, et al. TSH-receptor autoimmunity in Graves' disease after therapy with anti-thyroid drugs, surgery, or radioiodine: a 5-year prospective randomized study. Eur J Endocrinol 2008;158(1):69–75.
38. Sosa JA, Mehta PJ, Wang TS, et al. A population-based study of outcomes from thyroidectomy in aging Americans: at what cost? J Am Coll Surg 2008;206(3): 1097–105.
39. Sosa JA, Bowman HM, Tielsch JM, et al. The importance of surgeon experience for clinical and economic outcomes from thyroidectomy. Ann Surg 1998;228(3): 320–30.
40. Werner MC, Romaldini JH, Bromberg N, et al. Adverse effects related to thionamide drugs and their dose regimen. Am J Med Sci 1989;297(4):216–9.
41. Nayak B, Hodak SP. Hyperthyroidism. Endocrinol Metab Clin North Am 2007; 36(3):617–56, v.
42. Cooper DS. Antithyroid drugs. N Engl J Med 2005;352(9):905–17.
43. Siegel RD, Lee SL. Toxic nodular goiter. Toxic adenoma and toxic multinodular goiter. Endocrinol Metab Clin North Am 1998;27(1):151–68.
44. Führer D, Krohn K. Toxic adenoma and toxic multinodular goiter. In: Braverman LE, Utiger RD, editors. Werner's and Ingbar's the thyroid. 9th edition. Philadelphia: Lippincott Williams & Wilkins; 2005. p. 508–17.
45. Hamburger JI. Evolution of toxicity in solitary nontoxic autonomously functioning thyroid nodules. J Clin Endocrinol Metab 1980;50(6):1089–93.
46. Marsden P, Facer P, Acosta M, et al. Serum triiodothyronine in solitary autonomous nodules of the thyroid. Clin Endocrinol 1975;4(3):327–30.
47. Laurberg P, Pedersen KM, Vestergaard H, et al. High incidence of multinodular toxic goitre in the elderly population in a low iodine intake area vs. high incidence of Graves' disease in the young in a high iodine intake area: comparative surveys of thyrotoxicosis epidemiology in East-Jutland Denmark and Iceland. J Intern Med 1991;229(5):415–20.
48. Vanderpump MP. The epidemiology of thyroid diseases. In: Braverman LE, Utiger RD, editors. Werner's and Ingbar's the thyroid. 9th edition. Philadelphia: Lippincott Williams & Wilkins; 2005. p. 398–405.
49. Krohn K, Fuhrer D, Bayer Y, et al. Molecular pathogenesis of euthyroid and toxic multinodular goiter. Endocr Rev 2005;26(4):504–24.
50. Wiest PW, Hartshorne MF, Inskip PD, et al. Thyroid palpation versus high-resolution thyroid ultrasonography in the detection of nodules. J Ultrasound Med 1998;17(8):487–96.
51. van Soestbergen MJ, van der Vijver JC, Graafland AD. Recurrence of hyperthyroidism in multinodular goiter after long-term drug therapy: a comparison with Graves' disease. J Endocrinol Invest 1992;15(11):797–800.
52. Roti E, Vagenakis AG. Effect of excess iodide: clinical aspects. In: Braverman LE, Utiger RD, editors. Werner's and Ingbar's the thyroid. 9th edition. Philadelphia: Lippincott Williams & Wilkins; 2005. p. 290–300.

53. Martins MC, Lima N, Knobel M, et al. Natural course of iodine-induced thyrotoxicosis (Jodbasedow) in endemic goiter area: a 5 year follow-up. J Endocrinol Invest 1989;12(4):239–44.

54. Stanbury JB, Ermans AE, Bourdoux P, et al. Iodine-induced hyperthyroidism: occurrence and epidemiology. Thyroid 1998;8(1):83–100.

55. Goodwin TM, Hershman JM. Hyperthyroidism due to inappropriate production of human chorionic gonadotropin. Clin Obstet Gynecol 1997;40(1):32–44.

56. Hershman JM, Lee HY, Sugawara M, et al. Human chorionic gonadotropin stimulates iodide uptake, adenylate cyclase, and deoxyribonucleic acid synthesis in cultured rat thyroid cells. J Clin Endocrinol Metab 1988;67(1):74–9.

57. Yamazaki K, Sato K, Shizume K, et al. Potent thyrotropic activity of human chorionic gonadotropin variants in terms of 125I incorporation and de novo synthesized thyroid hormone release in human thyroid follicles. J Clin Endocrinol Metab 1995;80(2):473–9.

58. Yoshimura M, Hershman JM. Thyrotropic action of human chorionic gonadotropin. Thyroid 1995;5(5):425–34.

59. Goodwin TM, Montoro M, Mestman JH. Transient hyperthyroidism and hyperemesis gravidarum: clinical aspects. Am J Obstet Gynecol 1992;167(3):648–52.

60. Goodwin TM, Montoro M, Mestman JH, et al. The role of chorionic gonadotropin in transient hyperthyroidism of hyperemesis gravidarum. J Clin Endocrinol Metab 1992;75(5):1333–7.

61. Tan JY, Loh KC, Yeo GS, et al. Transient hyperthyroidism of hyperemesis gravidarum. BJOG 2002;109(6):683–8.

62. Walkington L, Webster J, Hancock BW, et al. Hyperthyroidism and human chorionic gonadotrophin production in gestational trophoblastic disease. Br J Cancer 2011;104(11):1665–9.

63. Lockwood CM, Grenache DG, Gronowski AM. Serum human chorionic gonadotropin concentrations greater than 400,000 IU/L are invariably associated with suppressed serum thyrotropin concentrations. Thyroid 2009;19(8):863–8.

64. Moskovitz JB, Bond MC. Molar pregnancy-induced thyroid storm. J Emerg Med 2010;38(5):e71–6.

65. Chowdhury TA, Tanchel BM, Jaganathan RS, et al. A toxic testicle. Lancet 2000; 355(9220):2046.

66. Oosting SF, de Haas EC, Links TP, et al. Prevalence of paraneoplastic hyperthyroidism in patients with metastatic non-seminomatous germ-cell tumors. Ann Oncol 2010;21(1):104–8.

67. Goodarzi MO, Van Herle AJ. Thyrotoxicosis in a male patient associated with excess human chorionic gonadotropin production by germ cell tumor. Thyroid 2000;10(7):611–9.

68. Giralt SA, Dexeus F, Amato R, et al. Hyperthyroidism in men with germ cell tumors and high levels of beta-human chorionic gonadotropin. Cancer 1992; 69(5):1286–90.

69. Beck-Peccoz P, Persani L, Mannavola D, et al. Pituitary tumours: TSH-secreting adenomas. Best Pract Res Clin Endocrinol Metab 2009;23(5):597–606.

70. Beck-Peccoz P, Persani L. Thyrotropin-induced thyrotoxicosis. In: Braverman LE, Utiger RD, editors. Werner's and Ingbar's the thyroid. 9th edition. Philadelphia: Lippincott Williams & Wilkins; 2005. p. 501–7.

71. Mixson AJ, Friedman TC, Katz DA, et al. Thyrotropin-secreting pituitary carcinoma. J Clin Endocrinol Metab 1993;76(2):529–33.

72. Arnason T, Clarke DB, Imran SA. Hyperthyroidism caused by a pituitary adenoma. CMAJ 2011;183(11):E757.

73. Socin HV, Chanson P, Delemer B, et al. The changing spectrum of TSH-secreting pituitary adenomas: diagnosis and management in 43 patients. Eur J Endocrinol 2003;148(4):433–42.

74. Brucker-Davis F, Oldfield EH, Skarulis MC, et al. Thyrotropin-secreting pituitary tumors: diagnostic criteria, thyroid hormone sensitivity, and treatment outcome in 25 patients followed at the National Institutes of Health. J Clin Endocrinol Metab 1999;84(2):476–86.

75. Beck-Peccoz P, Persani L. Medical management of thyrotropin-secreting pituitary adenomas. Pituitary 2002;5(2):83–8.

76. Suzuki S, Shigematsu S, Inaba H, et al. Pituitary resistance to thyroid hormones: pathophysiology and therapeutic options. Endocrine 2011;40(3):366–71.

77. Lee S, Young BM, Wan W, et al. A mechanism for pituitary-resistance to thyroid hormone (PRTH) syndrome: a loss in cooperative coactivator contacts by thyroid hormone receptor (TR)beta2. Mol Endocrinol 2011;25(7):1111–25.

78. Refetoff S. Resistance to thyroid hormone. In: Braverman LE, Utiger RD, editors. Werner's and Ingbar's the thyroid. 9th edition. Philadelphia: Lippincott Williams & Wilkins; 2005. p. 1110–28.

79. Guran T, Turan S, Bircan R, et al. 9 years follow-up of a patient with pituitary form of resistance to thyroid hormones (PRTH): comparison of two treatment periods of D-thyroxine and triiodothyroacetic acid (TRIAC). J Pediatr Endocrinol Metab 2009;22(10):971–8.

80. Alberobello AT, Congedo V, Liu H, et al. An intronic SNP in the thyroid hormone receptor beta gene is associated with pituitary cell-specific over-expression of a mutant thyroid hormone receptor beta2 (R338W) in the index case of pituitary-selective resistance to thyroid hormone. J Transl Med 2011;9:144.

81. Nicholson WK, Robinson KA, Smallridge RC, et al. Prevalence of postpartum thyroid dysfunction: a quantitative review. Thyroid 2006;16(6):573–82.

82. Vargas MT, Briones-Urbina R, Gladman D, et al. Antithyroid microsomal autoantibodies and HLA-DR5 are associated with postpartum thyroid dysfunction: evidence supporting an autoimmune pathogenesis. J Clin Endocrinol Metab 1988;67(2):327–33.

83. Shi X, Li C, Li Y, et al. Circulating lymphocyte subsets and regulatory T cells in patients with postpartum thyroiditis during the first postpartum year. Clin Exp Med 2009;9(4):263–7.

84. Stuckey BG, Kent GN, Ward LC, et al. Postpartum thyroid dysfunction and the long-term risk of hypothyroidism: results from a 12-year follow-up study of women with and without postpartum thyroid dysfunction. Clin Endocrinol 2010;73(3):389–95.

85. Stagnaro-Green A, Schwartz A, Gismondi R, et al. High rate of persistent hypothyroidism in a large-scale prospective study of postpartum thyroiditis in southern Italy. J Clin Endocrinol Metab 2011;96(3):652–7.

86. Stagnaro-Green A. Clinical review 152: postpartum thyroiditis. J Clin Endocrinol Metab 2002;87(9):4042–7.

87. Anderson PO. Drugs and breast milk. Pediatrics 1995;95(6):957 [author reply: 957–8].

88. Ghanem FA, Movahed A. Use of antihypertensive drugs during pregnancy and lactation. Cardiovasc Ther 2008;26(1):38–49.

89. Pearce EN, Farwell AP, Braverman LE. Thyroiditis. N Engl J Med 2003;348(26): 2646–55.

90. Lazarus JH. Sporadic and postpartum thyroiditis. In: Braverman LE, Utiger RD, editors. Werner's and Ingbar's the thyroid. 9th edition. Philadelphia: Lippincott Williams & Wilkins; 2005. p. 526–36.

91. Nikolai TF, Brosseau J, Kettrick MA, et al. Lymphocytic thyroiditis with spontaneously resolving hyperthyroidism (silent thyroiditis). Arch Intern Med 1980;140(4): 478–82.
92. Nakamura S, Isaji M, Ishimori M. Familial occurrence of silent thyroiditis. Endocr J 2005;52(5):617–21.
93. Pichert G, Jost LM, Zobeli L, et al. Thyroiditis after treatment with interleukin-2 and interferon alpha-2a. Br J Cancer 1990;62(1):100–4.
94. Faris JE, Moore AF, Daniels GH. Sunitinib (sutent)-induced thyrotoxicosis due to destructive thyroiditis: a case report. Thyroid 2007;17(11):1147–9.
95. Miller KK, Daniels GH. Association between lithium use and thyrotoxicosis caused by silent thyroiditis. Clin Endocrinol 2001;55(4):501–8.
96. Nikolai TF, Coombs GJ, McKenzie AK, et al. Treatment of lymphocytic thyroiditis with spontaneously resolving hyperthyroidism (silent thyroiditis). Arch Intern Med 1982;142(13):2281–3.
97. Mittra ES, McDougall IR. Recurrent silent thyroiditis: a report of four patients and review of the literature. Thyroid 2007;17(7):671–5.
98. Fatourechi V, Aniszewski JP, Fatourechi GZ, et al. Clinical features and outcome of subacute thyroiditis in an incidence cohort: Olmsted County, Minnesota, study. J Clin Endocrinol Metab 2003;88(5):2100–5.
99. Farwell AP. Subacute thyroiditis and acute infectious thyroiditis. In: Braverman LE, Utiger RD, editors. Werner's and Ingbar's the thyroid. 9th edition. Philadelphia: Lippincott Williams & Wilkins; 2005. p. 537–47.
100. Pearce EN, Bogazzi F, Martino E, et al. The prevalence of elevated serum C-reactive protein levels in inflammatory and noninflammatory thyroid disease. Thyroid 2003;13(7):643–8.
101. Walsh CH, Dunne C. Hyperthyroidism associated with acute suppurative thyroiditis. Ir J Med Sci 1992;161(5):137.
102. Fukata S, Miyauchi A, Kuma K, et al. Acute suppurative thyroiditis caused by an infected piriform sinus fistula with thyrotoxicosis. Thyroid 2002;12(2):175–8.
103. McLaughlin SA, Smith SL, Meek SE. Acute suppurative thyroiditis caused by *Pasteurella multocida* and associated with thyrotoxicosis. Thyroid 2006;16(3): 307–10.
104. Paes JE, Burman KD, Cohen J, et al. Acute bacterial suppurative thyroiditis: a clinical review and expert opinion. Thyroid 2010;20(3):247–55.
105. Fernandez JF, Anaissie EJ, Vassilopoulou-Sellin R, et al. Acute fungal thyroiditis in a patient with acute myelogenous leukaemia. J Intern Med 1991;230(6):539–41.
106. Olin R, LeBien WE, Leigh JE. Acute suppurative thyroiditis. Report of two cases including one caused by *Mycobacterium intracellulare* (*Battey bacillus*). Minn Med 1973;56(7):586–8.
107. Yu EH, Ko WC, Chuang YC, et al. Suppurative *Acinetobacter baumanii* thyroiditis with bacteremic pneumonia: case report and review. Clin Infect Dis 1998; 27(5):1286–90.
108. Moinuddin S, Barazi H, Moinuddin M. Acute blastomycosis thyroiditis. Thyroid 2008;18(6):659–61.
109. Goel MM, Budhwar P. Fine needle aspiration cytology and immunocytochemistry in tuberculous thyroiditis: a case report. Acta Cytol 2008;52(5):602–6.
110. Iwama S, Kato Y, Nakayama S. Acute suppurative thyroiditis extending to descending necrotizing mediastinitis and pericarditis. Thyroid 2007;17(3):281–2.
111. Kim KH, Sung MW, Koh TY, et al. Pyriform sinus fistula: management with chemocauterization of the internal opening. Ann Otol Rhinol Laryngol 2000;109(5): 452–6.

112. Nishiyama K, Kozuka T, Higashihara T, et al. Acute radiation thyroiditis. Int J Radiat Oncol Biol Phys 1996;36(5):1221–4.

113. Pearce EN. Thyrotoxicosis of extrathyroid origin. In: Braverman LE, Utiger RD, editors. Werner's and Ingbar's the thyroid. 9th edition. Philadelphia: Lippincott Williams & Wilkins; 2005. p. 549–51.

114. Mittra ES, Niederkohr RD, Rodriguez C, et al. Uncommon causes of thyrotoxicosis. J Nucl Med 2008;49(2):265–78.

115. Ioos V, Das V, Maury E, et al. A thyrotoxicosis outbreak due to dietary pills in Paris. Ther Clin Risk Manag 2008;4(6):1375–9.

116. Mariotti S, Martino E, Cupini C, et al. Low serum thyroglobulin as a clue to the diagnosis of thyrotoxicosis factitia. N Engl J Med 1982;307(7):410–2.

117. Chow E, Siddique F, Gama R. Thyrotoxicosis factitia: role of thyroglobulin. Ann Clin Biochem 2008;45(Pt 4):447–8 [author reply: 448].

118. Kung AW, Ma JT, Wang C, et al. Hyperthyroidism during pregnancy due to coexistence of struma ovarii and Graves' disease. Postgrad Med J 1990;66(772):132–3.

119. Simkin PH, Ramirez LA, Zweizig SL, et al. Monomorphic teratoma of the ovary: a rare cause of triiodothyronine toxicosis. Thyroid 1999;9(9):949–54.

120. Joja I, Asakawa T, Mitsumori A, et al. I-123 uptake in nonfunctional struma ovarii. Clin Nucl Med 1998;23(1):10–2.

121. Haq M, Hyer S, Flux G, et al. Differentiated thyroid cancer presenting with thyrotoxicosis due to functioning metastases. Br J Radiol 2007;80(950):e38–43.

122. Salvatori M, Saletnich I, Rufini V, et al. Severe thyrotoxicosis due to functioning pulmonary metastases of well-differentiated thyroid cancer. J Nucl Med 1998; 39(7):1202–7.

123. Naito Y, Sone T, Kataoka K, et al. Thyroid storm due to functioning metastatic thyroid carcinoma in a burn patient. Anesthesiology 1997;87(2):433–5.

124. Wartofsky L. Management of subclinical hyperthyroidism. J Clin Endocrinol Metab 2011;96(1):59–61.

125. Auer J, Scheibner P, Mische T, et al. Subclinical hyperthyroidism as a risk factor for atrial fibrillation. Am Heart J 2001;142(5):838–42.

126. Sawin CT. Subclinical hyperthyroidism and atrial fibrillation. Thyroid 2002;12(6): 501–3.

127. Sawin CT, Geller A, Wolf PA, et al. Low serum thyrotropin concentrations as a risk factor for atrial fibrillation in older persons. N Engl J Med 1994;331(19):1249–52.

128. Vadiveloo T, Donnan PT, Cochrane L, et al. The Thyroid Epidemiology, Audit, and Research Study (TEARS): morbidity in patients with endogenous subclinical hyperthyroidism. J Clin Endocrinol Metab 2011;96(5):1344–51.

129. Klein I. Thyroid and the heart: the intimacy is strained. Thyroid 2011;21(5):469–70.

130. Abdulrahman RM, Delgado V, Hoftijzer HC, et al. Both exogenous subclinical hyperthyroidism and short-term overt hypothyroidism affect myocardial strain in patients with differentiated thyroid carcinoma. Thyroid 2011;21(5):471–6.

131. Bensenor IM, Lotufo PA, Menezes PR, et al. Subclinical hyperthyroidism and dementia: the Sao Paulo Ageing & Health Study (SPAH). BMC Public Health 2010;10:298.

132. Gussekloo J, van Exel E, de Craen AJ, et al. Thyroid status, disability and cognitive function, and survival in old age. JAMA 2004;292(21):2591–9.

133. Lee JS, Buzkova P, Fink HA, et al. Subclinical thyroid dysfunction and incident hip fracture in older adults. Arch Intern Med 2010;170(21):1876–83.

134. Vadiveloo T, Donnan PT, Cochrane L, et al. The Thyroid Epidemiology, Audit, and Research Study (TEARS): the natural history of endogenous subclinical hyperthyroidism. J Clin Endocrinol Metab 2011;96(1):E1–8.

135. Basaria S, Cooper DS. Amiodarone and the thyroid. Am J Med 2005;118(7): 706–14.
136. Bogazzi F, Bartalena L, Gasperi M, et al. The various effects of amiodarone on thyroid function. Thyroid 2001;11(5):511–9.
137. Ahmed S, Van Gelder IC, Wiesfeld AC, et al. Determinants and outcome of amiodarone-associated thyroid dysfunction. Clin Endocrinol 2011;75(3):388–94.
138. Martino E, Safran M, Aghini-Lombardi F, et al. Environmental iodine intake and thyroid dysfunction during chronic amiodarone therapy. Ann Intern Med 1984; 101(1):28–34.
139. Martino E, Bartalena L, Bogazzi F, et al. The effects of amiodarone on the thyroid. Endocr Rev 2001;22(2):240–54.
140. Bogazzi F, Bartalena L, Brogioni S, et al. Color flow Doppler sonography rapidly differentiates type I and type II amiodarone-induced thyrotoxicosis. Thyroid 1997;7(4):541–5.
141. Bogazzi F, Bartalena L, Martino E. Approach to the patient with amiodarone-induced thyrotoxicosis. J Clin Endocrinol Metab 2010;95(6):2529–35.
142. Eskes SA, Wiersinga WM. Amiodarone and thyroid. Best Pract Res Clin Endocrinol Metab 2009;23(6):735–51.
143. Johnson RS, Moore WG. Fatal aplastic anaemia after treatment of thyrotoxicosis with potassium perchlorate. Br Med J 1961;1(5236):1369–71.
144. Weetman AP. Chronic autoimmune thyroiditis. In: Braverman LE, Utiger RD, editors. Werner's and Ingbar's the thyroid. 9th edition. Philadelphia: Lippincott Williams & Wilkins; 2005. p. 702–12.
145. Nabhan ZM, Kreher NC, Eugster EA. Hashitoxicosis in children: clinical features and natural history. J Pediatr 2005;146(4):533–6.
146. Sheth S. Role of ultrasonography in thyroid disease. Otolaryngol Clin North Am 2010;43(2):239–55, vii.
147. Surks MI, Sievert R. Drugs and thyroid function. N Engl J Med 1995;333(25): 1688–94.
148. Calvi L, Daniels GH. Acute thyrotoxicosis secondary to destructive thyroiditis associated with cardiac catheterization contrast dye. Thyroid 2011;21(4):443–9.
149. Chadha C, Pritzker M, Mariash CN. Effect of epoprostenol on the thyroid gland: enlargement and secretion of thyroid hormone. Endocr Pract 2009;15(2): 116–21.

Hypothyroidism: Etiology, Diagnosis, and Management

Jaime P. Almandoz, MB, BCh[a,b], Hossein Gharib, MD, MACP, MACE[b,*]

KEYWORDS

- Hypothyroidism • Thyroid-stimulating hormone
- Subclinical hypothyroidism • Thyrotropin-releasing hormone

Hypothyroidism is the result of inadequate production of thyroid hormone or inadequate action of thyroid hormone in target tissues. Hypothyroidism is commonly seen in outpatient practice, and improvements in assays and increased awareness of the condition has led to the evaluation of more patients. The wide array of symptoms of hypothyroidism indicates an effect on metabolism and dysfunction in multiple organ systems. Primary hypothyroidism is the principal manifestation of hypothyroidism, but other causes include central deficiency of thyrotropin-releasing hormone (TRH) or thyroid-stimulating hormone (TSH), or consumptive hypothyroidism from excessive inactivation of thyroid hormone. Subclinical hypothyroidism (SCH) is present when there is laboratory evidence of primary hypothyroidism with an elevated TSH but a normal free thyroxine (FT_4) level. Treatment in most cases involves oral administration of exogenous synthetic thyroid hormone.

This review presents an update on the etiology and types of hypothyroidism, including subclinical disease; drugs and thyroid function; and diagnosis and treatment of hypothyroidism, with a glance at some controversial issues.

EPIDEMIOLOGY

Hypothyroidism is a common condition and is more prevalent in women, the elderly, and certain ethnic groups. Hypothyroidism may be either clinical/overt, whereby there is an elevation in the TSH and low levels of FT_4, or subclinical, whereby the levels of FT_4 are normal with an elevated serum TSH. For this interpretation to be valid there must be an intact hypothalamic-pituitary-thyroid axis, an absence of concurrent illness, and reproducibility of this trend over at least a 4-week period. Studies in the

[a] Mayo School of Graduate Medical Education, College of Medicine, Mayo Clinic, 200 First Street SW, Rochester, MN 55905, USA
[b] Division of Endocrinology, Diabetes, Metabolism, and Nutrition, Mayo Clinic, 200 First Street SW, Rochester, MN 55905, USA
* Corresponding author. Division of Endocrinology, Diabetes, Metabolism, and Nutrition, Mayo Clinic, 200 First Street SW, Rochester, MN 55905.
E-mail address: gharib.hossein@mayo.edu

Med Clin N Am 96 (2012) 203–221
doi:10.1016/j.mcna.2012.01.005
0025-7125/12/$ – see front matter © 2012 Elsevier Inc. All rights reserved.

United States, Europe, and Japan have reported the prevalence of hypothyroidism to be between 0.6 and 12 per 1000 in women and between 1.3 and 4.0 per 1000 in men.[1] The National Health and Nutrition Examination Survey III data estimate the prevalence of overt hypothyroidism (OH) in the American population at 0.3% and prevalence of SCH at 4.3%.[2] The Colorado Thyroid Disease Prevalence Survey revealed a similar prevalence of hypothyroidism of 0.4% in a self-selected group not taking thyroid hormone, but a much higher prevalence of SCH at 8.5%.[3] The Colorado survey involved individuals voluntarily seeking screening, so the estimated prevalence might be expected to be higher. In the Wickham cohort, 20-year survivor follow-up data indicate the mean annual incidence of hypothyroidism to be 3.5 per 1000 in women and 0.6 per 1000 in men.[4] The odds ratio of developing hypothyroidism were increased from 8 in women and 44 in men with an elevated TSH, to 38 in women and 173 in men for those that had both an elevation in TSH and positive antibodies.[4]

ETIOLOGY

Hypothyroidism can arise as primary from the thyroid gland, when there is a defect in thyroid hormone synthesis and release; or centrally from the hypothalamic-pituitary-thyroid axis, when there is a defect in either TRH or TSH signaling to the thyroid (**Table 1**). The condition may also be transient or permanent.

Primary Hypothyroidism

Chronic autoimmune (Hashimoto) thyroiditis is the most common cause of hypothyroidism in iodine-sufficient areas. It is characterized by diffuse lymphocytic infiltration of the thyroid gland associated primarily with circulating antithyroid peroxidase (TPO)

Table 1 Causes of hypothyroidism	
Primary (Thyroid)	**Secondary (Pituitary)**
Autoimmune	Tumors, infarcts, or trauma
Chronic autoimmune thyroiditis (Hashimoto)	Surgery
Subacute, silent, postpartum thyroiditis	Infiltrative disorders (eg, sarcoidosis, histiocytosis, lymphoma, hemochromatosis)
Iatrogenic	Lymphocytic hypophysitis
Thyroidectomy/thyroid surgery	Infection
Radioactive iodine therapy	Medications
Antithyroid medications	
Miscellaneous	Tertiary (hypothalamus)
Iodine deficiency or excess	Infiltrative disorders (eg, sarcoidosis, histiocytosis, lymphoma, hemochromatosis)
Medications	Medications
Radiation exposure	
Systemic illness (usually moderate or severe)	
Thyroid agenesis	
Defective hormone synthesis	
Thyroid hormone resistance	

antibodies; antibodies may also be present against other aspects of the thyroid (thyroglobulin [Tg], TSH receptor, TSH-blocking antibodies).[5–7] This process seems to be due to an inherited defect in immune surveillance that leads to dysregulation and subsequent destruction of the thyroid gland.[8] As such, patients may present with or without a goiter.

Detecting serum thyroid autoantibodies is a vital component in diagnosing autoimmune thyroid disease. Positive serum autoantibodies in the absence of abnormalities in the testing of thyroid function should be interpreted with caution, as more than 20% of women older than 50 years in the general population have positive TPO antibodies, and thus antibody positivity does not equal clinical disease,[2] although these individuals are more likely than antibody-negative individuals to develop thyroid dysfunction.

Iodine deficiency remains the most common cause of hypothyroidism worldwide, but is uncommon in North America because of the widespread use of iodized table salt and other fortified foods.[9] A study of bread and cows' milk in the Boston area revealed that the average slice of bread contained 10 μg of iodine, whereas some brands provided more than 300 μg per slice. This study also showed that all cows' milk samples contained at least 88 μg per 250 mL.[10] As recently at 1990, 28.9% of the world's population was at risk for iodine deficiency. The recommended daily intake for iodine is 150 μg for the general population and 225 to 350 μg during pregnancy and lactation.[11] Radioactive iodine (^{131}I) therapy is the most common treatment modality for hyperthyroidism in the United States. It is also used for treatment of thyroid remnant ablation following thyroidectomy and treatment of iodine-avid thyroid cancers. The principal side effect of ^{131}I is hypothyroidism, requiring lifelong thyroid hormone replacement therapy.[12]

Excess exposure to iodine can lead to transient hypothyroidism, referred to as the Wolff-Chaikoff effect.[13] This effect is sometimes used in preparing patients with Graves disease for surgery or treating thyroid storm. Patients with underlying organification defects, for example, Hashimoto thyroiditis, or following ^{131}I therapy can suffer from prolonged hypothyroidism when exposed to excess iodide.[14,15] This situation also occurs in patients on amiodarone therapy and is likely caused by a failure to escape the Wolff-Chaikoff effect.[16] Escape or adaptation to the Wolff-Chaikoff effect occurs approximately 2 days after initial iodine exposure, and in rats has been shown to be due to a transcriptional decrease in sodium/iodide symporter messenger RNA and protein expression, which results in decreased iodide transport into the thyroid.[17]

External radiation exposure from treatment of nonthyroid cancer increases the chances of hypothyroidism. The prevalence of hypothyroidism following radiation for head and neck cancer ranges between 10% and 45% in the literature.[18] A recent systematic review looking at risk factors for developing hypothyroidism after radiation therapy identified female sex, white race, and concomitant thyroid or neck surgery as notable factors.[19] Considerable variation was seen between studies, but there was a radiation–dose response relationship, with a 50% risk of hypothyroidism with a dose of 45 Gy. Chemotherapy and age were not associated with an increased risk of hypothyroidism.

Tyrosine kinase inhibitors have been shown to cause hypothyroidism in 36% to 71% of patients in prospective data.[20] This class of medication has also been shown to increase the requirement of levothyroxine replacement in those already on thyroid hormone replacement, by an average dose of 50 μg per day in one study looking at vandetanib.[21] It has been suggested by several investigators that this increase in thyroid hormone requirement is attributable to an induction in type 3 deiodinase activity.[22,23]

The evidence linking low-dose environmental radiation exposure to autoimmune thyroid disease and hypothyroidism is inconclusive.[24] The Japanese Adult Health

Survey, when examining 50-year survivors of the Hiroshima and Nagasaki atomic bombs, found an increase in spontaneous OH with a prevalence of 5.6%.[25] There does not appear to be a link between radiation exposure and positive antithyroid antibody status or antibody-positive hypothyroidism in this cohort. The Hanford Thyroid Disease Study also failed to find an association between hypothyroidism, autoimmune thyroiditis, and prolonged ^{131}I exposure in infancy and childhood.[26]

Infiltrative processes can lead to primary hypothyroidism, and causes include hemochromatosis, lymphoma, sarcoidosis, and Riedel thyroiditis.[27–30] Infections of the thyroid with pathogens such as *Pneumocystis jiroveci* can cause inadequate production of thyroid hormone if enough of the gland is damaged. However, infections of the thyroid are rare because of its encapsulation, high iodide content, and lymphatic drainage.[30]

Inflammatory destruction of the thyroid as occurs in thyroiditis leads to transient thyrotoxicosis by release of thyroid hormone from the injured gland. As hormone stores are depleted, a transient hypothyroid phase follows until the inflammation has subsided. Postpartum thyroiditis (PPT) is caused by lymphocytic infiltration and may occur in 5% to 7% of women worldwide. PPT is more common in women with thyroid autoantibodies, and those with positive TPO antibodies early in pregnancy have a 30% to 52% chance of developing PPT. Other autoimmune conditions increase the incidence of PPT, which is at least 15% in women with type 1 diabetes mellitus.[31] It is widely believed that most women with PPT will recover before the end of the first postpartum year.[32] A recent large-scale prospective study of women in southern Italy challenged this, showing that 1 in 25 developed the condition and that 54% had persistent hypothyroidism at the end of the first postpartum year.[33]

Consumptive hypothyroidism results from excessive production of type 3 deiodinase by vascular endothelium, resulting in conversion of thyroxine (T_4) to reverse triiodothyronine (T_3) and T_3 to diiodothyronine. This rare condition is usually associated with hemangiomas, and surgical resection is curative.[34]

Medications

In addition to amiodarone, which contains a high concentration of iodine and causes hyperthyroidism or hypothyroidism, many other drugs can lead to hypothyroidism (**Box 1**). Medications such as iron and calcium salts can impair absorption of ingested exogenous thyroid hormone. Kelp supplements and perchlorate can impair iodine uptake. Thionamides, commonly used antithyroid medications, primarily interfere with thyroid hormone production. Secretion of thyroid hormone by the gland can be blocked by medications such as lithium. The hypothalamic-pituitary axis can be interrupted by glucocorticoids and dopamine. Barbiturates can lead to increased clearance of the thyroid hormone from the circulation.

Subclinical Hypothyroidism

SCH is used to describe an asymptomatic patient who has an elevated serum TSH and a normal serum FT_4 level. This description is only accurate if the hypothalamic-pituitary-thyroid axis is intact, there is no ongoing or recent severe illness, and the pattern is reproducible through time. It suggests a compensated early state of primary thyroid failure whereby an increased level of TSH is required to maintain levels of thyroid hormone within the normal range. SCH can occur in the setting of Hashimoto thyroiditis, prior thyroid surgery, radioiodine therapy, or external beam radiation. Transient SCH has also been reported following an episode of thyroiditis.[39]

DIAGNOSIS
Symptoms and Presentations

The symptoms of hypothyroidism are often very subjective, and vary according to the degree of biochemical hypothyroidism. Symptoms typically include fatigue, cold intolerance, dry skin, constipation, vocal changes, and muscle aches. These symptoms, including proposed scoring systems for the diagnosis of hypothyroidism, have poor sensitivity and specificity for the condition.[40] On physical examination prolonged ankle-jerk reflex time appears to correlate best with the degree of hypothyroidism; however, much of the clinical evaluation in current clinical practice has been overshadowed by the use of sensitive assays.[40,41]

The decrease in circulating thyroid hormones has a negative effect on basal metabolic rate, which has a negative effect on multiple organ systems. The accumulation of glycosaminoglycans from increased synthesis of hyaluronic acid along with the decreased metabolic rate can explain many of the presenting features of the affected patient.

Lipid Metabolism

Some investigators recommend that thyroid function be measured in all patients with lipid abnormalities, as more than 90% of patients with OH will have abnormal serum lipid values.[42] OH is characterized by increased low-density lipoproteins (LDL) and apolipoprotein B because of reduced hepatic clearance from a decreased number of hepatic LDL receptors. A decrease in cholesterylester transfer protein can increase the levels of high-density lipoproteins (HDL) in hypothyroidism.[43] Although there is a tendency toward elevated cholesterol in hypothyroidism, it seems to arise from an increase in large-LDL and large-HDL subtypes, which are thought to be less atherogenic.[44]

Cardiovascular and Other Changes

The most common cardiovascular findings in OH include bradycardia, systemic hypertension with decreased pulse pressure, and exercise impairment. Hypothyroid patients are prone to ventricular arrhythmias, and from a delayed cardiomyocyte action-potential may manifest a variety of electrocardiographic abnormalities including prolonged QT-interval and nonspecific ST changes.[45]

Hyponatremia may occur from plasma dilution, as there is a reduction in free water clearance in hypothyroidism. Combined with an excess of tissue mucopolysaccharides, decreased glomerular filtration rate, and a reduced cardiac ejection fraction, this may cause puffiness or frank edema.[46] The frequency of hyponatremia is increased with the concomitant use of thiazide diuretics.

Changes in the skin depend on the degree of hypothyroidism and the ethnicity of the patient. Findings include xerosis, decreased sweating, thickening of the skin, brittle hair, hair loss, loss of the lateral eyebrows (Queen Anne sign), livedo reticularis, and vitiligo.[47]

Neurologic manifestations of hypothyroidism include carpal tunnel syndrome, sensorimotor polyneuropathy, and myopathy. The myopathic symptoms usually consist of proximal weakness and are associated with a modest elevation in serum creatine kinase, which will respond to thyroid hormone replacement.[48,49] With the use of functional imaging studies, researchers have documented a decrease in cerebral blood flow and glucose metabolism in patients with hypothyroidism.[50] These changes may account for the increased prevalence of depression, anxiety, and psychomotor retardation.

Box 1
Medications that contribute to hypothyroidism

Certain agents may have more than 1 mechanism.

Medications decreasing TSH secretion

    Glucocorticoids

    Opiates

    Dopamine

    Bromocriptine

    Phentolamine

    Octreotide

    Growth hormone

Drugs affecting thyroid hormone synthesis and secretion

    Iodine

    Amiodarone

    Thionamides

    Thiocyanate

    Aminogluthemide

    Perchlorate

    Lithium

    Cytokines (IFN-γ, IL-2, GM-CSF)

Drugs altering thyroid hormone metabolism

    Rifampicin

    Phenytoin

    Carbamazepine

    Barbiturates

    Tyrosine kinase inhibitors

    Growth hormone

    Glucocorticoids

    Propylthiouracil

    β-Blockers

    Iodinated contrast agents

    Clomipramine

Drugs that increase thyroxine-binding globulin

    Estrogen

    SERMs

    Opiates

    Mitotane

    Clofibrate

    Perphenazine

    5-Fluorouracil

Drugs that affect exogenous thyroid hormone absorption

    Calcium compounds

    Sucralfate

    Aluminum hydroxide

    Ferrous compounds

    Cholestyramine

    Colesevelam

    Acid-reducing agents: proton pump inhibitors, H_2 blockers

    Coffee

Abbreviations: IFN-γ, interferon-gamma; IL-2, interleukin-2; GM-CSF, granulocyte-macrophage colony stimulating factor; SERMs, selective estrogen receptor modulators; TSH, thyroid-stimulating hormone.
    Data from Refs.[35–38]

Gastrointestinal symptoms and signs may be due to dysfunctional motility of the hollow viscera or associated autoimmune conditions in autoimmune thyroid disease. Decreased motility can lead to dyspepsia, gastroesophageal reflux, and constipation. Small bowel bacterial overgrowth can be seen in more than half of patients with hypothyroidism. Coexisting autoimmune conditions may lead to a decrease in production of gastric acid and malabsorption from celiac disease.[51]

Oligomenorrhea and menorrhagia are the most frequently seen menstrual disturbances in hypothyroidism and are related to severity of the condition. Some women present with amenorrhea and elevated prolactin levels from hypothyroidism, which will resolve with thyroid hormone replacement. The menorrhagia is probably the result of breakthrough bleeding associated with anovulation in conjunction with hemostasis defects seen with hypothyroidism.[52] Men with hypothyroidism may have lower concentrations of sex hormone–binding globulin and free testosterone than euthyroid men. The hyperprolactinemia associated with hypothyroidism may lead to hypogonadotropic hypogonadism, but it should be noted that only a small number of men presenting with hypothyroidism complain of sexual dysfunction.[53]

Diagnosis

Laboratory testing is required for the diagnosis of hypothyroidism because the symptoms and examination findings lack sensitivity and specificity. Accordingly, clinical scoring systems correlate poorly with hypothyroidism and should not be used for diagnosis. Nonthyroid serum testing such as elevated creatine kinase, hyperlipidemia, and physical findings such as basal metabolic rate should not be used to diagnose thyroid dysfunction, but should prompt more specific thyroid testing.

Primary hypothyroidism is manifested by an elevated serum TSH with a low serum FT_4. SCH is present when there is an elevation in TSH but the FT_4 is within the normal reference range. In secondary (pituitary) or tertiary (hypothalamic) hypothyroidism, the FT_4 is low and the TSH is not appropriately elevated. Imaging of the hypothalamus and pituitary gland should be performed on patients in whom central hypothyroidism is suspected.

TSH is widely measured using a third-generation chemiluminometric assay. There is controversy regarding the appropriate upper limit of normal for the reference range. The authors' laboratory currently uses a reference range of 0.3 to 5.0 mIU/L. A monograph by the National Academy of Clinical Biochemistry revealed that 95% of screened euthyroid volunteers had a serum TSH between 0.4 and 2.5 mIU/L.[54] Epidemiologic data from the National Health and Nutrition Examination Survey III shows a trend toward increasing TSH values with age, even when correcting for antithyroid antibodies.[2] Lowering the upper limit of normal for the reference range to 2.5 mIU/L would incorrectly diagnose up to 35% of older people as hypothyroid, prompting perhaps unnecessary therapy without a demonstrable benefit in outcome.[55,56]

Serum T_4 and T_3 are extensively bound to plasma proteins, which include thyroxine-binding globulin, albumin, and transthyretin. The bound thyroid hormones are considered to be biologically unavailable until they are dissociated from their carrier proteins. Conditions such as pregnancy, illness, and medications can affect levels of binding proteins, thus confounding interpretation of the total results. The measurement of FT_4 is used more often than total (bound) thyroxine, in conjunction with TSH, to assess the status of thyroid function.

FT_4 levels are measured by a direct FT_4 assay after ultrafiltration; equilibrium dialysis following addition of an anti-T_4 antibody to the serum; or FT_4 index, which is a calculation based on the total T_4 and the T_3 uptake. The T_3 uptake represents the concentration of unoccupied sites on carrier proteins.[57]

TPO antibodies are positive in almost all cases of Hashimoto thyroiditis. Measuring TPO antibodies in hypothyroid patients can help to determine the etiology, and also has prognostic value in assessing the risk of progression to OH for patients with a goiter or SCH. Antibody-positive individuals have been shown to have a much higher risk of developing hypothyroidism, and measuring TPO antibodies also identifies patients who may be at risk for other autoimmune conditions.[58] As much as 20% to 30% of the population with type 1 diabetes mellitus expresses TPO antibodies,[59] and in one study 83% of patients with idiopathic Addison disease expressed such antibodies.[60]

Radionuclide-uptake studies do not have a role in the diagnosis of hypothyroidism and are primarily used in the evaluation of hyperthyroidism.

Two-dimensional ultrasound imaging can be used in the evaluation of patients with hypothyroidism. In Hashimoto thyroiditis, a heterogeneous pattern is often seen and the degree of hypoechogenicity of the gland seems to correlate with the stage of the disease.[61] Ultrasonography findings correlate highly with TPO-antibody positivity and the presence of autoimmune thyroid dysfunction.[62]

Multinodular goiter is not usually associated with hypothyroidism arising from destruction of functioning thyroid tissue. In some patients with nodular disease, fine-needle aspiration biopsy may play a limited role in identifying disease if the patient has an autoimmune-mediated nodular thyroid and is at risk of developing hypothyroidism.

SCREENING

Universal screening of the general population is controversial, and there is disagreement between professional societies about who should be screened for thyroid hypofunction and when. The United States Preventive Services Task Force does not recommend routine screening for thyroid disease in adults,[63] whereas the American Thyroid Association (ATA) recommends screening for adults beginning at age 35 years and every 5 years thereafter.[64] The American Association of Clinical Endocrinologists (AACE) recommends screening in older patients of an unspecified age, particularly if female.[65]

Because of the lack of data supporting screening on a population-based level, a consensus group of representatives from the Endocrine Society, ATA, and AACE recommended aggressive case finding in pregnant women, those older than 60 years, and people at risk for thyroid dysfunction. Patients thought to be at risk included those with a family history of thyroid dysfunction or a personal history of autoimmune disease.[66] Other patients who could fall into the at-risk group include those on medications that affect thyroid function, those with presence of a goiter, those who have had prior neck surgery, or those with a history of radiation exposure.

Treatment

Hypothyroidism is permanent in most patients with the condition, therefore requiring lifelong thyroid hormone replacement. Therapy should begin once a diagnosis of hypothyroidism has been confirmed, and it is generally accepted that those with TSH levels greater than 10 mIU/L should be treated. For nonpregnant individuals, there are no clear outcome data showing a benefit to treating those with TSH levels between 5.0 and 10 mIU/L.[66]

Replacement with synthetic levothyroxine (LT4) is the mainstay of therapy, and provided that there is an intact hypothalamic-pituitary-thyroid axis, the dose can be titrated every 4 to 6 weeks to a normal TSH level. Thyroxine has a plasma half-life of about 1 week, and it is generally recommended that dose adjustments be made every 4 to 6 weeks so that the new dose has achieved a steady state at 6 half-lives.

Recent evidence suggests that the dose of LT4 replacement is dependent on sex and body mass, but not age as was previously thought.[67,68] Also, patients with central hypothyroidism or those who have had a total thyroidectomy or radioactive-iodine ablation of the thyroid may require higher doses than those with residual functioning thyroid tissue.[69] A full replacement dosage of LT4 is typically 1.6 μg/kg/d, and the calculations should be made using the ideal body weight.[70,71]

It is recommended that caution be exercised when initiating and titrating LT4 replacement in those with known or suspected coronary artery disease. A report from 1961[72] suggests that 2% of patients with hypothyroidism developed new-onset angina with initiation of LT4 replacement, and in those with preexisting angina, 16% had worsening symptoms.

A starting dosage of 25 to 50 μg per day is typically recommended in those at risk of adverse cardiovascular effects, with slow dose titration every 4 to 6 weeks. A study comparing initiation of a full calculated replacement dose versus starting with 25 μg daily and titrating every 4 weeks did not show any difference in improvement of symptoms, signs, or quality of life, although a biochemically euthyroid state was more quickly achieved with the full replacement dose.[73]

For patients who are not pregnant, the authors recommend that the dose of LT4 is adjusted to maintain the TSH level within the normal reference range for the performing laboratory. Current data suggest that aiming for a TSH within the lower half of the reference range (0.4–2.0 mIU/L) does not have any marked clinical impact, improvement in symptoms, or better quality-of-life scores.[74,75]

Many factors affect the absorption of LT4; thus it should be taken on an empty stomach, without other medications, supplements, or food for 1 hour, or in a similar fashion 4 hours after the last meal. A fasting regimen of administration helps to ensure that the TSH remains within a narrow target range.[76] There is evidence from a crossover trial that taking LT4 at bedtime instead of in the morning leads to higher levels of thyroid hormone but no change in quality-of-life measures.[77] Better nocturnal absorption may be facilitated by higher basal secretion of stomach acid and slower intestinal motility overnight combined with the fasting state.[78]

For patients who have difficulty with adherence to a daily regimen, or those on an alternative feeding regimen such as continuous enteral feeding, it may be difficult to achieve euthyroidism because of the timing of doses. A randomized crossover trial demonstrated that euthyroidism can probably be achieved with once-weekly dosing of LT4, at a dose slightly higher than 7 times the normal daily dose, without ill effects.[79]

Generic LT4 tablets are available from several manufacturers, and there can be considerable variation in the content of the active ingredient between formulations.[80] Imprecise methods of determining bioequivalence may put patients at risk for incorrect supplementation if different preparations are used interchangeably.[81] As a result, a joint statement from the Endocrine Society, ATA, and AACE has recommended monitoring of thyroid function tests when a change in LT4 preparation has occurred.[82] When a change in LT4 preparation has occurred, as with other dose modifications, serum TSH should be checked 4 to 6 weeks later, with dose adjustment as necessary.

Despite achieving a biochemically euthyroid state, some patients continue to complain of significant fatigue, weight issues, and diminished neurocognitive function, perceived to be due to inadequately treated hypothyroidism[83]; this has prompted some practitioners and investigators to advocate supplementation with T_3. Thyroid hormone replacement with T_3 alone is not generally used because of the short half-life, which requires multiple daily doses and causes fluctuations in plasma T3 and TSH levels.

A recent crossover study[84] compared a thrice-daily dosing regimen of liothyronine with LT4, titrated to a TSH of 0.5 to 1.5 mIU/L. The investigators demonstrated a small but significant decrease in body weight, total cholesterol, and LDL cholesterol in the liothyronine-treated group. There was no significant difference seen in heart rate, blood pressure, exercise tolerance, or insulin sensitivity. The dosing schedule would typically preclude this regimen for the general population, and these data need to be confirmed.

Desiccated animal thyroid is sometimes promoted to patients as a natural source of thyroid hormone replacement. These preparations contain a mixture of T_4 and T_3, which is not easily monitored or regulated. There are also occasional interruptions in the availability of these preparations from suppliers. There are currently no randomized controlled trials that would support the use of desiccated thyroid hormone over the current standard of care using exogenous levothyroxine.

A study looking at LT4 monotherapy versus combination therapy with liothyronine noted a more favorable response on the General Health Questionnaire 12 in patients on combination therapy who also had an alternative type 2 deiodinase subtype. This subtype was present in 16% of the study population, and there was no apparent difference in serum thyroid hormone levels.[85] This finding suggests a potential future role for genotyping in determining the type of hypothyroidism replacement regimen.

Looking at a wider pool of patients, a meta-analysis including more than 1200 patients randomized to LT4 monotherapy or combination therapy with liothyronine showed no difference in body pain, depression, anxiety, fatigue, quality of life, body weight, or lipids.[86] The authors believe that LT4 monotherapy should currently remain the treatment of choice for patients requiring thyroid hormone replacement.

Hypothyroidism in Pregnancy

Pregnancy is a time of increased metabolic need which, together with alterations in plasma-binding proteins, leads to a variation in results of thyroid tests in comparison with the standard nonpregnant reference ranges.[87] Thyroid autoantibodies are found frequently in women of childbearing age, and autoimmune thyroiditis is the primary cause of hypothyroidism in pregnancy.[71]

Prevalence of hypothyroidism in pregnancy is approximately 0.3% for OH and 2.5% for SCH.[88] The prevalence increases with age and in areas of iodine deficiency. At present there is insufficient evidence to recommend either for or against universal TSH screening at the first-trimester visit.[89] Isolated hypothyroxinemia is defined as a normal maternal TSH level with an FT_4 level in the lower 5th or 10th percentile of the reference range.

If the Endocrine Society and the ATA recommendations are combined, there are many factors to consider for hypothyroidism screening: age older than 30 years, body mass index 40 kg/m² or more, TPO-antibody positivity (if known), history of thyroid dysfunction, family history of thyroid disease, goiter, prior thyroid surgery, prior head and neck irradiation, use of amiodarone or lithium, recent iodinated contrast administration, symptoms of hypothyroidism, type 1 diabetes mellitus, coexisting autoimmune conditions, prior miscarriage, preterm delivery, and infertility.[90,91]

Screening only those in the high-risk group will miss approximately one-third of pregnant women with SCH/OH.[92] Current practice for screening varies, and a recent survey of members in the European Thyroid Association revealed that 42% screened all pregnant women, 43% performed targeted screening, and 17% did not carry out systematic screening.[93]

During pregnancy there is an increase in thyroxine-binding globulin, which confounds interpretation of total T_4 results when using a standard nonpregnant reference range. The measurement and interpretation of FT_4 is made difficult by high levels of thyroxine-binding globulin, which leads to elevated levels of total T_4, and low levels of albumin which, in turn, leads to lower levels of FT_4.[94] If available, FT_4 quantification in pregnancy is optimally assessed using serum dialysate or ultrafiltrate in online extraction/liquid chromatography/tandem mass spectrometry.[95] In the absence of this expensive and complicated method, each laboratory should have its own trimester-specific reference range for thyroid blood tests in pregnancy.[96]

The current ATA guidelines for pregnancy and postpartum management of thyroid disease recommend that if a laboratory does not have trimester-specific TSH reference ranges, the following be used: first trimester, 0.1 to 2.5 mIU/L; second trimester, 0.2 to 3.0 mIU/L; third trimester, 0.3 to 3.0 mIU/L.[91] The LT4 dose should be adjusted with a goal TSH level within the normal range for the respective stage of pregnancy.

It has been suggested by one study that TSH and total T_4 measurements are monitored every 4 weeks through mid-pregnancy and then again at week 30, as this identified more than 90% of abnormal values in a prospective randomized trial looking at different augmentation strategies for LT4 replacement in pregnancy.[97] This proposal is reflected in the current ATA guideline, which recommends maternal TSH monitoring every 4 weeks until mid-pregnancy and then at least once between weeks 26 and 32.[91]

An increase in LT4 supplementation of approximately 30% is required during pregnancy for the mother to remain biochemically euthyroid. There is an early increase in requirement at around 5 weeks, which increases through the mid-trimester and is then sustained through to delivery. Alexander and colleagues[98] suggest compensating for this higher demand by increasing the current LT4 regimen by 2 extra doses per week as soon as pregnancy is confirmed, and this is also recommended by the current ATA guideline.[91]

Untreated OH in pregnancy has been associated with a multitude of adverse maternal and fetal outcomes, including early miscarriage, intrauterine fetal demise, placental abruption, low birth weight, gestational hypertension, increased rate of operative delivery, and postpartum hemorrhage.[87,99,100] In mothers with low maternal FT_4 but a normal TSH, an association with macrosomia, gestational diabetes, and preterm labor has been identified.[101]

The developing fetus depends on maternal production and regulation of thyroid hormone until 18 weeks of gestation.[102] Thyroid hormone is important for in utero neurocognitive development, and Haddow and colleagues[103] demonstrated that progeny of mothers with untreated OH had an IQ score 7 points less than healthy or thyroxine-treated counterparts.

Treating thyroid autoantibody-positive women with LT4 significantly reduces the rate of preterm delivery when compared with untreated antibody-positive women whose thyroid function declined into SCH during pregnancy.[104] A study by Negro and colleagues[105] suggested that selenium supplementation with 200 µg per day significantly reduced levels of TPO antibodies compared with the placebo group during pregnancy, and resulted in fewer cases of postpartum thyroid dysfunction. In the authors' view, this single study is insufficient evidence to recommend routine selenium supplementation in TPO-positive women in pregnancy, and needs to be confirmed in an iodine-sufficient area.

There is evidence in the literature suggesting that untreated SCH in the first trimester is associated with an increase in miscarriage and fetal demise.[106] The effect of SCH on neurocognitive function later in life remains unclear. Two studies[107,108] suggest that there is neurocognitive impairment in the offspring of mothers with normal TSH and FT_4 levels below the 10th percentile, yet there has not been a randomized interventional study to evaluate this finding further. However, there is plausibility to a spectrum of psychomotor impairment that may occur as a result of varying degrees of insufficiency of fetal thyroid hormone.[109]

The ATA 2011 guideline[91] recommends that OH should be treated in pregnancy based on trimester-specific reference ranges in the presence of a low FT_4 or in all women with TSH levels greater than 10 mIU/L, regardless of the FT_4 level. The ATA considers that there is insufficient evidence for or against treating SCH in the absence of TPO antibodies because of a lack of randomized controlled trials, but acknowledges that it is reasonable to consider treatment. For the same reason, it is recommended that isolated hypothyroxinemia is not treated in pregnancy.

Congenital Hypothyroidism

Universal screening for congenital hypothyroidism (CH) is performed in most industrialized countries within the first few days of life. The purpose of this population-based screening is to prevent intellectual disability in those affected, previously estimated at 1 in 4000 live births in iodine-sufficient regions.[110] There are several screening strategies including an initial T_4 with a reflex TSH for those below a defined T_4 threshold, a TSH-only test, and a combined TSH and T_4 test. Congenital central hypothyroidism can be missed by TSH-only screening methods, and the estimated birth prevalence of this disorder is approximately 1 in 29,000.[111]

Thyroid dysgenesis accounts for 85% of the cases of CH, and of those, two-thirds are caused by an ectopic thyroid gland, followed by agenesis and hypoplasia. Most of these cases are sporadic and only 2% of cases are found to have known genetic mutations. Thyroid dyshormonogenesis is responsible for almost 15% of CH cases and includes defects in functional thyroid peroxidase, the sodium/iodide symporter. Transient CH is associated with conditions such as maternal iodine insufficiency or acute ingestion, and maternal TSH-blocking antibodies.[112]

In 2007, an article by Harris and Pass[113] raised concern that the birth prevalence of CH had doubled over the previous 2 decades. A 20-year retrospective study from Quebec determined that their stated increase in birth prevalence of CH was attributable to a lowering of the upper limit of normal in the confirmatory test, from 15 mIU/L to 5 mIU/L. The lowering of this diagnostic threshold identified an additional 49 cases that would not otherwise have been detected, out of a total of 620 cases. Although these additional cases were considered to be mild, 86% had permanent hypothyroidism.[114] There are no randomized controlled studies demonstrating a therapeutic benefit in these milder cases of CH, which would have been previously missed, but it would seem prudent to treat them.

REFERENCES

1. Vanderpump MP. The epidemiology of thyroid disease. Br Med Bull 2011;99: 39–51.
2. Hollowell JG, Staehling NW, Flanders WD, et al. Serum TSH, T(4), and thyroid antibodies in the United States population (1988 to 1994): National Health and Nutrition Examination Survey (NHANES III). J Clin Endocrinol Metab 2002; 87(2):489–99.
3. Canaris GJ, Manowitz NR, Mayor G, et al. The Colorado thyroid disease prevalence study. Arch Intern Med 2000;160(4):526–34.
4. Vanderpump MP, Tunbridge WM, French JM, et al. The incidence of thyroid disorders in the community: a twenty-year follow-up of the Whickham Survey. Clin Endocrinol (Oxf) 1995;43(1):55–68.
5. Rapoport B. Pathophysiology of Hashimoto's thyroiditis and hypothyroidism. Annu Rev Med 1991;42:91–6.
6. Nordyke RA, Gilbert FI Jr, Miyamoto LA, et al. The superiority of antimicrosomal over antithyroglobulin antibodies for detecting Hashimoto's thyroiditis. Arch Intern Med 1993;153(7):862–5.
7. Endo T, Kaneshige M, Nakazato M, et al. Autoantibody against thyroid iodide transporter in the sera from patients with Hashimoto's thyroiditis possesses iodide transport inhibitory activity. Biochem Biophys Res Commun 1996; 228(1):199–202.
8. Ban Y, Greenberg DA, Davies TF, et al. 'Linkage analysis of thyroid antibody production: evidence for shared susceptibility to clinical autoimmune thyroid disease. J Clin Endocrinol Metab 2008;93(9):3589–96.
9. Vanderpump MP, Tunbridge WM. Epidemiology and prevention of clinical and subclinical hypothyroidism. Thyroid 2002;12(10):839–47.
10. Pearce EN, Pino S, He X, et al. Sources of dietary iodine: bread, cows' milk, and infant formula in the Boston area. J Clin Endocrinol Metab 2004;89(7): 3421–4.
11. Delange F. Iodine requirements during pregnancy, lactation and the neonatal period and indicators of optimal iodine nutrition. Public Health Nutr 2007; 10(12A):1571–80 [discussion: 1581–3].
12. Singer PA, Cooper DS, Levy EG, et al. Treatment guidelines for patients with hyperthyroidism and hypothyroidism. Standards of Care Committee, American Thyroid Association. JAMA 1995;273(10):808–12.
13. Wolff J, Chaikoff IL, et al. The temporary nature of the inhibitory action of excess iodine on organic iodine synthesis in the normal thyroid. Endocrinology 1949; 45(5):504–13 illust.
14. Braverman LE, Ingbar SH, Vagenakis AG, et al. Enhanced susceptibility to iodide myxedema in patients with Hashimoto's disease. J Clin Endocrinol Metab 1971;32(4):515–21.
15. Braverman LE, Woeber KA, Ingbar SH. Induction of myxedema by iodide in patients euthyroid after radioiodine or surgical treatment of diffuse toxic goiter. N Engl J Med 1969;281(15):816–21.

16. Martino E, Bartalena L, Bogazzi F, et al. The effects of amiodarone on the thyroid. Endocr Rev 2001;22(2):240–54.
17. Eng PH, Cardona GR, Fang SL, et al. Escape from the acute Wolff-Chaikoff effect is associated with a decrease in thyroid sodium/iodide symporter messenger ribonucleic acid and protein. Endocrinology 1999;140(8):3404–10.
18. Grande C. Hypothyroidism following radiotherapy for head and neck cancer: multivariate analysis of risk factors. Radiother Oncol 1992;25(1):31–6.
19. Vogelius IR, Bentzen SM, Maraldo MV, et al. Risk factors for radiation-induced hypothyroidism: a literature-based meta-analysis. Cancer 2011;117(23): 5250–60.
20. Torino F, Corsello SM, Longo R, et al. Hypothyroidism related to tyrosine kinase inhibitors: an emerging toxic effect of targeted therapy. Nat Rev Clin Oncol 2009;6(4):219–28.
21. Brassard M, Neraud B, Trabado S, et al. Endocrine effects of the tyrosine kinase inhibitor vandetanib in patients treated for thyroid cancer. J Clin Endocrinol Metab 2011;96(9):2741–9.
22. Abdulrahman RM, Verloop H, Hoftijzer H, et al. Sorafenib-induced hypothyroidism is associated with increased type 3 deiodination. J Clin Endocrinol Metab 2010;95(8):3758–62.
23. Kappers MH, van Esch JH, Smedts FM, et al. Sunitinib-induced hypothyroidism is due to induction of type 3 deiodinase activity and thyroidal capillary regression. J Clin Endocrinol Metab 2011;96(10):3087–94.
24. Eheman CR, Garbe P, Tuttle RM. Autoimmune thyroid disease associated with environmental thyroidal irradiation. Thyroid 2003;13(5):453–64.
25. Imaizumi M, Usa T, Tominaga T, et al. Radiation dose-response relationships for thyroid nodules and autoimmune thyroid diseases in Hiroshima and Nagasaki atomic bomb survivors 55-58 years after radiation exposure. JAMA 2006; 295(9):1011–22.
26. Davis S, Kopecky KJ, Hamilton TE, et al. Thyroid neoplasia, autoimmune thyroiditis, and hypothyroidism in persons exposed to iodine 131 from the Hanford nuclear site. JAMA 2004;292(21):2600–13.
27. Edwards CQ, Kelly TM, Ellwein G, et al. Thyroid disease in hemochromatosis. Increased incidence in homozygous men. Arch Intern Med 1983;143(10):1890–3.
28. Thieblemont C, Mayer A, Dumontet C, et al. Primary thyroid lymphoma is a heterogeneous disease. J Clin Endocrinol Metab 2002;87(1):105–11.
29. Porter N, Beynon HL, Randeva HS. Endocrine and reproductive manifestations of sarcoidosis. QJM 2003;96(8):553–61.
30. Pearce EN, Farwell AP, Braverman LE. Thyroiditis. N Engl J Med 2003;348(26): 2646–55.
31. Muller AF, Drexhage HA, Berghout A. Postpartum thyroiditis and autoimmune thyroiditis in women of childbearing age: recent insights and consequences for antenatal and postnatal care. Endocr Rev 2001;22(5):605–30.
32. Stagnaro-Green A. Clinical review 152: postpartum thyroiditis. J Clin Endocrinol Metab 2002;87(9):4042–7.
33. Stagnaro-Green A, Schwartz A, Gismondi R, et al. High rate of persistent hypothyroidism in a large-scale prospective study of postpartum thyroiditis in southern Italy. J Clin Endocrinol Metab 2011;96(3):652–7.
34. Howard D, La Rosa FG, Huang S, et al. Consumptive hypothyroidism resulting from hepatic vascular tumors in an athyreotic adult. J Clin Endocrinol Metab 2011;96(7):1966–70.
35. Barbesino G. Drugs affecting thyroid function. Thyroid 2010;20(7):763–70.

36. Surks MI, Sievert R. Drugs and thyroid function. N Engl J Med 1995;333(25): 1688–94.
37. George J, Joshi SR. Drugs and thyroid. J Assoc Physicians India 2007;55: 215–23.
38. Benvenga S, Bartolone L, Pappalardo MA, et al. Altered intestinal absorption of L-thyroxine caused by coffee. Thyroid 2008;18(3):293–301.
39. Cooper DS. Clinical practice. Subclinical hypothyroidism. N Engl J Med 2001; 345(4):260–5.
40. Zulewski H, Muller B, Exer P, et al. Estimation of tissue hypothyroidism by a new clinical score: evaluation of patients with various grades of hypothyroidism and controls. J Clin Endocrinol Metab 1997;82(3):771–6.
41. Lawson JD. The free Achilles reflex in hypothyroidism and hyperthyroidism. N Engl J Med 1958;259(16):761–4.
42. O'Brien T, Dinneen SF, O'Brien PC, et al. Hyperlipidemia in patients with primary and secondary hypothyroidism. Mayo Clin Proc 1993;68(9):860–6.
43. Duntas LH. Thyroid disease and lipids. Thyroid 2002;12(4):287–93.
44. Pearce EN, Wilson PW, Yang Q, et al. Thyroid function and lipid subparticle sizes in patients with short-term hypothyroidism and a population-based cohort. J Clin Endocrinol Metab 2008;93(3):888–94.
45. Klein I, Ojamaa K. Thyroid hormone and the cardiovascular system. N Engl J Med 2001;344(7):501–9.
46. Hanna FW, Scanlon MF. Hyponatraemia, hypothyroidism, and role of arginine-vasopressin. Lancet 1997;350(9080):755–6.
47. Burman KD, McKinley-Grant L. Dermatologic aspects of thyroid disease. Clin Dermatol 2006;24(4):247–55.
48. Ridgway EC, McCammon JA, Benotti J, et al. Acute metabolic responses in myxedema to large doses of intravenous L-thyroxine. Ann Intern Med 1972; 77(4):549–55.
49. Scott KR, Simmons Z, Boyer PJ. Hypothyroid myopathy with a strikingly elevated serum creatine kinase level. Muscle Nerve 2002;26(1):141–4.
50. Bauer M, Silverman DH, Schlagenhauf F, et al. Brain glucose metabolism in hypothyroidism: a positron emission tomography study before and after thyroid hormone replacement therapy. J Clin Endocrinol Metab 2009;94(8): 2922–9.
51. Ebert EC. The thyroid and the gut. J Clin Gastroenterol 2010;44(6):402–6.
52. Krassas GE, Pontikides N, Kaltsas T, et al. Disturbances of menstruation in hypothyroidism. Clin Endocrinol (Oxf) 1999;50(5):655–9.
53. Bhasin S, Enzlin P, Coviello A, et al. Sexual dysfunction in men and women with endocrine disorders. Lancet 2007;369(9561):597–611.
54. Baloch Z, Carayon P, Conte-Devolx B, et al. Laboratory medicine practice guidelines. Laboratory support for the diagnosis and monitoring of thyroid disease. Thyroid 2003;13(1):3–126.
55. Surks MI, Hollowell JG. Age-specific distribution of serum thyrotropin and anti-thyroid antibodies in the US population: implications for the prevalence of subclinical hypothyroidism. J Clin Endocrinol Metab 2007;92(12):4575–82.
56. Fatourechi V, Klee GG, Grebe SK, et al. Effects of reducing the upper limit of normal TSH values. JAMA 2003;290(24):3195–6.
57. Midgley JE. Direct and indirect free thyroxine assay methods: theory and practice. Clin Chem 2001;47(8):1353–63.
58. Gharib H, Tuttle RM, Baskin HJ, et al. Subclinical thyroid dysfunction: a joint statement on management from the American Association of Clinical

Endocrinologists, the American Thyroid Association, and the Endocrine Society. J Clin Endocrinol Metab 2005;90(1):581–5 [discussion: 586–7].

59. Barker JM. Clinical review: type 1 diabetes-associated autoimmunity: natural history, genetic associations, and screening. J Clin Endocrinol Metab 2006; 91(4):1210–7.

60. Kasperlik-Zaluska A, Czarnocka B, Czech W. High prevalence of thyroid autoimmunity in idiopathic Addison's disease. Autoimmunity 1994;18(3):213–6.

61. Loy M, Cianchetti ME, Cardia F, et al. Correlation of computerized gray-scale sonographic findings with thyroid function and thyroid autoimmune activity in patients with Hashimoto's thyroiditis. J Clin Ultrasound 2004;32(3):136–40.

62. Raber W, Gessl A, Nowotny P, et al. Thyroid ultrasound versus antithyroid peroxidase antibody determination: a cohort study of four hundred fifty-one subjects. Thyroid 2002;12(8):725–31.

63. Helfand M. Screening for subclinical thyroid dysfunction in nonpregnant adults: a summary of the evidence for the U.S. Preventive Services Task Force. Ann Intern Med 2004;140(2):128–41.

64. Ladenson PW, Singer PA, Ain KB, et al. American Thyroid Association guidelines for detection of thyroid dysfunction. Arch Intern Med 2000;160(11):1573–5.

65. Baskin HJ, Cobin RH, Duick DS, et al. American Association of Clinical Endocrinologists medical guidelines for clinical practice for the evaluation and treatment of hyperthyroidism and hypothyroidism. Endocr Pract 2002; 8(6):457–69.

66. Surks MI, Ortiz E, Daniels GH, et al. Subclinical thyroid disease: scientific review and guidelines for diagnosis and management. JAMA 2004;291(2):228–38.

67. Devdhar M, Drooger R, Pehlivanova M, et al. Levothyroxine replacement doses are affected by gender and weight, but not age. Thyroid 2011;21(8):821–7.

68. Davis FB, LaMantia RS, Spaulding SW, et al. Estimation of a physiologic replacement dose of levothyroxine in elderly patients with hypothyroidism. Arch Intern Med 1984;144(9):1752–4.

69. Gordon MB, Gordon MS. Variations in adequate levothyroxine replacement therapy in patients with different causes of hypothyroidism. Endocr Pract 1999;5(5):233–8.

70. Fish LH, Schwartz HL, Cavanaugh J, et al. Replacement dose, metabolism, and bioavailability of levothyroxine in the treatment of hypothyroidism. Role of triiodothyronine in pituitary feedback in humans. N Engl J Med 1987;316(13): 764–70.

71. Santini F, Pinchera A, Marsili A, et al. Lean body mass is a major determinant of levothyroxine dosage in the treatment of thyroid diseases. J Clin Endocrinol Metab 2005;90(1):124–7.

72. Keating FR Jr, Parkin TW, Selby JB, et al. Treatment of heart disease associated with myxedema. Prog Cardiovasc Dis 1961;3:364–81.

73. Roos A, Linn-Rasker SP, van Domburg RT, et al. The starting dose of levothyroxine in primary hypothyroidism treatment: a prospective, randomized, double-blind trial. Arch Intern Med 2005;165(15):1714–20.

74. Boeving A, Paz-Filho G, Radominski RB, et al. Low-normal or high-normal thyrotropin target levels during treatment of hypothyroidism: a prospective, comparative study. Thyroid 2011;21(4):355–60.

75. Walsh JP, Ward LC, Burke V, et al. Small changes in thyroxine dosage do not produce measurable changes in hypothyroid symptoms, well-being, or quality of life: results of a double-blind, randomized clinical trial. J Clin Endocrinol Metab 2006;91(7):2624–30.

76. Bach-Huynh TG, Nayak B, Loh J, et al. Timing of levothyroxine administration affects serum thyrotropin concentration. J Clin Endocrinol Metab 2009;94(10): 3905–12.

77. Bolk N, Visser TJ, Nijman J, et al. Effects of evening vs morning levothyroxine intake: a randomized double-blind crossover trial. Arch Intern Med 2010; 170(22):1996–2003.

78. Vanderpump M. Pharmacotherapy: hypothyroidism-should levothyroxine be taken at bedtime? Nat Rev Endocrinol 2011;7(4):195–6.

79. Grebe SK, Cooke RR, Ford HC, et al. Treatment of hypothyroidism with once weekly thyroxine. J Clin Endocrinol Metab 1997;82(3):870–5.

80. Hennessey JV. Levothyroxine dosage and the limitations of current bio-equivalence standards. Nat Clin Pract Endocrinol Metab 2006;2(9):474–5.

81. Blakesley V, Awni W, Locke C, et al. Are bioequivalence studies of levothyroxine sodium formulations in euthyroid volunteers reliable? Thyroid 2004;14(3):191–200.

82. American Thyroid Association, The Endocrine Society, and American Association of Clinical Endocrinologists. Joint statement on the U.S. Food and Drug Administration's decision regarding bioequivalence of levothyroxine sodium. Thyroid 2004;14(7):486.

83. Wekking EM, Appelhof BC, Fliers E, et al. Cognitive functioning and well-being in euthyroid patients on thyroxine replacement therapy for primary hypothyroidism. Eur J Endocrinol 2005;153(6):747–53.

84. Celi FS, Zemskova M, Linderman JD, et al. Metabolic effects of liothyronine therapy in hypothyroidism: a randomized, double-blind, crossover trial of liothyronine versus levothyroxine. J Clin Endocrinol Metab 2011;96(11):3466–74.

85. Panicker V, Saravanan P, Vaidya B, et al. Common variation in the DIO2 gene predicts baseline psychological well-being and response to combination thyroxine plus triiodothyronine therapy in hypothyroid patients. J Clin Endocrinol Metab 2009;94(5):1623–9.

86. Grozinsky-Glasberg S, Fraser A, Nahshoni E, et al. Thyroxine-triiodothyronine combination therapy versus thyroxine monotherapy for clinical hypothyroidism: meta-analysis of randomized controlled trials. J Clin Endocrinol Metab 2006; 91(7):2592–9.

87. Glinoer D. The regulation of thyroid function in pregnancy: pathways of endocrine adaptation from physiology to pathology. Endocr Rev 1997;18(3):404–33.

88. Klein RZ, Haddow JE, Faix JD, et al. Prevalence of thyroid deficiency in pregnant women. Clin Endocrinol (Oxf) 1991;35(1):41–6.

89. Negro R, Schwartz A, Gismondi R, et al. Universal screening versus case finding for detection and treatment of thyroid hormonal dysfunction during pregnancy. J Clin Endocrinol Metab 2010;95(4):1699–707.

90. Abalovich M, Amino N, Barbour LA, et al. Management of thyroid dysfunction during pregnancy and postpartum: an Endocrine Society Clinical Practice Guideline. J Clin Endocrinol Metab 2007;92(Suppl 8):S1–47.

91. Stagnaro-Green A, Abalovich M, Alexander E, et al. Guidelines of the American Thyroid Association for the diagnosis and management of thyroid disease during pregnancy and postpartum. Thyroid 2011;21(10):1081–125.

92. Vaidya B, Anthony S, Bilous M, et al. Detection of thyroid dysfunction in early pregnancy: universal screening or targeted high-risk case finding? J Clin Endocrinol Metab 2007;92(1):203–7.

93. Vaidya B, Hubalewska-Dydejczyk A, Laurberg P, et al. Treatment and screening of hypothyroidism in pregnancy: results of a European survey. Eur J Endocrinol 2012;166(1):49–54.

94. Anckaert E, Poppe K, Van Uytfanghe K, et al. FT4 immunoassays may display a pattern during pregnancy similar to the equilibrium dialysis ID-LC/tandem MS candidate reference measurement procedure in spite of susceptibility towards binding protein alterations. Clin Chim Acta 2010;411(17-18):1348–53.

95. Kahric-Janicic N, Soldin SJ, Soldin OP, et al. Tandem mass spectrometry improves the accuracy of free thyroxine measurements during pregnancy. Thyroid 2007;17(4):303–11.

96. Soldin OP, Tractenberg RE, Hollowell JG, et al. Trimester-specific changes in maternal thyroid hormone, thyrotropin, and thyroglobulin concentrations during gestation: trends and associations across trimesters in iodine sufficiency. Thyroid 2004;14(12):1084–90.

97. Yassa L, Marqusee E, Fawcett R, et al. Thyroid hormone early adjustment in pregnancy (the THERAPY) trial. J Clin Endocrinol Metab 2010;95(7):3234–41.

98. Alexander EK, Marqusee E, Lawrence J, et al. Timing and magnitude of increases in levothyroxine requirements during pregnancy in women with hypothyroidism. N Engl J Med 2004;351(3):241–9.

99. Leung AS, Millar LK, Koonings PP, et al. Perinatal outcome in hypothyroid pregnancies. Obstet Gynecol 1993;81(3):349–53.

100. Davis LE, Leveno KJ, Cunningham FG. Hypothyroidism complicating pregnancy. Obstet Gynecol 1988;72(1):108–12.

101. Cleary-Goldman J, Malone FD, Lambert-Messerlian G, et al. Maternal thyroid hypofunction and pregnancy outcome. Obstet Gynecol 2008;112(1):85–92.

102. Contempre B, Jauniaux E, Calvo R, et al. Detection of thyroid hormones in human embryonic cavities during the first trimester of pregnancy. J Clin Endocrinol Metab 1993;77(6):1719–22.

103. Haddow JE, Palomaki GE, Allan WC, et al. Maternal thyroid deficiency during pregnancy and subsequent neuropsychological development of the child. N Engl J Med 1999;341(8):549–55.

104. Negro R, Formoso G, Mangieri T, et al. Levothyroxine treatment in euthyroid pregnant women with autoimmune thyroid disease: effects on obstetrical complications. J Clin Endocrinol Metab 2006;91(7):2587–91.

105. Negro R, Greco G, Mangieri T, et al. The influence of selenium supplementation on postpartum thyroid status in pregnant women with thyroid peroxidase autoantibodies. J Clin Endocrinol Metab 2007;92(4):1263–8.

106. Ashoor G, Maiz N, Rotas M, et al. Maternal thyroid function at 11 to 13 weeks of gestation and subsequent fetal death. Thyroid 2010;20(9):989–93.

107. Pop VJ, Brouwers EP, Vader HL, et al. Maternal hypothyroxinaemia during early pregnancy and subsequent child development: a 3-year follow-up study. Clin Endocrinol (Oxf) 2003;59(3):282–8.

108. Li Y, Shan Z, Teng W, et al. Abnormalities of maternal thyroid function during pregnancy affect neuropsychological development of their children at 25-30 months. Clin Endocrinol (Oxf) 2010;72(6):825–9.

109. de Escobar GM, Obregon MJ, del Rey FE. Maternal thyroid hormones early in pregnancy and fetal brain development. Best Pract Res Clin Endocrinol Metab 2004;18(2):225–48.

110. Gaudino R, Garel C, Czernichow P, et al. Proportion of various types of thyroid disorders among newborns with congenital hypothyroidism and normally located gland: a regional cohort study. Clin Endocrinol (Oxf) 2005;62(4):444–8.

111. Hanna CE, Krainz PL, Skeels MR, et al. Detection of congenital hypopituitary hypothyroidism: ten-year experience in the Northwest Regional Screening Program. J Pediatr 1986;109(6):959–64.

112. LaFranchi SH. Approach to the diagnosis and treatment of neonatal hypothyroidism. J Clin Endocrinol Metab 2011;96(10):2959–67.
113. Harris KB, Pass KA. Increase in congenital hypothyroidism in New York State and in the United States. Mol Genet Metab 2007;91(3):268–77.
114. Deladoey J, Ruel J, Giguere Y, et al. Is the incidence of congenital hypothyroidism really increasing? a 20-year retrospective population-based study in Quebec. J Clin Endocrinol Metab 2011;96(8):2422–9.

Subacute, Silent, and Postpartum Thyroiditis

Mary H. Samuels, MD

KEYWORDS

- Thyroiditis • Subacute thyroiditis • Silent thyroiditis
- Postpartum thyroiditis

Thyroiditis is a broad term that indicates thyroid gland inflammation. There are many types of thyroiditis, which can generally be divided into painful or painless categories.[1] Painful types include subacute and suppurative thyroiditis, as well as unusual cases induced by radioactive iodine administration, trauma, or other rare causes. Painless types include Hashimoto thyroiditis, the most common type of chronic thyroid disease, as well as silent, postpartum, drug-induced, and Riedel thyroiditis.

Thyroid function in patients with thyroiditis depends on the type of thyroiditis and, in certain cases, evolves from thyrotoxicosis to hypothyroidism and eventually to restoration of normal thyroid function. This classic triphasic course of thyroid dysfunction is characteristic of the 3 entities considered in this article: subacute, silent, and postpartum thyroiditis. The other types of thyroiditis are not discussed further, except in the context of the differential diagnosis. **Table 1** provides a comprehensive summary of the text of this article and can be referenced throughout the discussion that follows.

SUBACUTE THYROIDITIS
Clinical Findings and Course

Subacute thyroiditis, also called subacute granulomatous or de Quervain thyroiditis, is the most common cause of thyroid pain.[1,2] This condition usually presents as a prodrome of low-grade fever, fatigue, and pharyngitis symptoms. The thyroid gland becomes extremely painful and tender to palpation, with pain often radiating up to the jaw or ear and associated dysphagia. The pain can be unilateral or bilateral. The thyroid gland can be enlarged up to 3 to 4 times its normal size, but an extremely large or grossly nodular goiter is not characteristic of subacute thyroiditis and should raise the possibility of alternate diagnoses.

About 50% of patients with subacute thyroiditis have an initial thyrotoxic phase because of unregulated release of preformed thyroid hormone from damaged thyroid

Division of Endocrinology, Diabetes and Clinical Nutrition, Oregon Health & Science University, 3181 Southwest Sam Jackson Park Road, Portland, OR 97239, USA
E-mail address: samuelsm@ohsu.edu

Med Clin N Am 96 (2012) 223–233
doi:10.1016/j.mcna.2012.01.003

medical.theclinics.com

0025-7125/12/$ – see front matter © 2012 Elsevier Inc. All rights reserved.

Table 1
An overview of pertinent findings in subacute, silent, and postpartum thyroiditis

	Subacute Thyroiditis	Silent Thyroiditis	Postpartum Thyroiditis
Clinical findings	Viral URI prodrome, small painful goiter, symptoms and signs of thyroid dysfunction (variable)	Small painless goiter, symptoms and signs of thyroid dysfunction (variable)	Small painless goiter, symptoms and signs of thyroid dysfunction (variable)
Clinical course	Classic triphasic course (thyrotoxic, hypothyroid, recovery) but variable	Classic triphasic course (thyrotoxic, hypothyroid, recovery) but variable	Classic triphasic course (thyrotoxic, hypothyroid, recovery) but variable
Demographics	Incidence: approximately 3/100,000/y ♀:♂, 4:1 Peak age, 40–50 y Seasonal	♀:♂, 4:1 Peak age, 30–40 y More common in areas of iodine sufficiency	♀ only Occurs within 12 mo of pregnancy 8%–11% of pregnancies
Etiology	Probably viral	Probably autoimmune	Autoimmune
Laboratory findings	Elevated WBC, ESR, CRP level; approximately 25% have antithyroid antibodies, usually low titer; thyroid function varies with phase	Approximately 50% have antithyroid antibodies, thyroid function varies with phase	>80% have antithyroid antibodies, thyroid function varies with phase
Imaging	Decreased RaIU in thyrotoxic phase US: variable heterogeneous texture, hypoechogenic	Decreased RaIU in thyrotoxic phase US: variable heterogeneous texture, hypoechogenic	Decreased RaIU in thyrotoxic phase US: variable heterogeneous texture, hypoechogenic
Pathology	Granulomatous infiltrate	Lymphocytic infiltrate	Lymphocytic infiltrate
Differential diagnosis	Painful thyroid gland: rarely Hashimoto disease, Graves disease, RaI, amiodarone, contrast dye, suppurative thyroiditis, amyloid	Thyrotoxic phase: Graves disease Hypothyroid phase: Hashimoto disease	Thyrotoxic phase: Graves disease Hypothyroid phase: Hashimoto disease
Treatment	For pain: NSAIDs, glucocorticoids Thyrotoxic phase: β-blockers Hypothyroid phase: L-T_4	Thyrotoxic phase: β-blockers Hypothyroid phase: L-T_4	Thyrotoxic phase: β-blockers Hypothyroid phase: L-T_4
Long-term outcomes	5%–15% hypothyroid beyond a year	10%–20% hypothyroid beyond a year	15%–50% hypothyroid beyond a year
Recurrence rates	1%–4% after a year	5%–10% (much higher in Japan)	70% in subsequent pregnancies

Abbreviations: CRP, C-reactive protein; ESR, erythrocyte sedimentation rate; RaI, radioactive iodine; URI, upper respiratory illness; US, ultrasonography; WBC, white blood cell count.

follicular cells.[2] Therefore, if patients present early in the course of the disease, they may have clinical findings of thyrotoxicosis, although this is often mild. This phase usually lasts about 3 to 6 weeks, ending when the thyroid stores of preformed hormone are depleted. About one-third of patients subsequently enter a hypothyroid phase that can last up to 6 months. Thyroid pain has usually resolved by this time, and the predominant clinical features are those of hypothyroidism with a continued small goiter. Most patients return to euthyroidism within 12 months of onset of disease.

Demographics

The most comprehensive study of subacute thyroiditis analyzed 94 cases seen over 27 years in Olmsted County, Minnesota. The incidence rate was 3 cases per 100,000 per year in the most recent years of the survey.[2] Women seem to be more affected than men, in a 4:1 ratio.[2–5] The peak age of incidence is 40 to 50 years. Some studies suggest that there is a seasonal peak of cases during spring, summer, or fall, but this finding has not always been confirmed. There is no geographic or familial clustering.

Etiology

Subacute thyroiditis is probably caused by a viral infection of the thyroid gland. Implicated conditions include infections caused by Coxsackie virus, Epstein-Barr virus, adenoviruses, and influenza viruses; mumps; measles; primary human immunodeficiency virus infection; and a recent well-documented case occurring during an H1N1 influenza infection.[6]

Laboratory Findings

Patients with subacute thyroiditis have elevated erythrocyte sedimentation rates (often >50 mm/h) and C-reactive protein levels, consistent with acute inflammation.[2,3,5] The white blood cell count can be mildly elevated, although marked elevations raise the question of suppurative thyroiditis. During the thyrotoxic phase, thyrotropin (TSH) levels are low and free thyroxine (T_4) levels may be elevated, depending on the degree of thyrotoxicosis. During the hypothyroid phase, TSH levels are high and free T_4 levels may be low. Up to 25% of patients have low titers of antithyroid antibodies, although very high titers raise the question of painful autoimmune thyroiditis.[2–4,7]

Imaging Findings

A hallmark of subacute thyroiditis is low radioactive iodine uptake (RaIU) during the thyrotoxic phase, because the inflamed thyroid gland does not trap iodine.[7] As the thyrotoxic phase ends, the RaIU returns to normal or even becomes elevated during the hypothyroid phase. It is not necessary to obtain an ultrasonography of the thyroid in subacute thyroiditis, but, if ultrasonography is performed, it often shows inhomogeneous hypoechogenic texture, sometimes with nodules, because of the inflammatory process.[2,4,5,7,8]

Pathology

A biopsy of the thyroid gland is not usually necessary in subacute thyroiditis. However, if biopsy is performed due to uncertainty of the diagnosis, its result shows granulomatous infiltrate, sometimes with giant cells, consistent with a viral infection.[2]

Differential Diagnosis

In a patient who presents with a painful tender thyroid gland, by far the most common cause is subacute thyroiditis. However, there are other unusual causes of thyroid pain that must be considered if the patient has a consistent history, unusual symptoms, or a markedly enlarged gland.[9,10] These causes include Hashimoto disease, Graves disease, radioactive iodine administration, amiodarone-induced thyroiditis, contrast dye–induced thyroiditis, acute suppurative thyroiditis, or amyloid goiter.

During the thyrotoxic phase, the main differential diagnosis is between subacute thyroiditis and Graves disease. A recent history of neck pain indicates subacute thyroiditis, whereas the presence of ophthalmopathy or a thyroid bruit indicates Graves disease. Serum triiodothyronine (T_3) levels and T_3:T_4 ratios tend to be lower in subacute thyroiditis than in Graves disease, but there is significant overlap in thyroid hormone levels.[11] A definitive diagnosis can be made by RaIU measurement, because uptake is low in subacute thyroiditis and elevated in Graves disease.[7] Care must be taken to perform the RaIU test while the patient is still thyrotoxic, because RaIU increases as the patient enters the hypothyroid phase.

During the hypothyroid phase, the main differential diagnosis is between subacute thyroiditis and Hashimoto disease. A history of neck pain can be helpful but is often forgotten by patients if there was no obvious intervening thyrotoxic phase brought to medical attention earlier. Measurement of antithyroid antibodies may be helpful, because they tend to be absent or in low titer in subacute thyroiditis. In the absence of a definitive diagnosis, the patient may need monitoring or temporary treatment to see if the thyroid dysfunction resolves over time.

Treatment

Nonsteroidal antiinflammatory agents (NSAIDs) are the first-line treatment of thyroid pain in subacute thyroiditis. With NSAIDs alone, the median time for complete resolution of pain is 5 weeks, with a range of 1 to 20 weeks.[2] Glucocorticoids are used for severe cases or if NSAIDs are not effective. Typical prednisone dosages are 30 to 40 mg per day for 1 to 4 weeks, followed by tapering doses. Pain resolution is faster with glucocorticoids than with NSAIDs.[2] If glucocorticoids are stopped too soon, pain can recur and require restarting the drug for a longer course.[2,12]

β-Blockers are used for control of symptoms during the thyrotoxic phase, although often no treatment is needed if symptoms are mild. Thionamides (methimazole and propylthiouracil) are ineffective, because thyrotoxicosis is caused by the release of preformed thyroid hormone, rather than synthesis of new thyroid hormones. Once the patient enters the hypothyroid phase, levothyroxine (L-T_4) can be used to treat symptoms if needed. L-T_4 should also be administered if the patient is considering pregnancy regardless of symptoms. L-T_4 should be continued until 12 months have elapsed since the onset of subacute thyroiditis and can then be discontinued, because most patients would have fully recovered by that time.

Recurrence Rates and Long-Term Outcomes

Almost all patients with subacute thyroiditis recover full thyroid function, but about 5% to 15% have persistent hypothyroidism after 12 months.[2,4,5] In addition, recurrence rates of 1% to 4% have been described.[2] Recurrences are managed in the same manner as the initial occurrence, but, rarely, thyroidectomy has been used for repeated relapses.[2]

SILENT THYROIDITIS
Clinical Findings and Clinical Course

Silent thyroiditis, also called subacute lymphocytic thyroiditis, classically presents with the same triphasic course described earlier for subacute thyroiditis: thyrotoxicosis, followed by hypothyroidism, and eventual restoration of normal thyroid function.[1,13] The thyrotoxic phase occurs in 5% to 20% of patients and typically lasts 3 to 4 months. The hypothyroid phase is more common or at least is recognized more often. This phase typically lasts up to 6 months, before return to normal thyroid function, for a total duration of illness of up to 12 months. A small goiter is common but, unlike subacute thyroiditis, not painful.

Demographics

The incidence of silent thyroiditis is not well delineated, with reports that it accounts for 0% to 23% of thyrotoxicosis cases.[14–16] Silent thyroiditis seems to be more prevalent in areas of higher dietary iodine intake, accounting for up to 30% of cases of thyrotoxicosis in Japan.[17] Women are affected more commonly than men, in a 4:1 ratio.[13] The peak age of incidence is 30 to 40 years.

Etiology

Silent thyroiditis is probably autoimmune in nature, given the frequent presence of antithyroid antibodies and the characteristic pathologic findings of lymphocytic infiltration of the thyroid gland.[18]

Laboratory Findings

During the thyrotoxic phase of silent thyroiditis, TSH levels are low and free T_4 levels may be elevated, depending on the degree of thyrotoxicosis. During the hypothyroid phase, TSH levels are high and free T_4 levels may be low. About 50% of patients have antithyroid peroxidase (anti-TPO) antibodies.[1]

Imaging Findings

As in subacute thyroiditis, patients with silent thyroiditis have a low RaIU during the thyrotoxic phase.[1] Similarly, because the thyrotoxic phase ends, the RaIU returns to normal or becomes elevated during the hypothyroid phase. Ultrasonography of the thyroid often shows inhomogeneous hypoechogenic texture.[19]

Pathology

A thyroid gland affected by silent thyroiditis has a diffuse lymphocytic infiltrate that resembles Hashimoto disease but lacks Hürthle cells, lymphoid germinal center formation, or fibrosis of Hashimoto disease.[18,20]

Differential Diagnosis

During the thyrotoxic phase, the main differential diagnosis is between silent thyroiditis and Graves disease. The presence of ophthalmopathy or a thyroid bruit indicates Graves disease. Serum T_3 levels and T_3:T_4 (or free T_3 to free T_4) ratios tend to be lower in silent thyroiditis than in Graves disease, but there is significant overlap in thyroid hormone levels.[11,21,22] Titers of thyroid receptor antibodies (TRAb) or thyroid-binding inhibitory immunoglobulins are usually much higher in Graves disease than in silent thyroiditis,[11,19,23,24] although there is no cutoff with 100% accuracy. Doppler ultrasonography tends to show higher blood flow in Graves disease.[19,24] A definitive diagnosis can be made by RaIU measurement, because uptake is low in silent thyroiditis and elevated in Graves disease. Care must be taken to perform the RaIU test while the patient is still thyrotoxic, because RaIU increases as the patient enters the hypothyroid phase.

During the hypothyroid phase, the main differential diagnosis is between silent thyroiditis and Hashimoto disease. Measurement of antithyroid antibodies is often not helpful, because they may be present in either case. In the absence of a definitive diagnosis, the patient may need monitoring or temporary treatment to see if the thyroid dysfunction resolves over time.

Treatment

Treatment of silent thyroiditis is similar to that of subacute thyroiditis, except that NSAIDs or glucocorticoids are not used, because there is no neck pain. β-Blockers are used to control symptoms during the thyrotoxic phase, although often no treatment is needed if symptoms are mild. Thionamides are ineffective and not used. Once the patient enters the hypothyroid phase, L-T_4 can be used to treat symptoms if needed. L-T_4 should be administered if the patient is considering pregnancy regardless of symptoms. L-T_4 should be continued until 12 months have elapsed since the onset of silent thyroiditis and can then be discontinued.

Recurrence Rates and Long-Term Outcomes

Most patients with silent thyroiditis recover full thyroid function, but about 10% to 20% have persistent hypothyroidism after 12 months.[1] Recurrence rates are about 5% to 10% but may be much higher in Japan, with one study from Japan reporting a long-term recurrence rate of 65%.[20] Recurrences are managed in the same manner as in the initial occurrence, but some patients with multiple recurrences have opted for radioactive iodine ablation of the gland.[20]

POSTPARTUM THYROIDITIS
Clinical Findings and Clinical Course

Postpartum thyroiditis is defined as the development of thyroid dysfunction in a previously euthyroid woman within 12 months after pregnancy. Almost all cases occur after a term pregnancy, although there are reports of cases developing after a miscarriage. Like subacute and silent thyroiditis, the clinical course is classically triphasic, with an initial thyrotoxic phase followed by a hypothyroid phase and an eventual return to a euthyroid state, all within 12 months.[25] However, the pattern of thyroid dysfunction is quite variable; 25% to 40% of patients exhibit the classic triphasic course, whereas 20% to 30% develop only thyrotoxicosis and 40% develop only hypothyroidism.[25–27] The thyrotoxic phase occurs at 2 to 6 months post partum (median time of onset, 13 weeks) and is usually asymptomatic. However, irritability, heat intolerance, fatigue, and palpitations are more common in thyrotoxic women with postpartum thyroiditis.[28] This phase typically lasts 2 to 3 months. The hypothyroid phase occurs 3 to 12 months post partum (median time of onset, 19 weeks) and is often symptomatic, with cold intolerance, dry skin, loss of energy, and problems with concentration.[25,28] Most patients have a small painless goiter. Given the known effects of altered thyroid function on mood, investigators have questioned whether postpartum thyroiditis may play a role in the development of postpartum depression.[28] However, results from these studies have been mixed, and one randomized controlled trial of L-T_4 therapy in anti-TPO–positive postpartum women did not report a reduction in the incidence of postpartum depression.[29]

Demographics

Postpartum thyroiditis occurs in 8% to 11% of unselected pregnancies, with some variability owing to the population studied and the frequency of monitoring.[25,30–32]

There are several well-defined risk factors that greatly increase a woman's chance of developing postpartum thyroiditis. The best predictor is the presence of anti-TPO antibodies at the end of the first trimester of pregnancy, with 30% to 50% of these women progressing to postpartum thyroiditis.[25,28,30,33] Women with a past history of thyroid disease have a 40% risk of developing postpartum thyroiditis, whereas those with type 1 diabetes mellitus or a family history of thyroid disease have a 20% risk.[30]

Etiology

Postpartum thyroiditis is autoimmune in nature, with an HLA linkage, anti-TPO antibodies in most patients, laboratory findings of immune system activation, and dense lymphocytic infiltrates in affected thyroid glands.[28]

Laboratory Findings

Laboratory tests of thyroid function in postpartum thyroiditis are similar to those in subacute and silent thyroiditis. During the thyrotoxic phase, TSH levels are low and free T_4 levels may be elevated, depending on the degree of thyrotoxicosis. After the thyrotoxic phase, the American Thyroid Association recommends obtaining a serum TSH level test every 2 months in all women with postpartum thyroiditis until 1 year post partum, to monitor for the development of hypothyroidism.[28] During the hypothyroid phase, TSH levels are high and free T_4 levels may be low. More than 80% of patients have anti-TPO antibodies.[28]

Imaging Findings

As in subacute and silent thyroiditis, patients with postpartum thyroiditis have a low RaIU during the thyrotoxic phase.[1] Similarly, because the thyrotoxic phase ends, the RaIU returns to normal or becomes elevated during the hypothyroid phase. Ultrasonography of the thyroid almost always shows inhomogeneous hypoechogenic texture.[34]

Pathology

Pathology test results of the thyroid gland in postpartum thyroiditis show dense lymphocytic infiltration consistent with the autoimmune nature of the disease but without germinal centers or extensive Hürthle cell metaplasia that can be seen in Hashimoto disease.[1]

Differential Diagnosis

During the thyrotoxic phase, the main differential diagnosis is between postpartum thyroiditis and Graves disease. There may in fact be some overlap because both are autoimmune processes, and women with a history of 1 entity can eventually develop the other. The presence of ophthalmopathy, a thyroid bruit, or TRAb indicates Graves disease. T_3 levels and T_3:T_4 ratios are higher in Graves disease than in postpartum thyroiditis. A definitive diagnosis can be made by RaIU measurement because uptake is low in postpartum thyroiditis and elevated in Graves disease. However, it can be logistically difficult to perform an RaIU test on a postpartum woman because issues of breastfeeding and neonatal exposure to the radioactive iodine must be taken into account.

During the hypothyroid phase, the main differential diagnosis is between postpartum thyroiditis and Hashimoto disease. There is likely overlap, because a significant number of women with postpartum thyroiditis eventually develop permanent autoimmune hypothyroidism. Measurement of antithyroid antibodies is not helpful because these antibodies are usually present in either case. In the absence of a definitive diagnosis, the patient may need monitoring or temporary treatment to check if the thyroid dysfunction resolves over time (see caveats later).

Treatment

Treatment of postpartum thyroiditis is similar to that of silent thyroiditis, with extra caution indicated for breastfeeding women. β-Blockers are used for control of symptoms during the thyrotoxic phase, although often no treatment is needed if symptoms are mild. Once the patient enters the hypothyroid phase, L-T$_4$ can be used to treat symptoms if needed. L-T$_4$ should be administered if the patient is considering another pregnancy regardless of symptoms. If treatment is not started for hypothyroidism, TSH levels should be rechecked every 1 to 2 months until the patient is 12 months post partum.[28]

The issue of whether to continue L-T$_4$ after 12 months have elapsed since the onset of postpartum thyroiditis is complicated. Permanent hypothyroidism is common in postpartum thyroiditis, especially in certain high-risk subgroups (see later). Many of these women are still breastfeeding, and L-T$_4$ should be continued. Other women may be considering another pregnancy within a year, and intercurrent hypothyroidism would be detrimental to the pregnancy and developing fetus. Therefore, the decision to discontinue L-T$_4$ in women with postpartum thyroiditis should be individualized, based on the patient's likelihood of permanent hypothyroidism and personal situation.[28]

There have been 3 randomized controlled trials that attempted to prevent postpartum thyroiditis in high-risk women. Two trials of iodine or L-T$_4$ supplementation performed during or after pregnancy in women with anti-TPO antibodies failed to reduce the risk of postpartum thyroiditis.[35,36] In contrast, selenium administered to anti-TPO–positive women during and after pregnancy decreased the rate of postpartum thyroiditis from 50% in placebo-treated women to 29% in selenium-treated women.[37] The rate of permanent hypothyroidism decreased from 20% to 12%. However, the recent American Thyroid Association guidelines do not recommend treating high-risk women with selenium until its safety and efficacy can be further evaluated.[28]

Recurrent Rates and Long-Term Outcomes

In anti-TPO–positive women who recover from postpartum thyroiditis, there is a 70% recurrence rate in subsequent pregnancies.[25,28] In the long-term, 15% to 50% of women with a history of postpartum thyroiditis develop permanent hypothyroidism.[26,31,33,37–42] The longest study to date reported on more than 700 women who had postpartum thyroiditis 12 years earlier; 38% had hypothyroid.[31] Risks of permanent hypothyroidism increase in women with a hypothyroid phase of postpartum thyroiditis, high titers of anti-TPO antibodies, a hypoechogenic ultrasonography, or higher TSH levels at 6 months post partum.[31,33] Given these risks, all women with a history of postpartum thyroiditis should have TSH levels checked every year indefinitely.[28]

REFERENCES

1. Bindra A, Braunstein GD. Thyroiditis. Am Fam Physician 2006;73:1769–76.
2. Fatourechi V, Aniszewski JP, Fatourechi GZ, et al. Clinical features and outcome of subacute thyroiditis in an incidence cohort: Olmsted County, Minnesota, study. J Clin Endocrinol Metab 2003;88:2100–5.

3. Erdem N, Erdogan M, Ozbek M, et al. Demographic and clinical features of patients with subacute thyroiditis: results of 169 patients from a single university center in Turkey. J Endocrinol Invest 2007;30:546–50.
4. Benbassat CA, Olchovsky D, Tsvetov G, et al. Subacute thyroiditis: clinical characteristics and treatment outcome in fifty-six consecutive patients diagnosed between 1999 and 2005. J Endocrinol Invest 2007;30:631–5.
5. Nishihara E, Ohye H, Amino N, et al. Clinical characteristics of 852 patients with subacute thyroiditis before treatment. Intern Med 2008;47:725–9.
6. Dimos G, Pappas G, Akritidis N. Subacute thyroiditis in the course of novel H1N1 influenza infection. Endocrine 2010;37(3):440–1.
7. Espinoza PG, Guendelman CL, Quevedo, et al. A comparison between two imaging techniques for the diagnosis of subacute thyroiditis (de Quervain thyroiditis): brief communication. Clin Nucl Med 2010;35:862–4.
8. Omori N, Omori K, Takano K. Association of the ultrasonographic findings of subacute thyroiditis with thyroid pain and laboratory findings. Endocr J 2008; 55:583–8.
9. Kon YC, DeGroot LJ. Painful Hashimoto's thyroiditis as an indication for thyroidectomy: clinical characteristics and outcome in seven patients. J Clin Endocrinol Metab 2003;88:2667–72.
10. Calvi L, Daniels GH. Acute thyrotoxicosis secondary to destructive thyroiditis associated with cardiac catheterization contrast dye. Thyroid 2011;21:443–9.
11. Izumi Y, Hidaka Y, Tada H, et al. Simple and practical parameters for differentiation between destruction-induced thyrotoxicosis and Graves' thyrotoxicosis. Clin Endocrinol (Oxf) 2002;57:51–8.
12. Mizukoshi T, Noguchi S, Murakami T, et al. Evaluation of recurrence in 36 subacute thyroiditis patients managed with prednisolone. Intern Med 2001;40: 292–5.
13. Pearce EN, Farwell AP, Braverman LE. Thyroiditis. N Engl J Med 2003;348: 2646–55.
14. Nikolai TF, Brosseau J, Kettrick MA, et al. Lymphocytic thyroiditis with spontaneously resolving hyperthyroidism (silent thyroiditis). Arch Intern Med 1980;140: 478–82.
15. Schorr AB, Miller JL, Shtasel P, et al. Low incidence of painless thyroiditis in the Philadelphia area. Clin Nucl Med 1986;11:379–80.
16. Vitug AC, Goldman JM. Silent (painless) thyroiditis. Evidence of a geographic variation in frequency. Arch Intern Med 1985;145:473–5.
17. Nishimaki M, Isozaki O, Yoshihara A, et al. Clinical characteristics of frequently recurring painless thyroiditis: contributions of higher thyroid hormone levels, younger onset, male gender, presence of thyroid autoantibody and absence of goiter to repeated recurrence. Endocr J 2009;56:391–7.
18. Volpé R. Is silent thyroiditis an autoimmune disease? Arch Intern Med 1988;148: 1907–8.
19. Kamijo K. Study on cutoff value setting for differential diagnosis between Graves' disease and painless thyroiditis using the TRAb (Elecsys TRAb) measurement via the fully automated electrochemiluminescence immunoassay system. Endocr J 2010;57:895–902.
20. Mittra ES, McDougall IR. Recurrent silent thyroiditis: a report of four patients and review of the literature. Thyroid 2007;17:671–5.
21. Yanagisawa T, Sato K, Kato Y, et al. Rapid differential diagnosis of Graves' disease and painless thyroiditis using total T3/T4 ratio, TSH, and total alkaline phosphatase activity. Endocr J 2005;52:29–36.

22. Yoshimura Noh J, Momotani N, Fukada S, et al. Ratio of serum free triiodothyronine to free thyroxine in Graves' hyperthyroidism and thyrotoxicosis caused by painless thyroiditis. Endocr J 2005;52:537–42.
23. Izumi Y, Takeoka K, Amino N. Usefulness of the 2nd generation assay for anti-TSH receptor antibodies to differentiate relapse of Graves' thyrotoxicosis from development of painless thyroiditis after antithyroid drug treatment for Graves' disease. Endocr J 2005;52:493–7.
24. Ota H, Amino N, Morita S, et al. Quantitative measurement of thyroid blood flow for differentiation of painless thyroiditis from Graves' disease. Clin Endocrinol (Oxf) 2007;67:41–5.
25. Lazarus JH. The continuing saga of postpartum thyroiditis. J Clin Endocrinol Metab 2011;96:614–6.
26. Kita M, Goulis DG, Avramides A. Post-partum thyroiditis in a mediterranean population: a prospective study of a large cohort of thyroid antibody positive women at the time of delivery. J Endocrinol Invest 2002;25:513–9.
27. Lucas A, Pizarro E, Granada ML, et al. Postpartum thyroiditis: epidemiology and clinical evolution in a nonselected population. Thyroid 2000;10:71–7.
28. Stagnaro-Green A, Abalovich M, Alexander E, American Thyroid Association Taskforce on Thyroid Disease During Pregnancy and Postpartum, et al. Guidelines of the American Thyroid Association for the diagnosis and management of thyroid disease during pregnancy and postpartum. Thyroid 2011;21(10): 1081–125.
29. Harris B, Oretti R, Lazarus J, et al. Randomised trial of thyroxine to prevent postnatal depression in thyroid-antibody-positive women. Br J Psychiatry 2002;180: 327–30.
30. Nicholson WK, Robinson KA, Smallridge RC, et al. Prevalence of postpartum thyroid dysfunction: a quantitative review. Thyroid 2006;16:573–82.
31. Stuckey BG, Kent GN, Ward LC, et al. Postpartum thyroid dysfunction and the long-term risk of hypothyroidism: results from a 12-year follow-up study of women with and without postpartum thyroid dysfunction. Clin Endocrinol (Oxf) 2010;73: 389–95.
32. Guan H, Li C, Li Y, et al. High iodine intake is a risk factor of post-partum thyroiditis: result of a survey from Shenyang, China. J Endocrinol Invest 2005; 28:876–81.
33. Stagnaro-Green A, Schwartz A, Gismondi R, et al. High rate of persistent hypothyroidism in a large-scale prospective study of postpartum thyroiditis in southern Italy. J Clin Endocrinol Metab 2011;96:652–7.
34. Shahbazian HB, Sarvghadi F, Azizi F. Ultrasonographic characteristics and follow-up in post-partum thyroiditis. J Endocrinol Invest 2005;28:410–2.
35. Nøhr SB, Jørgensen A, Pedersen KM, et al. Postpartum thyroid dysfunction in pregnant thyroid peroxidase antibody-positive women living in an area with mild to moderate iodine deficiency: is iodine supplementation safe? J Clin Endocrinol Metab 2000;85:3191–8.
36. Kämpe O, Jansson R, Karlsson FA. Effects of L-thyroxine and iodide on the development of autoimmune postpartum thyroiditis. J Clin Endocrinol Metab 1990;70: 1014–8.
37. Negro R, Greco G, Mangieri T, et al. The influence of selenium supplementation on postpartum thyroid status in pregnant women with thyroid peroxidase autoantibodies. J Clin Endocrinol Metab 2007;92:1263–8.
38. Nikolai TF, Turney SL, Roberts RC. Postpartum lymphocytic thyroiditis. Prevalence, clinical course, and long-term follow-up. Arch Intern Med 1987;147:221–4.

39. Azizi F. The occurrence of permanent thyroid failure in patients with subclinical postpartum thyroiditis. Eur J Endocrinol 2005;153:367–71.
40. Premawardhana LD, Parkes AB, Ammari F, et al. Postpartum thyroiditis and long-term thyroid status: prognostic influence of thyroid peroxidase antibodies and ultrasound echogenicity. J Clin Endocrinol Metab 2000;85:71–5.
41. Lucas A, Pizarro E, Granada ML, et al. Postpartum thyroiditis: long-term follow-up. Thyroid 2005;15:1177–81.
42. Tachi J, Amino N, Tamaki H, et al. Long term follow-up and HLA association in patients with postpartum hypothyroidism. J Clin Endocrinol Metab 1988;66:480–4.

Thyroid Disorders During Pregnancy

Cynthia F. Yazbeck, MD[a], Shannon D. Sullivan, MD, PhD[b],*

KEYWORDS

- Pregnancy • Hypothyroidism • Isolated hypothyroxinemia
- Hyperthyroidism • Gestational transient thyrotoxicosis
- Postpartum thyroiditis • Thyroid nodules • Thyroid cancer

Thyroid disorders are common in pregnancy and in nonpregnant women of childbearing age, but can be missed because of nonspecific symptoms and normal changes in the physiology of the thyroid gland during pregnancy. The prevalence of overt hyperthyroidism complicating pregnancy has been reported to range between 0.4% and 1.7%,[1] and an estimated 2% to 3% of women are hypothyroid during pregnancy.[2,3] Abnormalities in maternal thyroid function are associated with complications during pregnancy, and can affect maternal and fetal outcomes. Therefore, it is important to identify thyroid disorders before pregnancy or early in pregnancy so that appropriate treatment can be initiated.

PHYSIOLOGY OF THYROID GLAND IN PREGNANCY

Normal pregnancy entails complex changes in thyroid physiology.[4] Indeed, in pregnant women with hypothyroidism, exogenous thyroid hormone replacement requirements typically increase by 25% to 47% to maintain normal serum thyroid-stimulating hormone (TSH) concentrations.[5–7] Several factors account for this. First, high estrogen states such as pregnancy increase hepatic thyroid-binding globulin (TBG) synthesis[8,9] and prolong TBG half-life because of estrogen-induced sialylation.[10] In pregnancy, TBG levels begin to increase after a few weeks, reach a plateau around mid-gestation, and remain 2- to 3-fold higher than preconception values until term.[11] The increased concentration of TBG leads to an elevation of total T_4 (TT_4) and total T_3 (TT_3) levels.[12] Levels of serum TT_4 increase sharply between 6 and 12 weeks of gestation, progress more slowly thereafter, and stabilize around mid-gestation. The

[a] Division of Endocrinology, University of Pittsburgh Medical Center, 200 Lothrop Street, E1140 BST, Pittsburgh, PA 15261, USA
[b] Department of Endocrinology, Washington Hospital Center, 110 Irving Street, NW, Suite 2A-72, Washington, DC 20010, USA
* Corresponding author.
E-mail address: Shannon.d.sullivan@medstar.net

Med Clin N Am 96 (2012) 235–256
doi:10.1016/j.mcna.2012.01.004
0025-7125/12/$ – see front matter © 2012 Elsevier Inc. All rights reserved.

increase in TT_3 concentration is more progressive. Both TT_4 and TT_3 reach their plateau by 20 weeks and are maintained until term.[4]

Second, human chorionic gonadotropin (hCG) is a thyroid regulator in normal pregnancy because the hormone-specific β subunits and the extracellular receptor-binding domains of human chorionic gonadotropin (hCG) and TSH share multiple similarities.[13] Consequently, high concentrations of hCG during pregnancy stimulate TSH receptors. In pathologic conditions such as molar pregnancy or choriocarcinoma, this may lead to gestational hyperthyroidism. In normal pregnancy, the placenta produces hCG in the first week after conception and the levels peak at week 10, before decreasing and reaching a plateau by week 20.[12] Between 8 and 14 weeks' gestation, the changes in hCG and TSH levels are mirror images of each other, with a significant negative correlation between the two. Conversely, there is a positive linear relationship between hCG and free T_4 concentrations during early gestation.[12]

Third, the maternal glomerular filtration rate increases in pregnancy, resulting in increased renal clearance of iodide, an indirect stimulus to the maternal thyroid machinery.[14] Later in gestation, transplacental passage of iodide and placental metabolism of iodothyronines further contribute to relative maternal iodine deprivation and stimulation of the maternal thyroid.[15]

In the nonpregnant condition, an adequate iodine intake is estimated to be 100 to 150 µg per day. Because of the increased iodine demands in pregnancy, all women who are planning pregnancy, are pregnant, or are lactating should ingest a minimum of 250 µg of iodine daily. In North America, this could be achieved by adding a daily multivitamin or prenatal vitamin that contains 150 µg of potassium iodide to an iodine-sufficient diet.[16]

Because thyroid hormone economy differs between healthy pregnant women and healthy nonpregnant women, laboratory-dependent, pregnancy-specific, and ideally trimester-specific reference intervals for thyroid function tests (TFTs) are required. Compared with preconception levels, TSH concentrations are lower throughout pregnancy. TSH is lowest in the first trimester, then increases during the second and third trimesters.[12] Among euthyroid pregnant women additional factors, including smoking status[17] and ethnicity,[18] also contribute to TSH differences. According to recent American Thyroid Association (ATA) guidelines, if laboratory-dependent, trimester-specific ranges for TSH are not available, the recommended reference ranges for TSH are 0.1 to 2.5 mIU/L in the first trimester, 0.2 to 3.0 mIU/L in the second trimester, and 0.3 to 3.0 mIU/L in the third trimester.[16]

The interpretation of levels of free thyroid hormone in pregnancy is more challenging. At least in part, this is due to the use of different assays and differences in dietary iodine intake among study participants.[19] The optimal method to assess serum free T_4 (fT_4) during pregnancy is measurement of T_4 in the dialysate or ultrafiltrate of serum samples by liquid chromatography coupled with tandem mass spectrometry (LC/MS/MS).[20] Unfortunately, this method is too technically complex and expensive for routine use. If LC/MS/MS is not available other assays can be used, as long as the limitations are considered. Method-specific and trimester-specific reference ranges for fT_4 are required. In general, fT_4 and free T_3 (fT_3) levels increase slightly during the first trimester. fT_4 levels subsequently decrease as pregnancy progresses, with a nadir in the third trimester.[19]

It has been suggested that TT_4 measurements are more reliable than fT_4 measurements during pregnancy. TT_4 levels are higher in pregnancy compared with the nonpregnant state, thus, in general, normal TT_4 reference ranges can be adjusted by a factor of 1.5 in pregnancy.[19] The fT_4 index may also be used in pregnancy, as the fT_4 index corrects TT_4 for TBG. Changes in the fT_4 index correspond to the changes in fT_4 measured by equilibrium dialysis and tandem mass spectrometry.[21]

FINDING THYROID DISORDERS IN PREGNANCY: UNIVERSAL SCREENING VERSUS TARGETED HIGH-RISK CASE FINDING

Thyroid disorders are much more common in women than in men. In the last decade, there has been more attention paid to thyroid dysfunction during pregnancy and its effects on maternal and fetal well-being. As a result, there has been a debate regarding the use of universal screening versus targeted high-risk case finding for thyroid dysfunction during pregnancy. Different studies have shown that targeted high-risk screening failed to detect 28% to 36% of women with hypothyroidism.[22–24] A recent study at an academic medical center in the Boston area revealed that targeted thyroid testing in high-risk patients would have missed 80% of pregnant women with either overt or subclinical hypothyroidism. However, the investigators were unable to advocate for universal screening, in the absence of data demonstrating that levothyroxine (LT$_4$) treatment improved outcomes in women with subclinical hypothyroidism.[25]

Screening for subclinical hypothyroidism in pregnancy has been shown to be a cost-effective strategy under a wide range of circumstances,[26] and universal screening has been supported by some investigators.[27] However, there are few prospective randomized trials to substantiate the benefits of universal screening. Negro and colleagues[24] showed that universal screening in comparison with case finding did not result in a decrease in adverse outcomes, but treatment of hypothyroidism or hyperthyroidism identified by screening a low-risk group was associated with a lower rate of adverse outcomes.

Data from 2 large, randomized controlled trials are currently pending. Preliminary results from the Controlled Antenatal Thyroid Study (CATS) have not shown a difference in neuropsychological development among the offspring of women screened and treated for subclinical thyroid disease or isolated hypothyroxinemia before 16 weeks' gestation, compared with control women.[28] The National Institutes of Health Maternal Fetal Medicine Thyrotropin Study (TSH Study), to be completed in 2015, is screening pregnant women for thyroid dysfunction, and is comparing maternal and fetal outcomes in women with subclinical hypothyroidism or isolated hypothyroxinemia treated with LT$_4$ versus placebo.[29] Because of a lack of consistent evidence to date demonstrating that universal screening improves population outcomes, several clinical organizations, including the ATA, recommend obtaining serum TSH early in pregnancy only in women at high risk for overt hypothyroidism (**Box 1**).

HYPOTHYROIDISM DURING PREGNANCY

Thyroid hormone deficiency is found in approximately 3% to 7% of women of child-bearing age,[2] and an estimated 2% to 3% of women are hypothyroid during pregnancy.[2,3] In iodine-sufficient areas, the most common cause is Hashimoto thyroiditis. Other causes include prior radioactive iodine (RAI) and/or surgical ablation of Graves disease,[30] surgical removal of the thyroid because of multinodular goiter or thyroid cancer, overtreatment of hyperthyroidism with thionamides, medications that alter the absorption or metabolism of levothyroxine, and central defects that inhibit the hypothalamic-pituitary-thyroid axis.

The fetal thyroid gland starts producing small amounts of thyroid hormone at approximately 10 weeks' gestation, until production plateaus at approximately 35 weeks.[12] Therefore, particularly in the first trimester of pregnancy, the fetus is entirely dependent on thyroid hormone from the mother. Maternal hypothyroidism can have devastating consequences if left untreated.

Box 1
Screening for serum TSH in early pregnancy in high-risk patients

Risk Factors for Overt Hypothyroidism

History of thyroid dysfunction or prior thyroid surgery

Age >30 years

Symptoms of thyroid dysfunction or the presence of goiter

Thyroid peroxidase antibody positivity

Type 1 diabetes mellitus or other autoimmune disorders

History of miscarriage or preterm delivery

History of head and neck radiation

Family history of thyroid dysfunction

Morbid obesity (body mass index $\geq$40 kg/m^2)

Use of amiodarone or lithium, or recent administration of iodinated radiologic contrast

Infertility

Residing in an area of known moderate to severe iodine sufficiency

Adapted from Stagnaro-Green A, Abalovich M, Alexander E, et al. Guidelines of the American Thyroid Association for the diagnosis and management of thyroid disease during pregnancy and postpartum. Thyroid 2011;21(10):1081–125; with permission.

Diagnosis

Overt hypothyroidism is defined by a serum TSH higher than the upper limit of the trimester-specific range and serum fT$_4$ below the trimester-specific reference range, or serum TSH level of 10 mIU/L or more, irrespective of fT$_4$ levels. Subclinical hypothyroidism is diagnosed when serum TSH is elevated but less than 10 mIU/L, and fT$_4$ is in the normal range. Differentiating between the two conditions is important because maternal and fetal outcomes are better established for overt maternal hypothyroidism than for subclinical hypothyroidism. Isolated hypothyroxinemia is defined as a normal TSH with an fT$_4$ in the lower 5th or 10th percentile of the reference range.[16]

Pregnancy Complications

Maternal hypothyroidism is associated with spontaneous abortion,[31] fetal death,[32] preterm delivery,[32,33] gestational hypertension,[34] anemia, postpartum hemorrhage,[35] placental abruption and preterm labor,[36] preeclampsia,[37] cesarean section,[38] and very early embryo loss.[39] In a study by Su and colleagues,[40] clinical hypothyroidism was associated with increased fetal loss (adjusted odds ratio [OR] 13.45, 95% confidence interval [CI] 2.54–71.20). Kuppens and colleagues[41] showed that breech position was significantly and independently related to high maternal TSH concentration ($\geq$2.5 mIU/L) at 36 weeks' gestation (OR 2.23, 95% CI 1.14–4.39). Higher TSH levels late in pregnancy also increased the risk of external cephalic version failure.[42]

Subclinical hypothyroidism has been associated with a 3-fold increased risk of placental abruption and a 1.8-fold increased risk of preterm labor.[36] In a cohort of euthyroid pregnant women without overt thyroid dysfunction, the risk of child loss attributable to miscarriage or fetal/neonatal death increased with higher levels of maternal TSH in early pregnancy, with an OR of 1.8 for every doubling in TSH concentration in multivariate analyses.[43] By contrast, other studies have failed to reveal an association between subclinical hypothyroidism and adverse pregnancy outcomes,[44,45] but interpretation of those data was limited because of the exclusion of a significant number of patients from final analyses.

Adverse Outcomes in Neonates and Offspring

Maternal hypothyroidism has been associated with increased risk of low birth weight, fetal distress, and impaired neuropsychological development.[31,36,46] Haddow and colleagues[46] described a 7-point IQ deficit in 7- to 9-year-old children born to untreated hypothyroid women when compared with age-matched children born to euthyroid women. Nineteen percent of children of hypothyroid mothers had IQ scores of less than 85, compared with 5% of controls. Su and colleagues[40] showed an increased risk of fetal loss (OR 13.45, 95% CI 2.54–71.20), low birth weight (OR 9.05, 95% CI 1.01–80.90), and congenital malformations of the circulation system (OR 10.44, 95% CI 1.15–94.62) in children of women with clinical hypothyroidism. Subclinical hypothyroidism was associated with increased fetal distress (OR 3.65, 95% CI 1.44–9.26), poor vision development (OR 5.34, 95% CI 1.09–26.16), and neurodevelopmental delay (OR 10.49, 95% CI 1.01–119.19). By contrast, a study by Behrooz and colleagues[47] showed that IQ levels and cognitive performance of children born to LT_4-treated hypothyroid mothers was similar between those whose mothers had high TSH levels (mean 11.3 ± 5.3 mIU/L) and those whose mothers achieved normal TSH concentrations during pregnancy.

Isolated Hypothyroxinemia

Isolated maternal hypothyroxinemia is identified in 1.3% of pregnant women. Some studies have failed to show a significant association between isolated hypothyroxinemia and adverse perinatal outcomes.[45,48] By contrast, other studies have shown an increased risk of fetal distress, musculoskeletal malformations, and small for gestational age (SGA) infants when hypothyroxinemia was diagnosed in the first 20 weeks of gestation,[40] and impaired mental and motor development at 1 to 2 years of age when hypothyroxinemia was diagnosed by 12 weeks of gestation.[49,50] Isolated hypothyroxinemia also predicted a higher risk of expressive language delay at 18 and 30 months of age as well as nonverbal cognitive delay in children.[51]

Treatment

All women with (1) overt hypothyroidism and (2) thyroid peroxidase (TPO) antibody–positive subclinical hypothyroidism should be treated with LT_4 during pregnancy to maintain serum TSH in the trimester-specific goal range. At present, there is insufficient evidence to recommend for or against LT_4 treatment in thyroid antibody–negative pregnant women with subclinical hypothyroidism.[16] Similarly, data demonstrating a benefit of LT_4 therapy in pregnant women with isolated hypothyroxinemia are not available, so routine LT_4 treatment is currently not recommended in these cases.[52] Nonetheless, the ongoing National Institutes of Health CATS and TSH studies will provide important data regarding the effects of LT_4 treatment in these special cases, and thereby help guide future evidence-based recommendations.

For women who require LT_4 treatment during pregnancy, it is crucial to adjust LT_4 doses appropriately to account for physiologic pregnancy-induced changes in economy of thyroid hormone. Adequate treatment with LT_4 to maintain TSH within the target ranges for pregnancy significantly decreases pregnancy-related complications that occur in inadequately treated hypothyroid women.[33] The etiology of hypothyroidism has a marked effect on the timing and magnitude of LT_4 dose adjustments. Women with primary hypothyroidism caused by Hashimoto thyroiditis require smaller dose increases, as do women treated for thyroid cancer, compared with women previously treated for Graves disease, who require the largest dose increases, indicating that a single recommendation might not apply to all patients. On average, among a large group of pregnant women with hypothyroidism of varying etiology, the required increase in LT$_4$ dose was 13% in the first trimester and 26% in the second and third trimesters.[53] Another study showed that an increase in LT$_4$ dose was required in 85% of hypothyroid pregnant women, starting as early as the fifth week of gestation and plateauing by week 16. The mean LT$_4$ requirement increased 47% during the first half of pregnancy in that study.[5]

The goal of treatment is to maintain TSH within trimester-specific reference ranges: 0.1 to 2.5 mIU/L in the first trimester, 0.2 to 3.0 mIU/L in the second trimester, and 0.3 to 3.0 mIU/L in the third trimester. At a minimum, serum TSH should be measured every 4 weeks during the first half of the pregnancy, then at least once between 26 and 32 weeks of gestation, so that appropriate dose adjustments can be made.[16] The recommended therapy is with oral LT$_4$, which should be taken on an empty stomach ($\geq$45 minutes before consumption of food, beverages, or other medications). In addition, calcium, iron, and prenatal vitamin supplements should be avoided within 4 hours of ingestion of LT$_4$, as these can decrease absorption and lead to inadequate circulating thyroxine levels.

A high proportion of pregnant women with hypothyroidism who are taking LT$_4$ have suboptimal TSH levels at 11 to 13 weeks of gestation.[37] Because most women do not have their first prenatal obstetric visit until the 8th to 12th week of pregnancy, one strategy is to empirically increase the levothyroxine dose as soon as pregnancy is confirmed. In the Thyroid Hormone Early Adjustment in Pregnancy (THERAPY) trial, an empiric increase by 2 additional LT$_4$ tablets per week (29% increase), when instituted immediately on confirmation of pregnancy, significantly reduced the risk of maternal hypothyroidism throughout pregnancy, with a safety profile superior to that of an increase of 3 additional tablets per week (43% increase).[54] Recent ATA guidelines endorse this recommendation, or the alternative option of empirically increasing LT$_4$ dose by approximately 25% to 30% on confirmation of pregnancy.[16] After delivery, the patient should be instructed to return to her prepregnancy dose of LT$_4$, and serum TSH should be checked again 6 weeks after delivery.

Iodine sufficiency is crucial in pregnancy. Indeed, maintaining the increased iodine requirements in pregnancy has been shown to prevent cretinism and improve motor skills in offspring. The recommended daily iodine dose in pregnancy and lactation is 250 µg of iodine daily. This dosage may be achieved by supplementing an iodine-sufficient diet with a daily oral prenatal multivitamin containing 150 µg of potassium iodide. Caution should be advised because supplemental iodine is not found in all prenatal multivitamins, so women should be advised to take a prenatal vitamin that provides iodine, in addition to ensuring adequate dietary iodine intake.

EUTHYROIDISM WITH AUTOIMMUNE THYROID DISEASE

Approximately 12% of women of child-bearing age have detectable circulating thyroid autoantibodies.[55] Several studies have shown an increased risk of pregnancy complications in euthyroid women with thyroid autoimmunity, including preterm delivery,[56] spontaneous miscarriage,[57] very preterm delivery (<34 weeks' gestation),[58] placental abruption,[59] postpartum thyroiditis, and postpartum depression.[60] Despite these findings, 2011 ATA guidelines state that there is insufficient evidence to recommend for or against screening all women for thyroid autoantibodies in the first trimester, or treating euthyroid women who are thyroid antibody–positive with LT$_4$.[16] That being said, at a minimum, serum TSH should be monitored throughout pregnancy in thyroid anti-body–positive euthyroid women, and LT_4 therapy should be initiated if serum TSH is greater than 2.5 mIU/L.

HYPERTHYROIDISM DURING PREGNANCY

Overt hyperthyroidism occurs in 0.4% to 1.7% of pregnant women, and Graves disease accounts for 85% to 90% of all cases.[61] Other causes of hyperthyroidism in pregnancy include subacute thyroiditis, toxic multinodular goiter, toxic thyroid adenoma, and excessive levothyroxine intake.[62] Maternal hyperthyroidism is defined as a low or suppressed serum TSH level in the presence of a high fT_4 level based on trimester-specific reference ranges. As described earlier, serum TSH levels are nor-mally suppressed in the first trimester of pregnancy because of the high levels of hCG, so it is necessary to evaluate fT_4 in conjunction with the TSH level for an appro-priate diagnosis.

Gestational Transient Thyrotoxicosis

Gestational transient thyrotoxicosis (GTT) is a transient period of hyperthyroidism that occurs in 1% to 3% of pregnancies[63] and is caused by elevated hCG levels. GTT is often associated with hyperemesis gravidarum, defined as severe nausea and vomit-ing that results in weight loss, dehydration, and ketonuria in early pregnancy. Risk factors for GTT include multiple gestations, hydatiform mole, and choriocarcinoma.[62] It is important to distinguish GTT from Graves disease because the course, fetal outcomes, management, and follow-up are different. GTT usually resolves spontane-ously by 20 weeks' gestation when hCG levels decline. Treatment with antithyroid drugs is not indicated unless the diagnosis is uncertain. Supportive management for hyperemesis gravidarum is the mainstay of therapy, and hospitalization may be required in severe cases.

Graves Disease in Pregnancy

Diagnosis

Clinical features of hyperthyroidism may be mistaken for normal symptoms of preg-nancy, such as palpitations, heat intolerance, dyspnea, and nervousness. Graves disease may present as a new diagnosis during pregnancy in a woman with no history of hyperthyroidism, as a recurrence from previous Graves disease that was in remis-sion, or as an exacerbation of stable disease treated with antithyroidal drugs (ATD). Exacerbations of Graves disease being treated with ATDs typically occur early in preg-nancy or soon after delivery.[64]

On physical examination, women with Graves disease usually have a palpable goiter, with or without a bruit. In some instances, Graves ophthalmopathy is present. Graves dermopathy may rarely be seen. On laboratory evaluation, TSH is usually sup-pressed or lower than the trimester-specific reference range and fT_4 is high. Women with Graves disease usually have positive TSH receptor antibodies (TRAb), which helps differentiate Graves disease from other causes of hyperthyroidism. Ultrasonog-raphy of the thyroid may also be helpful in certain circumstances, for example, to differentiate between toxic multinodular goiter, a single toxic nodule, or the heteroge-neous thyroid echotexture that is consistent with Graves disease. Use of radiolabeled iodine for diagnosis is contraindicated in pregnancy and lactation.

Outcomes

Lack of control of hyperthyroidism significantly increases the risk of pregnancy compli-cations and poor fetal outcomes. Millar and colleagues[65] showed that, compared with the risk in nonhyperthyroid women, the risk of low birth weight infants was 9.24 (95% CI 5.5–15.6) among women with uncontrolled hyperthyroidism during pregnancy, 2.36 (95% CI 1.4–4.1) in women whose hyperthyroidism was controlled at some point during pregnancy, and 0.74 (95% CI 0.2–3.1) in women whose hyperthyroidism was controlled at presentation so that euthyroidism was maintained throughout pregnancy. The risk of severe preeclampsia was also significantly higher among women with uncontrolled hyperthyroidism compared with hyperthyroid women with controlled thyroid levels during pregnancy (OR 4.7, 95% CI 1.1–19.7).[65] In addition, in a cohort of 60 women with overt hyperthyroidism in pregnancy, stillbirth was more common in untreated women (50%) than in partially treated (16%) and adequately treated hyperthyroid women (0%).[66] Overt untreated maternal hyperthyroidism is also associated with an increased risk of miscarriage,[67] maternal heart failure during pregnancy,[68] maternal gestational hypertension, and fetal growth restriction.[69] Uncontrolled maternal hyperthyroidism may cause central congenital hypothyroidism, due to impaired maturation of the fetal hypothalamic-pituitary thyroid system in a hyperthyroid fetal environment.[70]

TRAbs cross the placental barrier, and in high titers can stimulate the fetal thyroid gland, which may result in fetal hyperthyroidism.[71] Fetal thyrotoxicosis causes fetal tachycardia, goiter, oligohydramnios, intrauterine growth retardation, and accelerated bone maturation.[72] Neonatal hyperthyroidism may occur within 24 to 72 hours after delivery in cases of high maternal TRAb titers. Before delivery, the fetus is protected by ATDs that cross the placenta. Neonatal hyperthyroidism is usually a transient condition, lasting between 2 and 3 months. Treatment of the neonate with ATDs is indicated until resolution of the hyperthyroidism.[73]

Treatment

Preconception counseling As already described, uncontrolled hyperthyroidism affects maternal and fetal outcomes poorly. It is imperative to provide preconception counseling to women with hyperthyroidism so that the best therapeutic option to control the disease before pregnancy can be implemented. In the preconception period, treatment options for Graves disease include RAI ablation, total thyroidectomy, or ATDs. Surgery is a reasonable option in cases of high TRAb titers or in women planning to conceive in the subsequent 2 years, because TRAb titers tend to increase following RAI therapy and take longer to trend downwards.[74] RAI is absolutely contraindicated during pregnancy and lactation because of the high risk of transferring RAI to the fetus with resultant fetal thyroid ablation and congenital hypothyroidism. If RAI ablation is desired near pregnancy or lactation, special considerations should be kept in mind, and these are listed in **Box 2**.

Antithyroid drugs Two ATDs, methimazole (MMI) and propylthiouracil (PTU), are used to treat hyperthyroidism. Both drugs cross the placenta. The goal of ATD therapy in pregnant women with hyperthyroidism is to maintain maternal serum fT_4 at or just above the upper limit of normal for pregnancy using the smallest ATD dose possible. This treatment strategy minimizes the potential for overtreatment, which may result in fetal hypothyroidism[75] and goiter.[76] In this regard, Momotani and colleagues[77] showed a strong relationship between maternal and fetal thyroid function: the rates of transient neonatal hypothyroxinemia were 10% when maternal fT_4 was maintained in the upper one-third of the normal range, 36% when maternal fT_4 was maintained in the lower two-thirds of the normal range, and 100% when maternal fT_4 was maintained below the normal range. There was no relationship between the dose or the type of ATD used and neonatal thyroid function.

Box 2
Considerations for RAI therapy in women of child-bearing age

1. RAI is absolutely contraindicated during pregnancy and lactation

2. A pregnancy test should be performed on all women of child-bearing age before RAI

3. Conception should be delayed by a minimum of 6 months after RAI to allow adequate time for diagnosis and treatment of consequent hypothyroidism

4. Lactation should be delayed for at least 6 months following RAI therapy

5. RAI might increase TRAb titers and it may take up to 1 year for the titers to decline after RAI. Therefore, if TRAb titers are high before treatment, surgery might be a better option

6. Prepregnancy counseling regarding the need to adjust LT$_4$ dose at diagnosis of pregnancy is important

Adapted from Patil-Sisodia K, Mestman JH. Graves hyperthyroidism and pregnancy: a clinical update. Endocr Pract 2010;16(1):118–29; with permission.

In rare cases, use of MMI in the first trimester has been associated with congenital abnormalities, including fetal aplasia cutis,[78] choanal atresia, omphalocele, total situs invertus,[79] esophageal atresia,[80] tracheo-esophageal fistula, hypoplastic nipples, and psychomotor delay.[81] PTU, on the other hand, has not been associated with these fetal abnormalities. A major risk associated with PTU is acute liver failure, resulting in a need for liver transplant in approximately 1 in 10,000 treated adults.[82,83] To decrease the risk of congenital abnormalities associated with first-trimester MMI use, women taking MMI before pregnancy should be switched to PTU once pregnancy is confirmed, or alternatively, before conception. After the first trimester, consideration should be given to switching from PTU to an equivalent dose of MMI to avoid maternal liver injury.[16] Clinical experience has demonstrated an approximate conversion ratio from PTU to MMI of 10:1 to 15:1 (eg, 100 mg PTU = 7.5–10 mg MMI[84]).

After delivery, Graves disease may worsen or relapse, necessitating that ATDs are restarted or the dose increased. In the past, women taking ATDs were advised against breastfeeding because little was known about their effects on the newborn when delivered via breast milk. More recent studies, however, have demonstrated that ATDs are safe in lactating women. The use of PTU (as high as 750 mg daily) or methimazole (20–30 mg daily) have not been associated with an increased risk of infant hypothyroidism, and no adverse effects on physical or cognitive childhood development have been observed.[85,86]

Surgery Thyroidectomy during pregnancy is rarely indicated, but should be considered if a woman with severe hyperthyroidism is resistant to or intolerant of ATDs or if she requires high doses of ATDs to control her disease. If surgery is indicated during pregnancy, the optimal time is in the second trimester.[16] The use of β-blockers and a short course of cold iodine is recommended in preparation for surgery.[16] Determination of maternal TRAb titers before surgery is recommended, to assess the risk of fetal hyperthyroidism.[87]

β-Blockers β-Blockers can be used temporarily in pregnancy to help control adrenergic symptoms or in preparation for surgery. Long-term use should be avoided and has been associated with intrauterine growth retardation, fetal bradycardia, neonatal hypoglycemia, and spontaneous abortion.[88,89] Labetolol, a pregnancy category C medication, is the preferred β-blocker for use during pregnancy and lactation.

Cold iodine The use of cold (ie, nonradioactive) iodine during pregnancy should be limited to the acute management of thyroid storm or in preparation for thyroidectomy. Studies have reported neonatal hypothyroidism after maternal exposure to cold iodine, including instances in euthyroid women exposed to iodine-rich foods (such as seaweed), iodine-based medications (such as amiodarone), or contrast media, and reports of neonatal hypothyroidism in hypothyroid pregnant women treated simultaneously with ATD and cold iodine. By contrast, Momotani and colleagues[90] showed improved maternal thyroid function and normal neonatal outcomes after treatment of Graves disease with low doses of cold iodine in pregnancy, suggesting that careful, limited use of cold iodine in the management of Graves disease in pregnancy may be appropriate in select cases.

Radioactive iodine therapy As already discussed, RAI is absolutely contraindicated in pregnancy and lactation because of its potentially detrimental effects on the developing fetus, which primarily result from fetal thyroid ablation.

Monitoring Ultrasonography is the mainstay of monitoring for fetal hypothyroidism while treating maternal hyperthyroidism. Presence of a fetal goiter on ultrasonogram is highly suggestive of fetal hypothyroidism.[91] If fetal goiter is present, ATDs should be reduced or discontinued, keeping in mind that the risk of maternal hyperthyroidism in pregnancy is much less than the risk of fetal hypothyroidism, particularly with regard to fetal and neonatal growth and development. During pregnancy in women with Graves disease, TRAb levels often decrease because of a state of relative maternal immunosuppression. Decreased TRAb titers may permit decreased ATD doses in the second trimester and, possibly, discontinuation of ATDs in the third trimester. Maternal serum fT_4 and TSH levels should be monitored every 2 to 4 weeks at the initiation of ATD therapy, and every 4 to 6 weeks after achieving target levels. ATD dose adjustments should be based on fT_4 levels rather than on TSH, because TSH may remain suppressed throughout pregnancy. A combination of ATDs and LT_4 therapy is not recommended because this complicates monitoring of fetal thyroid function, thereby increasing the risk of fetal goiter and hypothyroidism.[89]

Indications for maternal TRAb measurement are listed in **Box 3**. TRAb titers should be measured at 20 to 28 weeks' gestation to determine the risk of fetal hyperthyroidism after delivery.[16] If TRAb titers are high ($\geq$3 times the upper limit of normal), close follow-up of the newborn's thyroid function, optimally in collaboration with a maternal-fetal-medicine specialist, is indicated. Serial fetal ultrasonography is also recommended in women with high TRAb titers and/or active Graves disease. The size of the fetal thyroid gland should be evaluated monthly starting at 22 weeks'

Box 3
Indications for TRAb measurement during pregnancy

1. Mothers with active hyperthyroidism

2. Previous history of treatment with RAI

3. Previous history of delivering an infant with hyperthyroidism

4. Thyroidectomy for treatment of hyperthyroidism in pregnancy

Adapted from Laurberg P, Nygaard B, Glinoer D, et al. Guidelines for TSH-receptor antibody measurements in pregnancy: results of an evidence-based symposium organized by the European Thyroid Association. Eur J Endocrinol 1998;139(6):584; with permission.

gestation to ensure early diagnosis of fetal thyroid dysfunction.[72] Sonographic features may be able to predict the nature of fetal thyroid dysfunction: the color Doppler pattern of fetal goiter typically has a peripheral vascular pattern in hypothyroidism and a central vascular pattern in hyperthyroidism. Additional clinical findings suggesting the nature of fetal thyroid dysfunction include heart rate (tachycardia may indicate hyperthyroidism and bradycardia may indicate hypothyroidism), bone maturation (advanced in hyperthyroidism and delayed in hypothyroidism), and intrauterine movement (increased in hyperthyroidism and decreased in hypothyroidism).[92]

In the later period of pregnancy, fetal thyroid function can be studied directly by measuring levels of fetal thyroid hormone in umbilical cord blood obtained by cordocentesis.[93] However, cordocentesis itself carries an increased risk of fetal morbidity and mortality, so this should be reserved for special circumstances, such as an inability to determine whether the fetus is hypothyroid or hyperthyroid, either clinically or based on fetal ultrasonography.[16]

Postpartum care Women with Graves disease may experience relapse or worsening of hyperthyroidism after delivery. Relapse of Graves disease usually occurs between 4 and 8 months after delivery,[94] so it is important to monitor thyroid function regularly postpartum. It is also necessary to distinguish Graves disease from postpartum thyroiditis (PPT) because treatments will differ. In women who choose not to breastfeed, RAI (^{123}I) uptake and scan may be performed to differentiate Graves disease from PPT. In lactating mothers RAI is contraindicated, and differentiating Graves disease from PPT may be achieved by measuring TRAb titers, assessing the time course of hyperthyroidism (ie, transient vs chronic), and prior history of maternal Graves disease.

POSTPARTUM THYROIDITIS

PPT is an autoimmune, destructive inflammation of the thyroid gland[95] that typically occurs within 1 year postpartum. The classic presentation of PPT starts with transient hyperthyroidism in the first 6 months postpartum, followed by transient hypothyroidism, then a return to the euthyroid state by 1 year postpartum. Not all women with PPT progress through all the phases of this classic presentation. Lazarus and colleagues[96] reported that, among a cohort of women diagnosed with PPT, 19.2% developed hyperthyroidism alone, 49.3% developed hypothyroidism alone, and 31.5% developed hyperthyroidism followed by hypothyroidism. One must keep in mind that PPT may occur in women with hypothyroidism caused by Hashimoto thyroiditis if the thyroid gland is not completely atrophic.[97] By convention, hypothyroidism with onset 1 year or more postpartum is not PPT.[98]

Prevalence

The reported prevalence of PPT varies widely across studies, from 1.1% to 16.7% (mean 7.5%) among parous women.[98] Women with a previous history of PPT have a 70% risk of developing recurrent PPT in future pregnancies.[99] PPT incidence is higher in women with autoimmune disease: 10% to 25% in women with type 1 diabetes mellitus,[98,100] 14% in women with systemic lupus erythamatosus,[101] and 25% in women with autoimmune hepatitis.[102] An estimated 30% to 50% of women with positive thyroid autoantibodies in the first trimester will develop PPT.[95,103,104]

Diagnosis

Screening for PPT is recommended in women with a history of thyroid disease, PPT, postpartum depression, or autoimmune disease, and in women with signs and/or symptoms of hyperthyroidism, hypothyroidism, or depression in the postpartum period. Screening should include measurement of TPO antibody titer, TSH, and fT_4. Clinical signs and symptoms of PPT are usually mild and transient, with the hypothyroid phase typically being the most symptomatic. In the hyperthyroid state, differentiating between Graves disease and PPT is important for guiding management. Clinical features unique to Graves disease include a goiter with bruit, ophthalmopathy, and elevated TRAb titers. Biochemically, the T_4/T_3 ratio is typically elevated in PPT. Thyroid ultrasound with Doppler flow measurements may be helpful in differentiating PPT from Graves disease (decreased vascular flow in PPT vs increased flow in Graves disease) and does not involve radiation that would necessitate an interruption in breastfeeding. RAI (^{123}I) uptake and scan can be performed to establish the diagnosis; thyroid ^{123}I uptake is elevated in Graves disease and low or absent in PPT. ^{123}I is preferred over ^{131}I for thyroid imaging during lactation because of its shorter half-life, allowing nursing to resume several days following administration of ^{123}I.[16]

Maternal Outcomes

PPT is associated with an increased risk of developing permanent hypothyroidism, which has been estimated to occur in 2% to 21% of affected women. Stagnaro-Green and colleagues[104] reported an even higher incidence of permanent hypothyroidism of 54%. The presence, but not the titers, of TPO antibody in the first trimester of pregnancy and the degree of hypothyroidism at 6 months postpartum were predictive of permanent hypothyroidism. Because of the increased risk of permanent hypothyroidism following PPT, yearly TSH monitoring is recommended, even in women who return to the euthyroid state.

Data remain inconclusive regarding the correlation between PPT and postpartum depression (PPD). TPO antibody positivity is associated with an increased risk of PPD, independent of maternal thyroid function.[105] Because the risk of PPT is also increased by TPO antibody positivity, one could predict that PPT and PPD are related entities. However, studies investigating a possible link between PPD and PPT have been unable to demonstrate a significant correlation, although studies to date are limited by small numbers of patients.[106]

Treatment of PPT

Most women with PPT do not require treatment in the hyperthyroid state, which is generally mild and transient. Propranolol, 10 to 20 mg daily, can be used as needed for adrenergic symptoms. ATDs are ineffective in the treatment of PPT because it is a destructive process and does not involve overproduction of thyroid hormone. In the hypothyroid phase, TSH should be tested every 4 to 8 weeks, even if the patient is asymptomatic. Levothyroxine treatment is indicated when TSH elevation persists longer than 6 months postpartum, or if symptoms of hypothyroidism are severe, the patient is breastfeeding, or another pregnancy is desired. Therapy should be continued for 6 to 12 months after initiation, followed by an attempt to wean the LT_4 by halving the dose every 6 to 8 weeks. If the patient is pregnant, breastfeeding, or trying to conceive, weaning LT_4 therapy is not indicated and therapy should be continued.[16]

Various attempts have been made to prevent PPT in women at risk. A single, randomized controlled trial by Negro and colleagues[107] showed that compared with placebo, selenium administration during pregnancy significantly decreased the prevalence of PPT in women with positive thyroid antibodies (28.6% vs 48.6%). In another study, the postpartum use of LT_4 in women with thyroid autoimmunity (defined as positive TPO antibody titers) did not prevent PPT but, as expected, reduced symptoms of hypothyroidism associated with PPT when it did occur.[108]

EVALUATION OF THYROID NODULES AND THYROID CANCER IN PREGNANCY

Not uncommonly, thyroid nodules and thyroid cancer are diagnosed in women during or around the time of pregnancy, posing important diagnostic and therapeutic dilemmas when considering the best interests of both the mother and her developing child. Differentiated thyroid cancer (DTC) occurs approximately 3-fold more frequently in women than in men, with peak onset in the female reproductive years.[109,110] Many women come under closer medical evaluation around pregnancies than at any other time in their lives, contributing to increased detection and diagnosis of thyroid nodules and DTC. In addition, normal physiologic changes in pregnancy include an increase in maternal thyroid volume, including increased size of thyroid nodules, which further increases detection rates.[111] Management of thyroid nodules and thyroid cancer diagnosed during pregnancy concerns both the affected mother and her fetus, therefore these cases require special consideration to ensure the best overall outcomes.

Because thyroid cancer is most commonly detected within thyroid nodules, thyroid nodules should be evaluated with neck ultrasonography and fine-needle aspiration (FNA), when indicated, to rule out malignancy. During pregnancy, both thyroid ultrasonography and FNA can be performed safely at any time, without risk of harm to the pregnancy. For this reason, thyroid nodules detected in pregnancy may be evaluated in the same way as in nonpregnant individuals. That being said, if a suspicious nodule is detected late in pregnancy and intervention will undoubtedly be delayed until after delivery, it is reasonable to postpone FNA until after delivery. Detection of a thyroid nodule in a pregnant woman should prompt measurement of levels of serum thyroid hormone (TSH, fT_4) so that maternal hypothyroidism or hyperthyroidism can be treated promptly and associated complications prevented.[108]

If thyroid malignancy is diagnosed in a pregnant woman, the recommended course of treatment differs from that in a nonpregnant individual. Despite these differences in management, however, most evidence suggests that DTC diagnosed during or around the time of pregnancy does not affect maternal or fetal morbidity or mortality. In the same regard, pregnancy does not increase a woman's risk for developing thyroid cancer.

When thyroid cancer is diagnosed during pregnancy, a decision must be made regarding performing total thyroidectomy during the pregnancy or postponing surgical resection until the postpartum period. In low-risk cases of DTC, postponing thyroidectomy until after delivery does not affect the course of disease and eliminates the risks associated with surgery during pregnancy.[108] Risks specific to thyroidectomy that may adversely affect a pregnancy include (1) difficulty resecting the thyroid because of increased gland volume in pregnancy, (2) uncontrolled maternal hypothyroidism postoperatively, and (3) transient or permanent maternal hypocalcemia caused by damage to the parathyroid glands. Anesthesia at any time during pregnancy is complicated by multiple factors, including increased maternal blood volume and cardiac output, and can result in maternal hypotension and fetal hypoperfusion.[112,113] In the majority of cases, for which thyroidectomy is not performed during pregnancy, monitoring should consist of a repeat neck ultrasonogram each trimester to rule out rapid growth of malignant tissue, with consideration of immediate surgical intervention if this should occur, and close monitoring of maternal TFTs (see later discussion).[108]

In cases of advanced DTC or in undifferentiated forms of thyroid cancer (eg, medullary, anaplastic, or insular variants), which are more aggressive and more likely to progress if intervention is delayed, thyroidectomy may be performed in the second trimester. This time point in gestation is the earliest at which organogenesis is complete and the risk to fetal development is lowest.[108]

In all cases of DTC diagnosed during pregnancy, whether or not thyroidectomy is performed during gestation, suppressive doses of LT_4 should be started, with goal TSH between 0.1 and 0.5 mIU/L. Neither surgery during the second trimester nor suppressive doses of LT_4 are recommended for pregnant women found to have nodules that are "suspicious for DTC" by FNA cytology, given that approximately 70% of these nodules are later proved to be benign.[108] RAI (^{131}I) ablation is often indicated following total thyroidectomy in patients with DTC to prevent disease recurrence. RAI is absolutely contraindicated during pregnancy and lactation because of the risk of transfer of RAI to the fetal thyroid gland. Exposure of the fetal thyroid to RAI results in fetal thyroid ablation, with resultant devastating effects on early development. If RAI is indicated in a woman who has been diagnosed with DTC during pregnancy, ^{131}I treatment should be begun as soon as possible in the postpartum period. Breastfeeding should not be initiated or continued for at least 6 months following RAI ablation, and for this reason many women will postpone RAI treatment until they have had an opportunity to breastfeed their infant for 3 to 6 months, a delay that does not worsen maternal outcomes.[108,114]

In women who have been diagnosed with DTC before pregnancy, most evidence suggests that pregnancy does not alter the course of disease. That is, long-term prognosis remains the same as the prognosis in cases of DTC diagnosed after pregnancies or in nulligravid women.[115–117] When DTC precedes a pregnancy, TSH suppression with LT_4 should be maintained at the same level as it was before pregnancy so as to minimize disease progression.[108] Most women on suppressive doses of LT_4 for DTC will require increased doses during pregnancy because of increased maternal and fetal demands (discussed previously).[55] Goal TSH in women with DTC during pregnancy does not change from that recommended for the nonpregnant state (TSH 0.1–0.5 mIU/L). In that regard, there are no clinically significant negative consequences to maternal subclinical hyperthyroidism during pregnancy, so maintaining prepregnancy TSH suppression is acceptable.[108]

Treatment of reproductive-aged women with DTC with RAI does not increase their future risk of infertility or adverse pregnancy outcomes, such as miscarriage. Furthermore, no differences have been demonstrated between children born to mothers or fathers who had previously received RAI ablation and those who had not, including physical or cognitive development and risk of childhood malignancies.[118]

In summary, thyroid cancer diagnosed during or around the time of pregnancy requires careful consideration of the health of both the mother and her developing child in order to determine the best course of treatment for optimization of maternal and fetal outcomes. These complex cases should be followed closely during pregnancy and lactation by a team of physicians that includes the patient's obstetrician, an endocrinologist, an endocrine surgeon, nuclear medicine specialists, and the baby's pediatrician. Most evidence suggests that long-term maternal outcomes are not adversely affected by delaying definitive treatment until the postpartum period. However, because of the theoretical potential that a delay in treatment may worsen maternal survival, very close clinical follow-up during and after pregnancy is paramount to making the optimal clinical decisions.

SUMMARY

- The physiology of the thyroid gland changes during pregnancy as a result of the effects of increased TBG and hCG levels and enhanced iodine metabolism. It is important to use trimester-specific reference ranges for TFTs during pregnancy. TSH reference ranges decrease during pregnancy, especially in the first trimester. Total T_4 and T_3 levels increase because of increased TBG levels. The interpretation of levels of free thyroid hormone in pregnancy is more challenging.

- Because of the lack of consistent evidence demonstrating that universal screening for thyroid disorders in pregnancy results in improved population outcomes, several clinical organizations recommend obtaining serum TSH early in pregnancy only in women at high risk for overt hypothyroidism.
- Iodine sufficiency is crucial in pregnancy. The recommended daily iodine intake in pregnancy and lactation is 250 μg of iodine daily, including 150 μg of supplemental iodine from prenatal vitamins in the form of potassium iodide.
- Hypothyroidism is associated with adverse maternal and fetal outcomes in pregnancy. The data on overt hypothyroidism are more conclusive than those on subclinical hypothyroidism. Adverse effects include spontaneous abortion, fetal death, preterm delivery, gestational hypertension, preeclampsia, postpartum hemorrhage, placental abruption and preterm labor, cesarean section, low birth weight, fetal distress, and impaired neuropsychological development.
- All women with overt hypothyroidism and TPO antibody–positive subclinical hypothyroidism should be treated with levothyroxine (LT_4) during pregnancy to maintain serum TSH levels within trimester-specific goal ranges. Some advocate empirically increasing the LT_4 dose by 25% to 30% when pregnancy is confirmed. At a minimum, serum TSH should be checked every 4 weeks during the first half of the pregnancy, then at least once between 26 and 32 weeks of gestation.
- There is not enough evidence to recommend for or against LT_4 treatment in thyroid antibody–negative pregnant women with subclinical hypothyroidism, women with isolated hypothyroxinemia, or euthyroid women who are thyroid antibody–positive. In these cases, close monitoring of TFTs during pregnancy is recommended.
- The most common cause of hyperthyroidism in pregnancy is GTT, which is caused by elevated hCG levels. It is important to distinguish GTT from Graves disease because the course, fetal outcomes, management, and follow-up are different.
- Uncontrolled hyperthyroidism during pregnancy is associated with adverse effects such as low birth weight, stillbirth, preeclampsia, miscarriage, maternal heart failure, maternal gestational hypertension, fetal growth restriction, central congenital hypothyroidism, fetal thyrotoxicosis, and neonatal hyperthyroidism.
- Thionamides are the treatment of choice for Graves disease during pregnancy. To decrease the risk of congenital abnormalities associated with first-trimester MMI use, women taking MMI before pregnancy should be switched to PTU once pregnancy is confirmed, or alternatively, before conception. After the first trimester, consideration should be given to switching from PTU to an equivalent dose of MMI to avoid maternal liver injury. Thionamide dose adjustments should be based on fT_4 levels, rather than on TSH, because TSH may remain suppressed throughout pregnancy. Surgery might be indicated in certain cases. β-Blockers and cold iodine can be given for a short duration in preparation for surgery. RAI ablation is contraindicated during pregnancy and lactation. Measurement of maternal TRAb titers is indicated before delivery to determine the risk of fetal hyperthyroidism.
- PPT is an autoimmune, destructive inflammation of the thyroid gland that typically occurs within 1 year postpartum. The classic presentation of PPT starts

with transient hyperthyroidism in the first 6 months postpartum, followed by transient hypothyroidism, then a return to the euthyroid state by 1 year postpartum. PPT has been associated with an increased risk of permanent hypothyroidism and a possible link to PPD. Most women with PPT do not require treatment in the hyperthyroid state, which is generally mild and transient. Levothyroxine is indicated in certain cases in the hypothyroid phase.

- Thyroid nodules detected in pregnancy may be evaluated with thyroid ultrasonography and FNA when necessary, which are both safe to perform at any time during pregnancy. When thyroid cancer is diagnosed during pregnancy, a decision regarding definitive treatment must be made. In most cases, delaying thyroidectomy and RAI ablation (if indicated) until postpartum does not alter maternal morbidity or mortality. In high-risk cases, thyroidectomy can be performed in the second trimester. RAI ablation is absolutely contraindicated during pregnancy and lactation. Similarly to nonpregnant individuals with thyroid cancer, TSH suppression with levothyroxine is indicated during pregnancy in women with thyroid cancer.

REFERENCES

1. Stagnaro-Green A. Overt hyperthyroidism and hypothyroidism during pregnancy. Clin Obstet Gynecol 2011;54(3):478–87.
2. Hollowell JG, Staehling NW, Flanders WD, et al. Serum TSH, T(4), and thyroid antibodies in the United States population (1988 to 1994): National Health and Nutrition Examination Survey (NHANES III). J Clin Endocrinol Metab 2002; 87(2):489–99.
3. Abalovich M, Amino N, Barbour LA, et al. Management of thyroid dysfunction during pregnancy and postpartum: an Endocrine Society Clinical Practice Guideline. J Clin Endocrinol Metab 2007;92(Suppl 8):S1–47.
4. Glinoer D. The regulation of thyroid function in pregnancy: pathways of endocrine adaptation from physiology to pathology. Endocr Rev 1997;18(3):404–33.
5. Alexander EK, Marqusee E, Lawrence J, et al. Timing and magnitude of increases in levothyroxine requirements during pregnancy in women with hypothyroidism. N Engl J Med 2004;351(3):241–9.
6. Kaplan MM. Monitoring thyroxine treatment during pregnancy. Thyroid 1992; 2(2):147–52.
7. Mandel SJ, Larsen PR, Seely EW, et al. Increased need for thyroxine during pregnancy in women with primary hypothyroidism. N Engl J Med 1990;323(2): 91–6.
8. Glinoer D, McGuire RA, Gershengorn MC, et al. Effects of estrogen on thyroxine-binding globulin metabolism in rhesus monkeys. Endocrinology 1977;100(1): 9–17.
9. Glinoer D, Gershengorn MC, Dubois A, et al. Stimulation of thyroxine-binding globulin synthesis by isolated rhesus monkey hepatocytes after in vivo beta-estradiol administration. Endocrinology 1977;100(3):807–13.
10. Ain KB, Mori Y, Refetoff S. Reduced clearance rate of thyroxine-binding globulin (TBG) with increased sialylation: a mechanism for estrogen-induced elevation of serum TBG concentration. J Clin Endocrinol Metab 1987;65(4):689–96.
11. Skjoldebrand L, Brundin J, Carlstrom A, et al. Thyroid associated components in serum during normal pregnancy. Acta Endocrinol (Copenh) 1982;100(4): 504–11.

12. Glinoer D, de Nayer P, Bourdoux P, et al. Regulation of maternal thyroid during pregnancy. J Clin Endocrinol Metab 1990;71(2):276–87.
13. Smits G, Govaerts C, Nubourgh I, et al. Lysine 183 and glutamic acid 157 of the TSH receptor: two interacting residues with a key role in determining specificity toward TSH and human CG. Mol Endocrinol 2002;16(4):722–35.
14. Dworkin HJ, Jacquez JA, Beierwaltes WH. Relationship of iodine ingestion to iodine excretion in pregnancy. J Clin Endocrinol Metab 1966;26(12):1329–42.
15. Burrow GN, Fisher DA, Larsen PR. Maternal and fetal thyroid function. N Engl J Med 1994;331(16):1072–8.
16. Stagnaro-Green A, Abalovich M, Alexander E, et al. Guidelines of the American Thyroid Association for the diagnosis and management of thyroid disease during pregnancy and postpartum. Thyroid 2011;21(10):1081–125.
17. Shields B, Hill A, Bilous M, et al. Cigarette smoking during pregnancy is associated with alterations in maternal and fetal thyroid function. J Clin Endocrinol Metab 2009;94(2):570–4.
18. La'ulu SL, Roberts WL. Ethnic differences in first-trimester thyroid reference intervals. Clin Chem 2011;57(6):913–5.
19. Mandel SJ, Spencer CA, Hollowell JG. Are detection and treatment of thyroid insufficiency in pregnancy feasible? Thyroid 2005;15(1):44–53.
20. Kahric-Janicic N, Soldin SJ, Soldin OP, et al. Tandem mass spectrometry improves the accuracy of free thyroxine measurements during pregnancy. Thyroid 2007;17(4):303–11.
21. Lee RH, Spencer CA, Mestman JH, et al. Free T4 immunoassays are flawed during pregnancy. Am J Obstet Gynecol 2009;200(3):260,e261–6.
22. Vaidya B, Anthony S, Bilous M, et al. Detection of thyroid dysfunction in early pregnancy: Universal screening or targeted high-risk case finding? J Clin Endocrinol Metab 2007;92(1):203–7.
23. Li Y, Shan Z, Teng W, et al. Abnormalities of maternal thyroid function during pregnancy affect neuropsychological development of their children at 25-30 months. Clin Endocrinol 2010;72(6):825–9.
24. Negro R, Schwartz A, Gismondi R, et al. Universal screening versus case finding for detection and treatment of thyroid hormonal dysfunction during pregnancy. J Clin Endocrinol Metab 2010;95(4):1699–707.
25. Chang DL, Leung AM, Braverman LE, et al. Thyroid testing during pregnancy at an academic Boston Area Medical Center. J Clin Endocrinol Metab 2011;96(9): E1452–6.
26. Thung SF, Funai EF, Grobman WA. The cost-effectiveness of universal screening in pregnancy for subclinical hypothyroidism. Am J Obstet Gynecol 2009;200(3): 267,e261–7.
27. Alexander EK. Here's to you, baby! A step forward in support of universal screening of thyroid function during pregnancy. J Clin Endocrinol Metab 2010;95(4):1575–7.
28. Lazarus J. Outcome of the CATS study in pregnant women. Presented at the 14th International Thyroid Congress. Paris, France, September 11–16, 2010.
29. Casey BM. A randomized trial of thyroxine therapy for subclinical hypothyroidism or hypothyroxinemia diagnosed during pregnancy. Thyroid dysfunction and pregnancy: miscarriage, preterm delivery and decreased IQ. Booklet of the Research Summit and Spring Symposium of the ATA. Washington, DC, April 16–17, 2009.
30. Neale D, Burrow G. Thyroid disease in pregnancy. Obstet Gynecol Clin North Am 2004;31(4):893–905, xi.

31. Abalovich M, Gutierrez S, Alcaraz G, et al. Overt and subclinical hypothyroidism complicating pregnancy. Thyroid 2002;12(1):63–8.
32. Allan WC, Haddow JE, Palomaki GE, et al. Maternal thyroid deficiency and pregnancy complications: implications for population screening. J Med Screen 2000; 7(3):127–30.
33. Stagnaro-Green A. Maternal thyroid disease and preterm delivery. J Clin Endocrinol Metab 2009;94(1):21–5.
34. Leung AS, Millar LK, Koonings PP, et al. Perinatal outcome in hypothyroid pregnancies. Obstet Gynecol 1993;81(3):349–53.
35. Davis LE, Leveno KJ, Cunningham FG. Hypothyroidism complicating pregnancy. Obstet Gynecol 1988;72(1):108–12.
36. Casey BM, Dashe JS, Wells CE, et al. Subclinical hypothyroidism and pregnancy outcomes. Obstet Gynecol 2005;105(2):239–45.
37. Ashoor G, Rotas M, Maiz N, et al. Maternal thyroid function at 11-13 weeks of gestation in women with hypothyroidism treated by thyroxine. Fetal Diagn Ther 2010;28(1):22–7.
38. Cohen N, Levy A, Wiznitzer A, et al. Perinatal outcomes in post-thyroidectomy pregnancies. Gynecol Endocrinol 2011;27(5):314–8.
39. De Vivo A, Mancuso A, Giacobbe A, et al. Thyroid function in women found to have early pregnancy loss. Thyroid 2010;20(6):633–7.
40. Su PY, Huang K, Hao JH, et al. Maternal thyroid function in the first twenty weeks of pregnancy and subsequent fetal and infant development: a prospective population-based cohort study in china. J Clin Endocrinol Metab 2011;96(10):3234–41.
41. Kuppens SM, Kooistra L, Wijnen HA, et al. Maternal thyroid function during gestation is related to breech presentation at term. Clin Endocrinol 2010; 72(6):820–4.
42. Kuppens SM, Kooistra L, Hasaart TH, et al. Maternal thyroid function and the outcome of external cephalic version: a prospective cohort study. BMC Pregnancy Childbirth 2011;11:10.
43. Benhadi N, Wiersinga WM, Reitsma JB, et al. Higher maternal TSH levels in pregnancy are associated with increased risk for miscarriage, fetal or neonatal death. Eur J Endocrinol 2009;160(6):985–91.
44. Cleary-Goldman J, Malone FD, Lambert-Messerlian G, et al. Maternal thyroid hypofunction and pregnancy outcome. Obstet Gynecol 2008;112(1):85–92.
45. Mannisto T, Vaarasmaki M, Pouta A, et al. Perinatal outcome of children born to mothers with thyroid dysfunction or antibodies: a prospective population-based cohort study. J Clin Endocrinol Metab 2009;94(3):772–9.
46. Haddow JE, Palomaki GE, Allan WC, et al. Maternal thyroid deficiency during pregnancy and subsequent neuropsychological development of the child. N Engl J Med 1999;341(8):549–55.
47. Behrooz HG, Tohidi M, Mehrabi Y, et al. Subclinical hypothyroidism in pregnancy: intellectual development of offspring. Thyroid 2011;21(10):1143–7.
48. Casey BM, Dashe JS, Spong CY, et al. Perinatal significance of isolated maternal hypothyroxinemia identified in the first half of pregnancy. Obstet Gynecol 2007;109(5):1129–35.
49. Pop VJ, Brouwers EP, Vader HL, et al. Maternal hypothyroxinaemia during early pregnancy and subsequent child development: a 3-year follow-up study. Clin Endocrinol 2003;59(3):282–8.
50. Pop VJ, Kuijpens JL, van Baar AL, et al. Low maternal free thyroxine concentrations during early pregnancy are associated with impaired psychomotor development in infancy. Clin Endocrinol 1999;50(2):149–55.

51. Henrichs J, Bongers-Schokking JJ, Schenk JJ, et al. Maternal thyroid function during early pregnancy and cognitive functioning in early childhood: the generation R study. J Clin Endocrinol Metab 2010;95(9):4227–34.

52. Negro R, Soldin OP, Obregon MJ, et al. Hypothyroxinemia and pregnancy. Endocr Pract 2011;17(3):422–9.

53. Loh JA, Wartofsky L, Jonklaas J, et al. The magnitude of increased levothyroxine requirements in hypothyroid pregnant women depends upon the etiology of the hypothyroidism. Thyroid 2009;19(3):269–75.

54. Yassa L, Marqusee E, Fawcett R, et al. Thyroid hormone early adjustment in pregnancy (the THERAPY) trial. J Clin Endocrinol Metab 2010;95(7):3234–41.

55. Negro R, Formoso G, Mangieri T, et al. Levothyroxine treatment in euthyroid pregnant women with autoimmune thyroid disease: effects on obstetrical complications. J Clin Endocrinol Metab 2006;91(7):2587–91.

56. Negro R. Thyroid autoimmunity and pre-term delivery: brief review and meta-analysis. J Endocrinol Invest 2011;34(2):155–8.

57. Chen L, Hu R. Thyroid autoimmunity and miscarriage: a meta-analysis. Clin Endocrinol 2011;74(4):513–9.

58. Negro R, Schwartz A, Gismondi R, et al. Thyroid antibody positivity in the first trimester of pregnancy is associated with negative pregnancy outcomes. J Clin Endocrinol Metab 2011;96(6):E920–4.

59. Abbassi-Ghanavati M, Casey BM, Spong CY, et al. Pregnancy outcomes in women with thyroid peroxidase antibodies. Obstet Gynecol 2010;116(2 Pt 1):381–6.

60. Pop VJ, de Rooy HA, Vader HL, et al. Microsomal antibodies during gestation in relation to postpartum thyroid dysfunction and depression. Acta Endocrinol (Copenh) 1993;129(1):26–30.

61. Glinoer D. Thyroid hyperfunction during pregnancy. Thyroid 1998;8(9):859–64.

62. Patil-Sisodia K, Mestman JH. Graves hyperthyroidism and pregnancy: a clinical update. Endocr Pract 2010;16(1):118–29.

63. Tan JY, Loh KC, Yeo GS, et al. Transient hyperthyroidism of hyperemesis gravidarum. BJOG 2002;109(6):683–8.

64. Amino N, Tanizawa O, Mori H, et al. Aggravation of thyrotoxicosis in early pregnancy and after delivery in Graves' disease. J Clin Endocrinol Metab 1982;55(1):108–12.

65. Millar LK, Wing DA, Leung AS, et al. Low birth weight and preeclampsia in pregnancies complicated by hyperthyroidism. Obstet Gynecol 1994;84(6):946–9.

66. Davis LE, Lucas MJ, Hankins GD, et al. Thyrotoxicosis complicating pregnancy. Am J Obstet Gynecol 1989;160(1):63–70.

67. Anselmo J, Cao D, Karrison T, et al. Fetal loss associated with excess thyroid hormone exposure. JAMA 2004;292(6):691–5.

68. Sheffield JS, Cunningham FG. Thyrotoxicosis and heart failure that complicate pregnancy. Am J Obstet Gynecol 2004;190(1):211–7.

69. Luewan S, Chakkabut P, Tongsong T. Outcomes of pregnancy complicated with hyperthyroidism: a cohort study. Arch Gynecol Obstet 2011;283(2):243–7.

70. Kempers MJ, van Tijn DA, van Trotsenburg AS, et al. Central congenital hypothyroidism due to gestational hyperthyroidism: detection where prevention failed. J Clin Endocrinol Metab 2003;88(12):5851–7.

71. Zakarija M, McKenzie JM. Pregnancy-associated changes in the thyroid-stimulating antibody of Graves' disease and the relationship to neonatal hyperthyroidism. J Clin Endocrinol Metab 1983;57(5):1036–40.

72. Polak M, Le Gac I, Vuillard E, et al. Fetal and neonatal thyroid function in relation to maternal Graves' disease. Best Pract Res Clin Endocrinol Metab 2004;18(2):289–302.

73. McKenzie JM, Zakarija M. Fetal and neonatal hyperthyroidism and hypothyroidism due to maternal TSH receptor antibodies. Thyroid 1992;2(2):155–9.
74. Laurberg P, Bournaud C, Karmisholt J, et al. Management of Graves' hyperthyroidism in pregnancy: focus on both maternal and foetal thyroid function, and caution against surgical thyroidectomy in pregnancy. Eur J Endocrinol 2009; 160(1):1–8.
75. Ibbertson HK, Seddon RJ, Croxson MS. Fetal hypothyroidism complicating medical treatment of thyrotoxicosis in pregnancy. Clin Endocrinol 1975;4(5):521–3.
76. Ochoa-Maya MR, Frates MC, Lee-Parritz A, et al. Resolution of fetal goiter after discontinuation of propylthiouracil in a pregnant woman with Graves' hyperthyroidism. Thyroid 1999;9(11):1111–4.
77. Momotani N, Noh J, Oyanagi H, et al. Antithyroid drug therapy for Graves' disease during pregnancy. Optimal regimen for fetal thyroid status. N Engl J Med 1986;315(1):24–8.
78. Martinez-Frias ML, Cereijo A, Rodriguez-Pinilla E, et al. Methimazole in animal feed and congenital aplasia cutis. Lancet 1992;339(8795):742–3.
79. Clementi M, Di Gianantonio E, Cassina M, et al. Treatment of hyperthyroidism in pregnancy and birth defects. J Clin Endocrinol Metab 2010;95(11):E337–41.
80. Di Gianantonio E, Schaefer C, Mastroiacovo PP, et al. Adverse effects of prenatal methimazole exposure. Teratology 2001;64(5):262–6.
81. Clementi M, Di Gianantonio E, Pelo E, et al. Methimazole embryopathy: delineation of the phenotype. Am J Med Genet 1999;83(1):43–6.
82. Bahn RS, Burch HS, Cooper DS, et al. The role of propylthiouracil in the management of Graves' disease in adults: report of a meeting jointly sponsored by the American Thyroid Association and the Food and Drug Administration. Thyroid 2009;19(7):673–4.
83. Kim HJ, Kim BH, Han YS, et al. The incidence and clinical characteristics of symptomatic propylthiouracil-induced hepatic injury in patients with hyperthyroidism: a single-center retrospective study. Am J Gastroenterol 2001;96(1):165–9.
84. Mandel SJ, Cooper DS. The use of antithyroid drugs in pregnancy and lactation. J Clin Endocrinol Metab 2001;86(6):2354–9.
85. Azizi F, Bahrainian M, Khamseh ME, et al. Intellectual development and thyroid function in children who were breast-fed by thyrotoxic mothers taking methimazole. J Pediatr Endocrinol Metab 2003;16(9):1239–43.
86. Momotani N, Yamashita R, Makino F, et al. Thyroid function in wholly breastfeeding infants whose mothers take high doses of propylthiouracil. Clin Endocrinol 2000;53(2):177–81.
87. Laurberg P, Nygaard B, Glinoer D, et al. Guidelines for TSH-receptor antibody measurements in pregnancy: results of an evidence-based symposium organized by the European Thyroid Association. Eur J Endocrinol 1998;139(6): 584–6.
88. Rubin PC. Current concepts: beta-blockers in pregnancy. N Engl J Med 1981; 305(22):1323–6.
89. Sherif IH, Oyan WT, Bosairi S, et al. Treatment of hyperthyroidism in pregnancy. Acta Obstet Gynecol Scand 1991;70(6):461–3.
90. Momotani N, Hisaoka T, Noh J, et al. Effects of iodine on thyroid status of fetus versus mother in treatment of Graves' disease complicated by pregnancy. J Clin Endocrinol Metab 1992;75(3):738–44.
91. Soliman S, McGrath F, Brennan B, et al. Color Doppler imaging of the thyroid gland in a fetus with congenital goiter: a case report. Am J Perinatol 1994; 11(1):21–3.

92. Huel C, Guibourdenche J, Vuillard E, et al. Use of ultrasound to distinguish between fetal hyperthyroidism and hypothyroidism on discovery of a goiter. Ultrasound Obstet Gynecol 2009;33(4):412–20.
93. Nachum Z, Rakover Y, Weiner E, et al. Graves' disease in pregnancy: prospective evaluation of a selective invasive treatment protocol. Am J Obstet Gynecol 2003;189(1):159–65.
94. Rotondi M, Cappelli C, Pirali B, et al. The effect of pregnancy on subsequent relapse from Graves' disease after a successful course of antithyroid drug therapy. J Clin Endocrinol Metab 2008;93(10):3985–8.
95. Stagnaro-Green A, Roman SH, Cobin RH, et al. A prospective study of lymphocyte-initiated immunosuppression in normal pregnancy: evidence of a T-cell etiology for postpartum thyroid dysfunction. J Clin Endocrinol Metab 1992;74(3):645–53.
96. Lazarus JH, Hall R, Othman S, et al. The clinical spectrum of postpartum thyroid disease. QJM 1996;89(6):429–35.
97. Caixas A, Albareda M, Garcia-Patterson A, et al. Postpartum thyroiditis in women with hypothyroidism antedating pregnancy? J Clin Endocrinol Metab 1999;84(11):4000–5.
98. Stagnaro-Green A. Postpartum thyroiditis. Best Pract Res Clin Endocrinol Metab 2004;18(2):303–16.
99. Lazarus JH, Ammari F, Oretti R, et al. Clinical aspects of recurrent postpartum thyroiditis. Br J Gen Pract 1997;47(418):305–8.
100. Alvarez-Marfany M, Roman SH, Drexler AJ, et al. Long-term prospective study of postpartum thyroid dysfunction in women with insulin dependent diabetes mellitus. J Clin Endocrinol Metab 1994;79(1):10–6.
101. Stagnaro-Green A, Akhter E, Yim C, et al. Thyroid disease in pregnant women with systemic lupus erythematosus: increased preterm delivery. Lupus 2011;20(7):690–9.
102. Elefsiniotis IS, Vezali E, Pantazis KD, et al. Post-partum thyroiditis in women with chronic viral hepatitis. J Clin Virol 2008;41(4):318–9.
103. Harris B, Othman S, Davies JA, et al. Association between postpartum thyroid dysfunction and thyroid antibodies and depression. BMJ 1992;305(6846):152–6.
104. Stagnaro-Green A, Schwartz A, Gismondi R, et al. High rate of persistent hypothyroidism in a large-scale prospective study of postpartum thyroiditis in southern Italy. J Clin Endocrinol Metab 2011;96(3):652–7.
105. Kuijpens JL, Vader HL, Drexhage HA, et al. Thyroid peroxidase antibodies during gestation are a marker for subsequent depression postpartum. Eur J Endocrinol 2001;145(5):579–84.
106. Lucas A, Pizarro E, Granada ML, et al. Postpartum thyroid dysfunction and postpartum depression: are they two linked disorders? Clin Endocrinol 2001;55(6):809–14.
107. Negro R, Greco G, Mangieri T, et al. The influence of selenium supplementation on postpartum thyroid status in pregnant women with thyroid peroxidase auto-antibodies. J Clin Endocrinol Metab 2007;92(4):1263–8.
108. Kampe O, Jansson R, Karlsson FA. Effects of L-thyroxine and iodide on the development of autoimmune postpartum thyroiditis. J Clin Endocrinol Metab 1990;70(4):1014–8.
109. Rahbari R, Zhang L, Kebebew E. Thyroid cancer gender disparity. Future Oncol 2010;6(11):1771–9.
110. Aschebrook-Kilfoy B, Ward MH, Sabra MM, et al. Thyroid cancer incidence patterns in the United States by histologic type, 1992-2006. Thyroid 2011;21(2):125–34.

111. Kung AW, Chau MT, Lao TT, et al. The effect of pregnancy on thyroid nodule formation. J Clin Endocrinol Metab 2002;87(3):1010–4.
112. Kuy S, Roman SA, Desai R, et al. Outcomes following thyroid and parathyroid surgery in pregnant women. Arch Surg 2009;144(5):399–406 [discussion: 406].
113. Mazzaferri EL. Approach to the pregnant patient with thyroid cancer. J Clin Endocrinol Metab 2011;96(2):265–72.
114. Sisson JC, Freitas J, McDougall IR, et al. Radiation safety in the treatment of patients with thyroid diseases by radioiodine [131]I: practice recommendations of the American Thyroid Association. Thyroid 2011;21(4):335–46.
115. Hirsch D, Levy S, Tsvetov G, et al. Impact of pregnancy on outcome and prognosis of survivors of papillary thyroid cancer. Thyroid 2010;20(10):1179–85.
116. Leboeuf R, Emerick LE, Martorella AJ, et al. Impact of pregnancy on serum thyroglobulin and detection of recurrent disease shortly after delivery in thyroid cancer survivors. Thyroid 2007;17(6):543–7.
117. Rosario PW, Barroso AL, Purisch S. The effect of subsequent pregnancy on patients with thyroid carcinoma apparently free of the disease. Thyroid 2007;17(11):1175–6.
118. Sioka C, Fotopoulos A. Effects of I-131 therapy on gonads and pregnancy outcome in patients with thyroid cancer. Fertil Steril 2011;95(5):1552–9.

Thyroid Hormone and the Cardiovascular System

Sara Danzi, PhD[a], Irwin Klein, MD[b],*

KEYWORDS

- Thyroid hormone • Cardiovascular system • Heart
- Hemodynamics

Studies of patients with spontaneously occurring hyperthyroidism and hypothyroidism indicate that thyroid hormone has profound effects on the heart and cardiovascular system.[1] This article describes the cellular mechanisms by which thyroid hormone acts at the level of the cardiac myocyte and the vascular smooth muscle cell to alter both phenotype and physiology.[2] Because it is well established that thyroid hormone, specifically T_3, acts on almost every cell and organ in the body, studies on the regulation of thyroid hormone transport into cardiac and vascular tissue take on added clinical significance (**Fig. 1**). The characteristic changes in cardiovascular hemodynamics and metabolism that accompany thyroid disease states can then be best understood at the cellular level.[3]

THYROID HORMONE METABOLISM

Thyroid hormones, tetraiodothyronine (T_4) and triiodothyronine (T_3), are produced in the thyroid gland in a molar ratio of approximately 7:1. All enzymatic steps in the synthesis and secretion of T_4 and T_3 are regulated by thyroid-stimulating hormone (TSH).[4] T_3, the physiologically active form of thyroid hormone, is produced primarily by 5'-monodeiodenation of T_4 in the liver, kidney, skeletal muscle, and pituitary gland.[5] Both T_4 and T_3 circulate in blood almost entirely (>95%) bound to a family of hormone binding proteins. The free hormone, specifically T_3, is transported through a variety of membrane transport proteins and, after transit to the cell nucleus, acts to regulate the expression of selected myocyte genes.[6,7] In addition to the classic regulation of thyroid hormone metabolism, it has been shown recently that 5'-monodeiodinase, which catalyzes the conversion of T_4 to T_3 in both the liver and pituitary, can be altered in a variety of cardiac disease states.[8]

[a] Department of Biological Sciences and Geology, Queensborough Community College, 222-05 56th Avenue, Bayside, NY 11364, USA
[b] Private Practice, 935 Northern Boulevard, Great Neck, NY 11021, USA
* Corresponding author.
E-mail address: iklein@nshs.edu

Med Clin N Am 96 (2012) 257–268
doi:10.1016/j.mcna.2012.01.006
0025-7125/12/$ – see front matter © 2012 Elsevier Inc. All rights reserved.

medical.theclinics.com

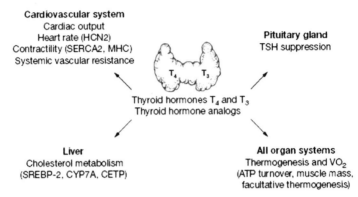

Fig. 1. Sites of action of thyroid hormone on the heart and cardiovascular system. CETP, cholesteryl ester transport protein; CYP7A, cholesterol 7α-hydroxylase; HCN2, hyperpolarization activated cyclic nucleotide-gated potassium channel 2; MHC, myosin heavy chains; SERCA2, sarcoplasmic reticulum (SR) Ca^{2+} ATPase; SREBP-2, sterol regulatory element binding protein 2; VO_2, maximal oxygen uptake.

CELLULAR MECHANISMS OF THYROID HORMONE ACTION ON THE HEART
Thyroid Hormone Transporters

Several families of thyroid hormone transporters have been identified, including the Na^+-taurocholate cotransporting polypeptide (NTCP), the Na^+-independent organic anion transporting polypeptides (OATPs), the heterodimeric L-type amino acid transporters (LAT), and the monocarboxylate transporters (MCTs).[6,9] These proteins transport a variety of ligands but only MCT8 and MCT10 are highly specific for iodothyronines and are expressed in heart (Danzi and Klein, unpublished data, 2011). Conversely, the cardiac plasma membrane transporters that are responsible for thyroid hormone uptake have not been well characterized. Both MCT8 and MCT10 were identified as monocarboxylate transporters and only recently found to be thyroid hormone transporters in an experimental cell system.[6] In humans, MCT8 gene mutations are the cause of Allan-Herndon-Dudley syndrome (AHDS), an X-linked syndrome with specific thyroid and neurologic abnormalities.[10]

Although both MCT8 and MCT10 facilitate uptake and efflux of both T_4 and T_3 in experimental cell systems, our recent data suggest that T_4 is not transported into the heart (Danzi and Klein, unpublished data, 2011). MCT10 has greater affinity for T_3 than T_4 and has a greater capacity to transport T_3 than MCT8.[11] As 1 of 2 thyroid hormone transporters shown to be expressed in rat or human heart, the MCT8 knockout mouse heart has not been characterized phenotypically.[12] The mechanism of transport for thyroid hormone via MCT8 and MCT10 in a variety of tissues seems to be via facilitative diffusion. Radiolabeled T_3 transport in rat neonatal ventricular myocytes is adenosine triphosphate (ATP) dependent, inhibited by excess unlabeled T_3, and Na^+-dependent. In that system, the magnitude of transport of T_3 is greater than 2.5-fold higher than T_4 (**Fig. 2**).[7]

Nuclear Receptors

The classic thyroid hormone effects on cardiac myocyte–specific gene transcription are mediated by thyroid hormone receptors (TRs), members of the steroid hormone superfamily of nuclear transcription factors.[13] Two genes encode the TRs and, in the mammalian heart, 2 splice variants of the TRα gene, TRα1 and TRα2, and 1 splice

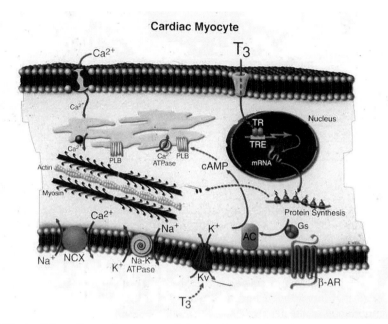

Fig. 2. Effects of T_3 on the cardiac myocyte. T_3 has both genomic and nongenomic effects on the cardiac myocyte. Genomic mechanisms involve T_3 binding to thyroid hormone receptor (TRs), which regulate transcription of specific cardiac genes. Nongenomic mechanisms include direct modulation of membrane ion channels as indicated by the dashed arrows. AC, adenylyl cyclase; β-AR, β-adrenergic receptor; Gs, guanine nucleotide binding protein; Kv, voltage-gated potassium channels; NCX, sodium calcium exchanger; PLB, phospholamban; TRE, thyroid hormone response element.

variant of the TRβ gene, TRβ1, are expressed. These receptor proteins are bound to thyroid hormone response elements (TREs) in the promoter region of certain T_3-responsive genes.[13,14] TRs activate transcription of positively regulated genes in the presence of T_3 by recruiting coactivator complexes, and repress transcription in the absence of ligand by recruiting corepressor complexes.[15]

It seems that the nuclear content of TRs are in turn regulated by T_3 such that, in the myocardium of hypothyroid animals, TRα-1 and α-2 mRNA levels are increased. After 72 hours of treatment with thyroid hormone, TRα-1 and TRα-2 mRNA levels decrease.[16] In a study of human hearts, comparison of TR mRNA in left ventricular tissue of patients with dilated cardiomyopathy showed decreased levels of TRα-1 and decreased TRα-1/TRα-2 ratios compared with normal donor hearts.[17] After heterotopic cardiac transplantation, the expression of TRα-1 and TRα-2 is altered in the rat heart.[18]

Transcriptional Regulation of Cardiac Myocyte Genes

T_3 regulates multiple myocyte genes intimately related to cardiac contractile function, including sarcoplasmic reticulum (SR) Ca^{2+} ATPase (SERCA2), phospholamban (PLB), and the myosin heavy chains (MHC), α and β (see **Fig. 2**; **Table 1**).[1,16] Some of these genes are positively regulated (SERCA2, α-MHC), whereas others are negatively regulated (PLB, β-MHC).[19] Cardiac muscle contraction and relaxation are regulated in turn by the intracellular free calcium concentration $[Ca^{2+}]_i$, which is largely

Table 1	
T$_3$-regulated cardiac genes	
Positively Regulated	**Negatively Regulated**
α-MHC	β-MHC
Voltage-gated K$^+$ channels (Kv1.5, Kv4.2)	Na$^+$/Ca^{2+} exchanger (NCX1)
SERCA2	Phospholamban
Na$^+$/K$^+$ ATPase	Adenylyl cyclase types V,VI
β1-Adrenergic receptor	Thyroid hormone receptor α1
Adenine nucleotide translocase 1	

determined by SR Ca^{2+} release via the ryanodine receptors,[20] and reuptake into the SR by the Ca^{2+} ATPase. PLB, an integral SR protein that regulates SERCA2 activity, is the mechanism by which β-adrenergic agonists exert positive inotropic action on the heart.[21] Varying degrees of impaired SR calcium uptake have been associated with human and experimental models of heart failure.[22] PLB-deficient transgenic mice showed increased contractility and knockout of PLB in the hypothyroid animal in the study by Kranias and colleagues,[23] which resulted in measures of contractility similar to that in wild-type animals treated with thyroid hormone, thus confirming the importance of the family of thyroid hormone–responsive genes in determining cardiac contractility.[1–3] Similarly, in a series of studies using transgenic overexpression of SERCA2 in hypothyroid mice, myocyte contractile function was restored to levels seen in euthyroid animals, confirming the role of SERCA2 in mediating the effects of thyroid disease on the heart.[24]

The cardiac phenotype is extremely sensitive to changes in serum T$_3$. In a rat model of thyroid hormone deficiency, administration of 5 μg/kg of T$_3$ induced transcription of the positively regulated, cardiac-specific, α-MHC within 30 minutes.[25] Maximal transcription, at more than euthyroid levels, occurred 6 hours after hormone administration, showing that the receptor saturating dose of T$_3$ is lower than previously suggested and the half-life of T$_3$ in vivo was 7 hours.[25] In experimental animal models of the low T$_3$ syndrome, when T$_4$ levels remain normal, the genotype, phenotype, and contractile function are those seen with more classic hypothyroidism.[26]

CARDIOVASCULAR HEMODYNAMICS
Hyperthyroidism

Cardiac contractility is enhanced including both systolic and diastolic function, and cardiac output and resting heart rate are increased in hyperthyroidism.[27] A decrease in systemic vascular resistance decreases afterload and improves myocardial efficiency.[28] An increase in blood volume and an increase in venous return cause the preload of the heart to increase, further augmenting cardiac output.[29] The increase in cardiovascular hemodynamics allows for increased blood flow leading to enhanced perfusion to provide for the substrate and oxygen demands of peripheral tissues (**Fig. 3, Table 2**).[1]

An increase in cardiac mass occurs in hyperthyroidism, both in animals and humans. Hypertrophy, usually increased left ventricular mass, results from sustained volume overload and the resulting increase in cardiac work and is a compensatory adaptation that, in turn, increases protein synthesis in the terminally differentiated cardiac myocyte.[30] Recent studies have shown that, in contrast with mean systemic pressures, pulmonary artery pressure is increased in hyperthyroidism, which in turn

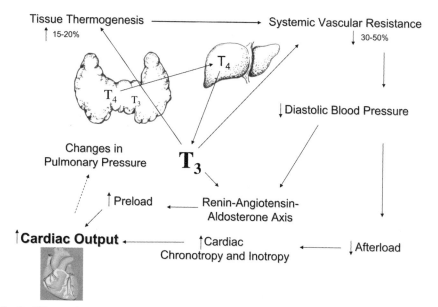

Fig. 3. Effects of thyroid hormone on cardiovascular hemodynamics. T_3 affects tissue thermogenesis, systemic vascular resistance, blood volume, cardiac contractility, heart rate, and cardiac output, as indicated by the arrows.

imparts an increase in right ventricular strain, increasing chamber size, mass, and filling pressure. The consequences of this may include the appearance of right heart or backward failure with neck vein distension and peripheral edema.[31,32]

Heterotopic cardiac transplantation into the abdominal cavity of a host animal provides a vascularly perfused, spontaneously beating, nonworking heart exposed to the same plasma thyroid hormone levels as the in situ working heart.[30] When these animals are exposed to excess amounts of thyroid hormone, only the in situ working heart became hypertrophic. This finding confirms the hypothesis that it is the excess workload resulting from the cardiovascular hemodynamics of hyperthyroidism that is responsible for the increase in cardiac mass.

The clinical manifestations of hyperthyroidism include characteristic cardiac-related signs and symptoms that are independent of the cause of the increased levels of

Table 2			
Changes in cardiovascular hemodynamics accompanying thyroid dysfunction			
Parameter	Normal	Hyperthyroid	Hypothyroid
Systemic vascular resistance (dyn-cm s^{-5})	1500–1700	700–1200	2100–2700
Heart rate (beats/min)	72–84	88–130	60–80
Pulmonary artery pressure	25	35–40	Unknown
% Ejection fraction	60	>60	<60
Isovolumic relaxation time (ms)	60–80	25–40	>80
Cardiac output (L/min)	5.8	>7.0	<4.5
Blood volume (% of normal)	100	105.5	84.5

thyroid hormone.[1,3,33] On physical examination, tachycardia is the most common finding. Heart rate is increased both at rest and with exercise and, commonly, rapid and forceful palpitations occur.[34] Occasionally atrial arrhythmias, including atrial fibrillation, can occur, but this is more common in older patients.[35] Other findings include widened pulse pressure, increased systolic and lowered diastolic pressure, dyspnea on exertion, and exercise intolerance with sustained activity.[36] Advanced disease may cause further exercise intolerance with limitations such as climbing 1 flight of stairs resulting from both skeletal muscle and respiratory weakness as well as a decrement in cardiac reserve capacity.[37,38]

Rarely, signs and symptoms of heart failure may occur in patients with thyrotoxicosis.[1,36] This condition usually occurs in the setting of prolonged and severe hyperthyroidism or after the onset of atrial fibrillation.[33] Because cardiac output at rest is increased in hyperthyroidism, the increased output that normally accompanies exercise is blunted.[38] Pulmonary and peripheral edema can occur as atrial filling pressure increases, causing a congested circulation. True heart failure in hyperthyroidism, characterized by decreased cardiac contractility, abnormal diastolic compliance, and pulmonary congestion, has been referred to as rate-related heart failure because sustained tachycardia impairs left ventricular contractility.[1,3,36] This finding should be confirmed by noninvasive cardiac measures such as echocardiography followed by the usual course of diuretics. β-Adrenergic blocking drugs are indicated to control the heart rate, and should be used within an intensive care unit setting if the degree of heart failure is significant enough to impair cardiovascular hemodynamics. Although propranolol is the most commonly used agent, intravenous use should be avoided and the short-acting agent esmolol can be used if concern about negative inotropy outweighs the goal of rate reduction. Attention to other potential medical comorbidities, such as infection, should also be addressed. Definitive treatment of the hyperthyroidism in almost all cases returns cardiac function to normal.[39–41]

Hypothyroidism

Overt hypothyroidism affects approximately 3% of the adult female population, with an increased prevalence in individuals more than 40 years of age. The cardiac manifestations of hypothyroidism are the result of decreased thyroid hormone action on both the heart and the peripheral vasculature.[1] The most common clinical signs are a narrowed pulse pressure, diastolic hypertension, low cardiac output with a decreased ejection fraction, impaired diastolic filling, and various degrees of bradycardia.[27] The increase in diastolic pressure is accompanied by a decrease in systolic pressure, so the pulse pressure is low. Hypothyroidism results in increased systemic vascular resistance, further contributing to the decrease in cardiac output.

Overt hypothyroidism is also associated with accelerated atherosclerosis and coronary artery disease, possibly caused by the higher incidence of hypercholesterolemia and hypertension (see **Fig. 1**).[42,43] Hypothyroidism, like hypertension and the effects of aging, leads to reduced SERCA2 activity and therefore, impaired calcium cycling, resulting in increased myocardial stiffness and left ventricular diastolic dysfunction.[3,24] Even mild (subclinical) hypothyroidism can increase the prevalence of heart failure and diastolic dysfunction.[44]

SPECIAL CONSIDERATIONS
Atrial Fibrillation

Sinus tachycardia is the most common rhythm disturbance in patients with hyperthyroidism.[45] However, atrial fibrillation caused by hyperthyroidism (especially subclinical hyperthyroidism) is more common with advancing age.[46] Although the yield of abnormal thyroid function testing, including a low serum TSH level, seems to be low in patients with new-onset atrial fibrillation, the benefit associated with the ability to restore thyrotoxic patients to a euthyroid state and sinus rhythm justifies TSH testing in most patients with recent onset of otherwise unexplained atrial fibrillation or other supraventricular arrhythmias.[47]

Symptomatic treatment of thyrotoxic atrial fibrillation includes β-adrenergic blockade.[48] This can be accomplished rapidly, whereas treatments leading to restoration of the euthyroid state require a longer time.[40] Digitalis has been used to control the ventricular response in hyperthyroidism-associated atrial fibrillation, but usually requires higher doses of this medication. Anticoagulation in patients with hyperthyroidism and atrial fibrillation is controversial because the potential for systemic or cerebral embolization must be weighed against the risk of bleeding and complications.[40] The major risk factor for systemic embolization in thyrotoxicosis seems to be age and not the presence of atrial fibrillation.[49] Therefore, unless there is a separate cardiac indication for warfarin or other forms of anticoagulation, aspirin can be safely used in this setting as an alternative in younger individuals.

Successful treatment of hyperthyroidism with radioiodine or antithyroid drugs to restore normal serum levels of T_4 and T_3 leads to reversion to sinus rhythm in most patients within a few months.[47] In the setting of atrial fibrillation of longer duration and in older patients, the rate of reversion to sinus rhythm is lower and electrical or pharmacologic cardioversion should therefore be attempted, but only after the patient has been rendered euthyroid.[47]

Pulmonary Artery Hypertension

There are reports of pulmonary artery hypertension in patients with thyrotoxicosis.[31,32,34] An apparent failure of pulmonary arterial resistance to decline, similar to that seen in the systemic circulation, results in significant increases of both mean and peak pulmonary artery pressures. These pressures usually normalized with a return to a chemically euthyroid state.[32] Although primary pulmonary hypertension is a rare, often fatal, disease of unknown cause that primarily affects young women, the frequency of both Graves disease (and chronic autoimmune thyroiditis, Hashimoto disease) is increased in this patient population as well, suggesting the value of routine thyroid function tests in all patients with pulmonary hypertension.[4,34]

Cholesterol Metabolism

Increased low-density lipoprotein (LDL) cholesterol occurs in the setting of hypothyroidism and in proportion to the increase in serum TSH levels.[42,50] Thyroid hormone alters cholesterol metabolism through a variety of mechanisms, including a decrease in LDL receptor expression but, perhaps more importantly, a decrease in biliary excretion. Further support for the role of thyroid hormone in the regulation of cholesterol metabolism comes from a recent study that describes a liver-selective thyroid hormone agonist, eprotirome, that can synergistically lower cholesterol levels in statin-treated patients.[50] Not only was high-density lipoprotein significantly decreased but a unique ability to lower Lp(a), an especially atherogenic lipid particle, was seen.

Amiodarone-Induced Thyroid Disease

Amiodarone is an iodine-rich antiarrhythmic agent effective for the treatment of ventricular and atrial tachyarrhythmias. Its iodine content and structural similarity to levothyroxine causes abnormalities in thyroid function tests in as many as 60% of patients treated with the drug.[51,52] Dronedarone, a recently approved noniodinated benzofuran antiarrhythmic, does not alter thyroid function and confirms this concept.[52,53] Amiodarone inhibits the 5'-monodeiodination of T_4 in the liver and pituitary, thereby decreasing serum T_3 and increasing serum T_4 levels. Serum TSH levels initially remain normal. In patients with underlying goiter, autoimmune thyroid disease, defects in thyroid hormone biosynthesis, and in some patients without any risk factors, there may be a progression to overt chemical and clinical hypothyroidism with a marked increase in serum TSH levels.[51,54]

Thyroid function should be measured every 3 months in all patients receiving amiodarone and for at least 6 months after stopping treatment because the effect on thyroid function can occur at any time after initiating treatment (and, because of the long half-life of the drug, alterations in thyroid function may still occur up to 1 year after discontinuing therapy).[52]

Less common than amiodarone-induced hypothyroidism, but perhaps more challenging, is the development of amiodarone-induced thyrotoxicosis. The development of this condition may be signaled by the new onset or recurrence of ventricular irritability, decreased warfarin sodium dose requirements, or the return or worsening of heart failure symptoms.[52] Early studies distinguished 2 forms of amiodarone-induced thyrotoxicosis. Type I occurs primarily in patients with preexisting thyroid disease and most commonly in iodine-deficient areas. These patients frequently have some measures of thyroid autoimmunity, including antithyroid antibodies.[51] In contrast, type II disease was identified as a form of thyroiditis, presumably mediated by a variety of proinflammatory cytokines. This process is destructive, causing release of preformed thyroid hormone, which may continue for weeks or months and most often is associated with low to absent radioiodine uptake.[54] Clinically important is the report that amiodarone-induced thyrotoxicosis is associated with a 3-fold increased risk for major adverse cardiovascular events.[55]

Therapy for these patients is especially challenging because the use of iodine 131 is almost always ineffective and treatment with antithyroid drugs has marginal effectiveness.[40,51,52,54] Treatment with corticosteroids may provide benefit and, in most cases, lowers serum levels of both T_4 and T_3 within 2 to 3 weeks.[54] In patients unresponsive to glucocorticoids with evidence of hyperthyroidism, including weight loss, tachycardia, palpitations, worsening angina, ventricular tachycardia, or other untoward cardiac effects, treatment with antithyroid therapy such as methimazole is variably effective.[54] Total thyroidectomy with preoperative treatment with β-blockers can be performed safely and is an effective means of reversing the hyperthyroidism rapidly.[55] Discontinuation of amiodarone is a cardiology decision.

ALTERATIONS IN THYROID HORMONE METABOLISM THAT ACCOMPANY HEART DISEASE

The prohormone T_4 is metabolized to T_3 primarily in the liver, kidney, and skeletal muscle by 5'-monodeiodination.[56] Altered thyroid hormone metabolism occurs in heart disease, after cardiac surgery, or after acute myocardial infarction, resulting in low serum T_3 levels despite normal TSH and T_4.[57] In patients with heart failure, the decrease in serum T_3 concentration is proportional to the severity of the heart disease as assessed by the New York Heart Association (NYHA) functional classification, and a low serum T_3 level is a powerful predictor of mortality in patients with NYHA Class III to IV heart failure.[58]

The heart failure phenotype is similar to the hypothyroid cardiac phenotype.[59] Hypothyroidism may also be associated with accelerated atherosclerosis and coronary artery disease.[43] The T_3-regulated genes that are altered in overt hypothyroidism are almost identical to the changes in gene expression in heart failure and include the genes that encode the contractile proteins, α-MHC and β-MHC, the sodium calcium exchanger (NCX1), SERCA2, PLB, and the β-adrenergic receptor (β-AR).[3] The net effect of these alterations in gene expression is to alter cardiac contractility, calcium cycling, and diastolic relaxation of the myocardium.[22,44]

Interleukin 6 (IL-6) and tumor necrosis factor-α (TNF-α) levels are increased in the low T_3 syndrome and can impair the expression and the activity of hepatic monodeiodinase, leading to decreased metabolism of T_4. The cardiac myocyte seems to transport T_3 in marked preference to T_4 and is exquisitely sensitive to changes in serum T_3.[60] Evidence is accumulating that suggests that low T_3 levels contribute to the heart failure phenotype and that normalization of T_3 might improve cardiac function in this setting. A recent study of T_3 treatment of humans with NYHA Class III or IV heart failure has shown beneficial effects.[8] Further studies are required to determine whether thyroid hormone–based treatments may be useful in selected patients with heart failure.[3,8]

REFERENCES

1. Klein I, Danzi S. Thyroid disease and the heart. Circulation 2007;116:1725–35.
2. Dillmann WH. Cardiac hypertrophy and thyroid hormone signaling. Heart Fail Rev 2010;15:125–30.
3. Klein I. Endocrine disorders and cardiovascular disease. In: Bonow RO, Mann DL, Zipes DP, et al, editors. Braunwald's heart disease. 9th edition. St Louis (MO): WB Saunders and Company; 2011. p. 1829–43. Chapter 86.
4. Demers LM, Spencer CA. Laboratory medicine practice guidelines. Laboratory support for the diagnosis and monitoring of thyroid disease. Thyroid 2003;13:3.
5. Koenig RJ. Regulation of type 1 iodothyronine deiodinase in health and disease. Thyroid 2005;15:835.
6. Visser WE, Wong WS, van Mullem AA, et al. Study of the transport of thyroid hormone by transporters of the SLC10 family. Mol Cell Endocrinol 2010; 315(1–2):138–45.
7. Everts ME, Verhoeven FA, Bezstarosti K, et al. Uptake of thyroid hormones in neonatal rat cardiac myocytes. Endocrinology 1996;137:4235–42.
8. Pingitore A, Galli E, Barison A, et al. Acute effects of triiodothyronine (T3) replacement therapy in patients with chronic heart failure and low-T3 syndrome: a randomized, placebo-controlled study. J Clin Endocrinol Metab 2008;93: 1351–8.
9. Visser WE, Friesema EC, Visser TJ. Minireview: thyroid hormone transporters: the knowns and the unknowns. Mol Endocrinol 2011;25:1–14.
10. Dumitrescu AM, Liao XH, Best TB, et al. A novel syndrome combining thyroid and neurological abnormalities associated with mutations in a monocarboxylate transporter gene. Am J Hum Genet 2004;74:168–75.
11. Friesema EC, Jansen J, Jachtenberg JW, et al. Effective cellular uptake and efflux of thyroid hormone by human monocarboxylate transporter 10. Mol Endocrinol 2008;22:1357–69.
12. Dumitrescu AM, Liao XH, Weiss RE, et al. Tissue-specific thyroid hormone deprivation and excess in monocarboxylate transporter (Mct) 8-deficient mice. Endocrinology 2009;150:4450–8.
13. Lazar M. Thyroid hormone receptors: multiple forms, multiple possibilities. Endocr Rev 1993;14:184–93.

14. Hodin R, Lazar M, Chin W. Differential and tissue-specific regulation of the multiple rat c-erbA messenger RNA species by thyroid hormone. J Clin Invest 1990;85:101–5.

15. Xu L, Glass CK, Rosenfeld MG. Coactivator and corepressor complexes in nuclear receptor function. Curr Opin Genet Dev 1999;9(2):140–7.

16. Balkman C, Ojamaa K, Klein I. Time course of the in vivo effects of thyroid hormone on cardiac gene expression. Endocrinology 1992;130:2001–6.

17. Sylven C, Jansson E, Sotonyi P, et al. Cardiac nuclear hormone receptor mRNA in heart failure in man. Life Sci 1996;599(22):1917–22.

18. Ojamaa K, Samarel A, Kupfer J, et al. Thyroid hormone effects on cardiac gene expression independent of cardiac growth and protein synthesis. Am J Physiol 1992;263:E534–40.

19. Danzi S, Klein S, Klein I. Differential regulation of myosin heavy chain genes α and β in the rat atria and ventricles: role of antisense RNA. Thyroid 2008;18(7):761–8.

20. Huang M, Knight PR, Izzo JL Jr. Ca^{2+} induced Ca^{2+} release involved in positive inotropic effect mediated by CGRP in ventricular myocytes. Am J Physiol 1999; 276:R259–64.

21. Koss KL, Kranias EG. Phospholamban, a prominent regulator of myocardial contractility. Circ Res 1996;79:1059–63.

22. Dipla K, Mattiello JA, Margulies KB, et al. The sarcoplasmic reticulum and the Na^+/Ca^{2+} exchanger both contribute to the Ca^{2+} transient of failing human ventricular myocytes. Circ Res 1999;84:435–44.

23. Kiss E, Brittsan AG, Edes I, et al. Thyroid hormone-induced alterations in phospholamban-deficient mouse hearts. Circ Res 1998;83:608–13.

24. Bluhm WF, Meyer M, Sayen MR, et al. Overexpression of sarcoplasmic reticulum Ca2+ ATPase improves cardiac contractile function in hypothyroid mice. Cardiovasc Res 1999;43:382–8.

25. Danzi S, Ojamaa K, Klein I. Triiodothyronine-mediated myosin heavy chain gene transcription in the heart. Am J Physiol Heart Circ Physiol 2003;284:H2255–62.

26. Katzeff H, Powell SR, Ojamaa K. Alterations in cardiac contractility and gene expression during the low T_3 syndrome. Am J Physiol 1997;273:E951–6.

27. Danzi S, Klein I. Thyroid hormone and blood pressure regulation. Curr Hypertens Rep 2003;5:513–20.

28. Bengel FM, Lehnert J, Ibrahim T, et al. Cardiac oxidative metabolism, function, and metabolic performance in mild hyperthyroidism: a noninvasive study using positron emission tomography and magnetic resonance imaging. Thyroid 2003;13:471–7.

29. Biondi B, Palmieri EA, Lombardi G, et al. Effects of thyroid hormone on cardiac function: the relative importance of heart rate, loading conditions, and myocardial contractility in the regulation of cardiac performance in human hyperthyroidism. J Clin Endocrinol Metab 2002;87:968–74.

30. Klein I, Hong C. Effects of thyroid hormone on cardiac size and myosin content of the heterotopically transplanted rat heart. J Clin Invest 1986;77:1694–8.

31. Ismail HM. Reversible pulmonary hypertension and isolated right-sided heart failure associated with hyperthyroidism. J Gen Intern Med 2007;22:148–50.

32. Di Giovambattista R. Hyperthyroidism as a reversible cause of right ventricular overload and congestive heart failure. Cardiovasc Ultrasound 2008;6:29.

33. Delit C, Silver S, Yohalem SB, et al. Thyrocardiac disease and its management with radioactive iodine I-131. JAMA 1961;176:262–7.

34. Klein I, Danzi S. The cardiovascular system in thyrotoxicosis. In: Braverman L, Utiger R, editors. Werner & Ingbar's the thyroid: a fundamental and clinical text. 10th edition. Philadelphia: Lippincott Williams & Wilkins; in press. Chapter 31.

35. Shimizu T, Koide S, Noh JY, et al. Hyperthyroidism and the management of atrial fibrillation. Thyroid 2002;12:489–93.
36. Dahl P, Danzi S, Klein I. Thyrotoxic cardiac disease. Curr Heart Fail Rep 2008; 5(3):170–6.
37. Olsen B, Klein I, Benner R, et al. Hyperthyroid myopathy and the response to treatment. Thyroid 1991;1:137–41.
38. Kahaly G, Kampmann C, Mohr-Kahaly S. Cardiovascular hemodynamics and exercise tolerance in thyroid disease. Thyroid 2002;12:473.
39. Mintz G, Pizzarello R, Klein I. Enhanced left ventricular diastolic function in hyperthyroidism: noninvasive assessment and response to treatment. J Clin Endocrinol Metab 1991;73:146–50.
40. Bahn RS, Burch HB, Cooper DS, et al. Hyperthyroidism and other causes of thyrotoxicosis: management guidelines of the American Thyroid Association and American Association of Clinical Endocrinologists. Endocr Pract 2011; 17(3):456–520.
41. Klein I, Becker D, Levey GS. Treatment of hyperthyroid disease. Ann Intern Med 1994;121:281–8.
42. Cappola AR, Ladenson PW. Hypothyroidism and atherosclerosis. J Clin Endocrinol Metab 2003;88:2438–44.
43. Biondi B, Klein I. Hypothyroidism as a risk factor for cardiovascular disease. Endocrine 2004;24:1–14.
44. Rodondi N, den Elzen WP, Bauer DC, et al, Thyroid Studies Collaboration. Subclinical hypothyroidism and the risk of coronary heart disease and mortality. JAMA 2010;304:1365–74.
45. Klein I, Ojamaa K. Mechanisms of disease: thyroid hormone and the cardiovascular system. N Engl J Med 2001;344:501–9.
46. Sawin CT, Geller A, Wolf PA, et al. Low serum thyrotropin levels as a risk factor for atrial fibrillation in older persons. N Engl J Med 1994;33:1249.
47. Nakazawa H, Lythall DA, Noh J, et al. Is there a place for the late cardioversion of atrial fibrillation? A long-term follow-up study of patients with post-thyrotoxic atrial fibrillation. Eur Heart J 2000;21:327.
48. Ventrella S, Klein I. Beta-adrenergic receptor blocking drugs in the management of hyperthyroidism. Endocrinologist 1994;4:391–9.
49. Petersen P, Hansen JM. Stroke in thyrotoxicosis with atrial fibrillation. Stroke 1988; 19:15.
50. Ladenson PW, Kristensen JD, Ridgway EC, et al. Use of the thyroid hormone analogue eprotirome in statin-treated dyslipidemia. N Engl J Med 2010;362:906–16.
51. Martino E, Bartalena L, Bogassi F, et al. The effects of amiodarone on the thyroid. Endocr Rev 2001;22:240.
52. Cohen-Lehman J, Dahl P, Danzi S, et al. Effects of amiodarone on thyroid function. Nat Rev Endocrinol 2010;6:34–41.
53. Kathofer S, Thomas D, Karle CA. The novel antiarrhythmic drug dronedarone: comparison with amiodarone. Cardiovasc Drug Rev 2005;23:217.
54. Bogazzi F, Bartalena L, Cosci C, et al. Treatment of type II amiodarone-induced thyrotoxicosis by either iopanoic acid or glucocorticoids: a prospective, randomized study. J Clin Endocrinol Metab 2003;88:1999.
55. Williams M, Lo Gerfo P. Thyroidectomy using local anesthesia in critically ill patients with amiodarone-induced thyrotoxicosis: a review and description of the technique. Thyroid 2002;12:523.
56. DeGroot LJ. Dangerous dogmas in medicine: the nonthyroidal illness syndrome. J Clin Endocrinol Metab 1999;84:151–64.

57. Ascheim DD, Hryniewicz K. Thyroid hormone metabolism in patients with congestive heart failure: the low triiodothyronine state. Thyroid 2002;12:511.

58. Iervasi G, Pingitore A, Landi P, et al. Low-T3 syndrome: a strong prognostic predictor of death in patients with heart disease. Circulation 2003;107:708–13.

59. Klein I, Danzi S. The cardiovascular system in hypothyroidism. In: Braverman L, Utiger R, editors. Werner & Ingbar's the thyroid: a fundamental and clinical text. 10th edition. Philadelphia: Lippincott Williams & Wilkins; in press. Chapter 53.

60. Danzi S, Klein I. Post-transcriptional regulation of myosin heavy chain expression in the heart by triiodothyronine. Am J Physiol Heart Circ Physiol 2005;288: H455–60.

The Effect of Thyroid Disorders on Lipid Levels and Metabolism

Leonidas H. Duntas, MD[a],*, Gabriela Brenta, MD[b]

KEYWORDS

- Thyroid • Cholesterol • Hypothyroidism • TSH
- Hyperthyroidism • Lipids

Thyroid hormones regulate cholesterol and lipoprotein metabolism, whereas thyroid disorders, including overt and subclinical hypothyroidism (SCH), considerably alter lipid profile and promote cardiovascular disease. Hypercholesterolemia in hypothyroidism is caused by a reduction in low-density lipoprotein (LDL) receptors and the diminishing control by T3 over sterol regulatory element-binding protein 2 (SREBP-2), crucial for the expression of LDL receptor. The action of thyroid hormone on bile acids has recently emerged as a discernible hypocholesterolemic effect. Increased flow of bile acids causes depletion of the hepatic cholesterol pool followed by an increase in the synthesis of cholesterol in the liver and the hepatic uptake of cholesterol from the circulation. Good evidence shows that high thyroid-stimulating hormone (TSH) is associated with a nonfavorable lipid profile, although TSH has no cutoff threshold for its association with lipids. L-T4 has a hypolipidemic effect in SCH, whereas the therapeutic benefit is greater with a higher initial value of cholesterol and TSH. Thyromimetics represent a new class of hypolipidemic drugs: their imminent application in patients with severe dyslipidemias, combined or not with statins, will improve the lipid profile, potentially accelerate energy expenditure and, as a consequence, vitally lessen the risk of cardiovascular disease.

More than a century ago, in 1900, von Noorden, working in Vienna, recognized the fact that the thyroid plays a key role in the development of "fatty disease." In 1918 researchers determined that blood cholesterol is related to the glands of internal secretion, particularly to the adrenals and thyroid, whereas studies in the early 1930s revealed the connection of cholesterol with thyroid function and disease.[1–3] At the beginning of that decade, specifically on Christmas day of 1930, a landmark

---

Disclosure: There is no conflict of interest for the authors.
[a] Endocrine Unit, Evgenidion Hospital, University of Athens, 20 Papadiamantopoulou Street, 11528 Athens, Greece
[b] Department of Endocrinology, Dr César Milstein Hospital, Buenos Aires, Argentina
* Corresponding author.
E-mail address: ledunt@otenet.gr

Med Clin N Am 96 (2012) 269–281
doi:10.1016/j.mcna.2012.01.012
0025-7125/12/$ – see front matter © 2012 Elsevier Inc. All rights reserved.
medical.theclinics.com

article published by Mason and colleagues[4] in the *New England Journal of Medicine* revealed the significance of cholesterol values in hyperthyroidism and hypothyroidism. Shortly thereafter, mainstream studies were published concerning the induction of hypothyroidism through cholesterol feeding to rabbits and the discovery that thyroid hormone supplementation inhibited the development of this lesion.[5] Subsequently, thyroid functioning has been firmly associated with cholesterol levels, whereas the incidence of hypothyroidism has consistently been reported to be significantly higher in patients with hypercholesterolemia.[6] The rise of cholesterol together with arterial hypertension, which is usually from the increased peripheral resistance, constitutes a major risk factor for atherosclerotic cardiovascular disease in hypothyroidism.[7]

In a multicenter study evaluating the prevalence of hypothyroidism in 752 hypercholesterolemic patients, primary hypothyroidism amounted to 3.7%, SCH to 2.4% and overt hypothyroidism to 1.4%.[8] The overall prevalence of hypothyroidism was calculated at 4.3% in patients with hypercholesterolemia. In contrast, in thyrotoxicosis cholesterol synthesis is increased, but this is simultaneously counterbalanced by an enhanced rate of degradation and excretion.[9] In addition, free fatty acid release and fatty acid oxidation have been described as being higher in hyperthyroidism, and this impairment may promote insulin resistance.[10]

The biochemical and molecular alterations induced by thyroid hormones in lipids during thyroid dysfunctions are variable, therefore constituting a complex field of study. This article updates the current knowledge concerning the impact of thyroid disease on lipid metabolism and pathophysiology and reviews the effect of thyromimetics on lipids and the controversy surrounding thyroxine treatment of SCH.

NOTES ON METABOLISM OF CHOLESTEROL AND LIPOPROTEINS

Cholesterol is generated within the body through hydrolysis of the molecules acetyl coenzyme A (CoA) and acetoacetyl-CoA, which form 3-hydroxy-3-methylglutaryl-CoA (HMG-CoA) that is then reduced to mevalonate by the rate-limiting enzyme HMG-CoA reductase. Cholesterol is transported within the blood by lipoproteins called, based on increasing density, chylomicrons, very low-density lipoprotein (VLDL), intermediate-density lipoprotein (IDL), LDL, and high-density lipoprotein (HDL). As shown by centrifugational analysis, cardioprotective HDL may be subdivided into HDL2 (lipid content, 59%–67%) and HDL3 (4%–44%).[11] Cholesterol synthesis is mediated by the sensing of intracellular cholesterol in the endoplasmic reticulum via SREBP 1 and 2, the transcription factor that positively regulates the expression of LDL receptor and cholesterol synthesis, and which is bound to two other proteins, SCAP (SREBP-cleavage-activating protein) and INSIG1 (insulin-induced gene 1).[12] The *SREBP-2* gene is regulated by thyroid hormone. After cleavage by specific proteases, namely S1P (sphingosine-1-phosphate) and S2P, SREBP migrates to the nucleus and acts as a transcription factor to bind to the sterol regulatory element, which stimulates the transcription of the low-density lipoprotein LDL receptor and HMG-CoA reductase genes. Increased serum triglycerides have been associated with proatherogenic changes in lipoproteins, for instance reduction of cardioprotective HDL and generation of small dense LDL.[13,14]

Reverse Cholesterol Transport

Cholesterol is removed from the extrahepatic tissues by HDL and is transferred back to the liver by a pathway named *reverse cholesterol transport*, the most important and effective antiatherogenic process of the human body.

Cholesterol is converted to cholesteryl esters by lecithin-cholesterol acyltransferase (LCAT) and is transported by cholesteryl ester transfer protein (CETP) from HDL2 to serum triglycerides, VLDL, and LDL, and vice versa. Subsequently LDL can be taken up by the liver LDL receptor (**Fig. 1**). The enzyme hepatic lipase regulates the hydrolysis of HDL2 to HDL3, whereas the lipoprotein lipase catabolizes serum triglycerides and transports free cholesterol into HDL.

THE ROLE OF THYROID HORMONES

Thyroid hormones have variable effects on lipid metabolism, because thyroid function regulates cholesterol synthesis and degradation and mediates the activity of key enzymes.[15] The cholesterol-lowering effect of thyroid hormones mainly occurs through an increased expression of LDL receptors at the hepatic and peripheral levels. The fact that T3 regulates LDL receptors was discovered more than 40 years ago after the observation that in conditions of hypothyroidism, LDL cholesterol elimination was reduced (**Fig. 2**).[9,16] It was subsequently shown that the number of LDL receptors in human murine fibroblasts and hepatocytes was regulated by T3,[17] and that in hypothyroid rats, the hepatic levels of LDL receptor mRNA were decreased (see **Fig. 2**).[18,19] The causative mechanisms consist of an indirect effect through the

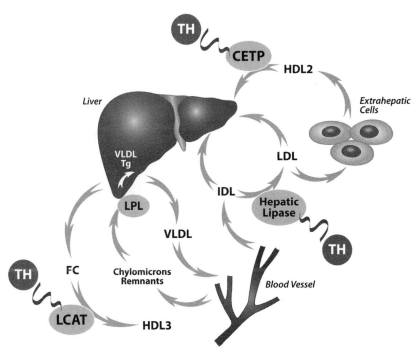

Fig. 1. The cholesterol transport from the peripheral tissues to the liver is mediated by HDL. LPL delipidates chylomicrons and VLDL, leading to production of IDL and transport of phospholipids into HDL, which carry cholesterol from extrahepatic tissues to the liver. Free cholesterol is esterified by LCAT to cholesteryl ester, which is transported by CETP from HDL2 to VLDL and IDL. CETP, cholesteryl-esters transfer protein; FC, free cholesterol; HDL, high density lipoproteins; HL, hepatic lipase; IDL, intermediate density lipoproteins; LCAT, lecithin-cholesterol acyltransferase; LPL, lipoprotein lipase; Tg, triglyceride; TH, thyroid hormones; VLDL, very low-density lipoproteins.

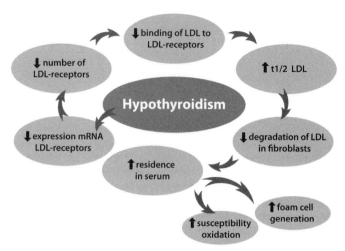

Fig. 2. Pathogenetic mechanism of increased low-density lipoprotein (LDL) in hypothyroidism. Hypothyroidism reduces the expression of LDL mRNA and the number of LDL receptors and the binding of LDL to LDL receptor, leading to increased half-life of LDL levels, reduced degradation of LDL in the fibroblasts, enhanced residence time in serum, and susceptibility to oxidation.

increased expression of SREBP-2[20] and a direct effect of T3 on the promoter of the LDL receptor gene.[21] Although T3 increases the expression of LDL membrane receptors, an increase of mRNA, protein, and activity of HMG-CoA occurs concomitantly.[22,23] Moreover, thyroid hormone to varying degrees increases the activity of the enzymes involved in the metabolism of lipoproteins and reverse cholesterol transport, such as hepatic lipase,[24] lipoprotein lipase,[25,26] CETP,[27] and LCAT[28] (see **Fig. 1**). The deranged binding of iodothyronines to lipoproteins in hypothyroidism manifests in their binding to small subfractions of HDL, thereby potentially altering the molecular structure.[29]

In hypothyroidism, if SREBP-2 nuclear protein levels are raised independently of thyroid hormones, activation of LDL receptor gene expression and reversal of the associated hypercholesterolemia are nonetheless achieved.[30] Researchers have therefore proposed that the reduced LDL receptor and the elevated serum cholesterol that have been linked to hypothyroidism may be considered to be consequential to the thyroid hormone impact on SREBP-2. These findings indicate that potential exists for reversal of hypercholesterolemia associated with hypothyroidism via agents capable of directly elevating SREBP-2. The same findings moreover imply that mutations or drugs that reduce nuclear SREBP-2 would cause hypercholesterolemia.

Another explanation for the cholesterol-lowering effect, as is shown with thyromimetics, is the accelerated clearance of cholesterol by the liver. This is achieved through increase of the HDL receptor, known as scavenger receptor B1,[31] and increasing bile acid synthesis via the upregulation of cholesterol 7alpha-hydroxylase,[32] the rate-limiting enzyme in the synthesis of bile acids.

The depletion of the intrahepatic cholesterol pool caused by increased flow of bile acids is followed by an increase in the synthesis of cholesterol in the liver and of the hepatic uptake of cholesterol from the circulation. Both processes are regulated by thyroid hormones and help to maintain the balance in hepatic cholesterol levels. Recently, bile acids have been implicated in thyroid-regulated energy metabolism because of its activation of the TGR-5/adenylate cyclase/type 2 deiodinase pathway.[33] It has also been suggested that bile acids interact with the thyroid set point axis, because the TSH decreases after a nutritional load is correlated to the bile acid increase.[33]

Recently, the carbohydrate response element-binding protein (ChREBP) that, together with SREBP-1c, controls hepatic lipogenesis, was found to be regulated by thyroid hormone in mamamals.[34] Researchers have also recently reported that ChREBP mRNA is positively controlled by T3 binding to thyroid receptor ß-1.[35] This novel observation indicates that TH fine-tunes hepatic lipogenesis through regulating SREBP-1c and ChREBP gene expression reciprocally.[35] T3 additionally has a lipogenic effect in white adipose tissue where both thyroid receptor isoforms are expressed.[36]

However, T3 upregulates apolipoprotein AV gene (APOAV), which is a major determinant of serum triglycerides metabolism.[37] The fact that T3 increases APOAV mRNA and protein levels in hepatocyte, thus leading to a decrease of triglyceride, points to a plausible mechanism of T3 action and a potential therapeutic target for control of triglyceride metabolism.

HYPOTHYROIDISM AND SECONDARY HYPERLIPIDEMIA

The lipid profile in hypothyroidism is characterized by increased total and LDL cholesterol levels with increased or normal HDL levels. Usually the HDL2 subfraction, and not the HDL3, is elevated.[38] Triglyceride levels are not markedly affected or are at most slightly elevated. However, it has been recorded that the levels of lipoprotein (a) may be increased.[39] All of these abnormalities are reversed by treatment with L-T4. The most frequent form of dyslipidemia, as shown in a study of 295 overt hypothyroid patients, is type IIA or pure hypercholesterolemia (56%), followed by type IIb (hypercholesterolemia and hypertriglyceridemia; 34%) and type IV (hypertriglyceridemia; 1.5%), whereas only 8.5% had no lipid abnormalities.[39]

The pathophysiologic mechanism behind these lipid abnormalities has been determined to be a decreased biosynthesis and degradation of lipoproteins, with a predominance in the reduction of catabolic pathways.[18] The reduction in the number of LDL receptors results in an excess of LDL particles, which circulate in plasma and are prone to oxidation (see **Fig. 2**). A lower activity of the enzymes lipoprotein lipase[25,26] and hepatic lipase[24] has been extensively described in overt hypothyroidism, together with a decrease in the activity of CETP.[27] These changes in enzymatic activity could account for the increased levels of lipoproteins possessing high atherogenic potential, such as VLDL and VLDL remnants/IDL, in plasma of hypothyroid patients. Similar to what occurs with LDL particles in excess, aberrant receptors of macrophages can also dispose of these remnants and initiate the transformation into foam cells and oxidation of LDL.[40,41] Paraoxonase 1 (PON1) activity, which is an HDL-associated lactonase that protects against macrophage-mediated LDL oxidation, is reportedly decreased in thyroid disorders,[42] and therefore researchers have postulated that the increased LDL oxidation in hypothyroidism is caused to some extent by the reduced PON1 activity.[43]

Regarding LDL size, except for one study,[44] most agree that there is an absence of small LDL in hypothyroidism.[45–47]

Although HDL particles may attain increased levels in hypothyroidism, the net effect of the impaired activity of the lipoprotein remodeling enzymes on HDL functional capacity remains to be determined.

Serum concentrations of non–HDL cholesterol (non–HDL-C) have also been reportedly increased in hypothyroidism, presumably caused by the disturbed metabolism of

LDL and remnants.[48,49] Replacement therapy with LT4 reduces non–HDL-C levels, thus potentially contributing to cardioprotection, taking into consideration that assessment of non–HDL-C, which constitutes a secondary target of therapy, was proposed in patients at increased risk for cardiovascular disease.[48,50]

IMPACT OF SUBCLINICAL HYPOTHYROIDISM ON THE LIPID PROFILE

Concerning SCH, several older studies, in the 1970s and 1980s, showed a lipoprotein derangement and hypothesized that this could be associated with increased cardiovascular risk.[51–53] Although 1% to 11% of all patients with dyslipidemia have SCH, the results of epidemiologic studies analyzing lipid levels according to thyroid status are highly controversial.[54] The U.S. Colorado study, with a population sample of 25,862 subjects,[55] showed that patients with SCH had higher levels of total cholesterol compared with the remaining euthyroid population. However, in an Austrian population study of 6014 subjects,[56] SCH was found to yield similar cholesterol levels to those of euthyroids, whereas cholesterol values were higher only in the group with overt hypothyroidism. Likewise, a cross-sectional analysis of a population sample[57] of the third U.S. National Health and Nutrition Examination Survey (NHANES III) showed that, although cholesterol and triglyceride levels were higher in patients with SCH than in euthyroid subjects, after adjusting for variables such as sex, race, age, and whether the patient was under lipid lowering drugs, SCH was not related to an abnormal lipid profile. In contrast, another study that distributed patients into groups according to severity of dyslipidemia[58] showed a larger incidence of SCH was found in the group with the highest levels of serum cholesterol. These findings are consistent with the results of a recent study showing a high prevalence of SCH in a population of 1610 women older than 50 years with dyslipidemia.[59]

A plausible explanation for the discrepancy between these study results may reside in the great heterogeneity of the populations studied. Among factors involved are differences in TSH levels used to define SCH and in selection criteria according to age, sex, race, degree of smoking,[60] or insulin resistance.[61] In fact, good evidence has been provided that the association of TSH with LDL cholesterol is modified by insulin sensitivity. Insulin-resistant patients with high normal TSH are more susceptible to higher cholesterol serum levels. These results have been replicated in the Fermantle study, a community-based observational study, including 117 women with type 2 diabetes mellitus.[62] Therefore, although hyperinsulinemia may determine an increased hepatic output of VLDL particles, hypothyroidism might meanwhile suppress their removal, resulting in the net effect of accumulation of modified lipoproteins. Moreover, researchers have reported that in SCH, LDL particles have an impaired composition and become triglyceride-rich lipoproteins.[62] VLDL remnants and IDL tend to accumulate in circulation.[49,63] Furthermore, both atherogenic alterations have been associated with a reduction of hepatic lipase activity.[63,64] However, fractional clearance rates of triglycerides and cholesteryl esters have been reportedly equal in patients with SCH and controls, indicating that lipolysis and remnant removal of triglyceride-rich lipoproteins were normal.[65] Nevertheless, transfer of triglycerides to HDL was reduced when compared with controls.

All of these findings have resulted in the hypothesis that TSH has no cutoff threshold for its association with lipids.

EFFECT OF L-T4 THERAPY ON LIPID PROFILE IN SUBCLINICAL HYPOTHYROIDISM

Treatment of severe hypothyroidism with L-T4 reverses lipid abnormalities. In subclinical forms of the disease, however, the results are less conclusive. Numerous intervention studies are being conducted to evaluate lipid changes in SCH. A frequently quoted meta-analysis[66] involving a selection of 13 intervention studies registered a reduction in lipids, especially in patients in whom the baseline total cholesterol level was greater than 240 mg/dL. After the publication of this meta-analysis, other placebo-controlled studies were performed. In 66 women with TSH greater than 5 mU/L treated over 50 weeks with L-T4, a significant reduction of 3.2% and 8% in total cholesterol and LDL, respectively, was seen at the end of the treatment period.[67] In another trial, subclinical hypothyroid patients were randomized to placebo or L-T4 for a 6 months.[68] A reduction of 9% and 13% in total cholesterol and LDL, respectively, was shown, although the results were criticized because no significant difference was seen between the levels of cholesterol in the placebo and treated groups by the end of the study. Nevertheless, in a subsequent study by this research group, carotid intima-media thickness values were found to be higher in the subclinical hypothyroid group, and cholesterol levels after treatment were clearly lower than those in the placebo group.[69]

L-thyroxine administration has exhibited a significant cholesterol-lowering effect in hypercholesterolemic patients with antibody-positive, high-normal (2.0–4.0 mIU/L) TSH levels compared with those with low-normal (0.40–1.99 μU/mL) TSH levels.[70] Thus, it has been suggested that the known associations of overt and SCH with hyperlipidemia may be extended into the normal range of thyroid function.[70]

This assumption was further confirmed in the large, population-based, fifth Tromsø study[71] recruiting 5143 Norwegian subjects in whom a slight but significant association between TSH levels and total cholesterol and LDL was reported. Further analysis of a subgroup of 84 patients with TSH levels between 3.5 and 10 mU/L also showed significantly higher levels of total cholesterol and LDL compared with the control group. The Nord-Trøndelag Health (HUNT) study,[72] another epidemiologic study, also conducted in Norway, enrolling 30,565 participants, similarly showed that a linear increase of total cholesterol, LDL-C, non–HDL-C, and triglycerides, and a decrease in HDL cholesterol is seen within the normal range of TSH.

A double-blind crossover study involving 100 subjects with TSH greater than 6.1 mU/L showed a significant decrease in total cholesterol and LDL after 12 weeks of treatment with 100 μg L-T4.[73] Similarly, in a trial using individually adjusted doses of L-T4, the authors noted a reduction of cholesterol levels, especially in patients with TSH greater than 8 mU/L.[74]

According to the results of most of the intervention studies, L-T4 has a hypolipemic effect in SCH, whereas the therapeutic benefit is greater with a higher initial value of cholesterol and TSH.

Cardiovascular Risk

Thyroid disorders have been associated with atherosclerotic cardiovascular disease. Although this finding is evidence-based in manifested hypothyroidism, questionable whether this association exists in SCH is questionable.[75–79] The association of thyroid disease with cardiovascular disease partly may be explained by thyroid hormone's regulation of lipid metabolism and its effects on blood pressure.[80,81] However, the impact of various degrees of thyroid dysfunction on these factors continues to be debated.[75,82,83] Most studies in SCH have exhibited a favorable effect in that they reduced the risk of cardiovascular disease and mortality.[75,84,85]

LIPID CHANGES IN HYPERTHYROIDISM

In hyperthyroidism, an increase is seen in the synthesis and degradation of lipids, with a predominance of the catabolic pathways. Consequently, plasma levels of cholesterol are reduced in hyperthyroid patients.[86,87] Although this finding can be partly attributed to malnutrition and weight loss, the high uptake of cholesterol into cells and its larger excretion in bile salts through the gut can all contribute to the hypolipemic effect observed in these patients.[16,17,39] Nevertheless, although LDL serum levels are low in hyperthyroidism, which may account for an antiatherogenic benefit, LDL particles are more prone to oxidation.[88,89] Furthermore, HDL, and more specifically subfraction HDL$_2$, has been found reduced in hyperthyroidism (43 to 27).

In adipose tissue, lipolysis is also augmented, with elevation of nonesterified fatty acids (NEFA) in plasma, with their consequent oxidization and enhanced ketogenesis in the liver.[90,91] However, mild hypertriglyceridemia has been paradoxically observed in hyperthyroidism. A plausible explanation for this phenomenon would be that hepatic lipogenesis is augmented, accompanied by an increased fatty acyl-CoA availability for hepatic reesterification, although evidence shows a direct stimulation of hepatic lipogenesis by thyroid hormones.[92]

Normalization of lipid changes on reversal of the thyrotoxic state has been noted by several authors, although the magnitude of the response depends on factors such as the duration and modality of treatment of the thyroid dysfunction and the characteristics of each individual.[93,94]

THYROMIMETICS: MODES OF ACTION AND PERSPECTIVES

The notion that the T3 effect on plasma cholesterol levels is mediated through TRβ1 has ignited research into the development of thyroid hormone receptor isoform β-selective analogs, the thyromimetics that specifically target TRβ1, either through selective hepatic uptake and/or through higher binding affinity to TRβ1, to treat hypercholesterolemia, while avoiding adverse effects in the heart or skeleton.[95] They may protect from atherosclerosis by promoting reverse cholesterol transport and activating hepatic lipase. They reduced serum cholesterol levels by 25% and serum triglycerides by 75% in chow-fed mice and also attenuated diet-induced hypercholesterolemia. Sobetirome reduced plasma HDL cholesterol levels, increased expression of the hepatic HDL receptor SR-BI, stimulated activity of cholesterol 7alpha-hydroxylase, and increased fecal excretion of bile acids.[96,97]

Eprotirome (KB2115), another TRβ1-selective agent, has been shown to be capable of lowering cholesterol, triglycerides, and lipoprotein(a) in hypercholesterolemic patients receiving statins.[98] Thus, a randomized, placebo-controlled, double-blind, multicenter trial showed that the addition of placebo or eprotirome at a dose of 25, 50, or 100 μg daily for 12 weeks to ongoing statin treatment significantly decreased the mean level of serum LDL cholesterol, apolipoprotein B, triglycerides, lipoprotein(a) up to a mean reduction from baseline of 7%, 22%, 28%, and 32%, respectively.[97] Eprotirome therapy was shown to be safe, TSH and T3 levels were not influenced, and it was not associated with adverse effects. New phase III studies with thyromimetics in dyslipidemic patients, combined or not with statins, are currently ongoing. It is reasonably expected that they will improve the lipid profile, potentially accelerate energy expenditure and, consequently, vitally lessen the risk of cardiovascular disease.

REFERENCES

1. Von Noorden CH. Die fettsucht. Wien; 1900.
2. Luden G. Collected papers of Mayo Clinic. Mayo Clin Proc 1918;10:482–7.
3. Epstein AA, Lande H. Studies on blood lipoids: I. The relation of cholesterol and protein deficiency to basal metabolism. Arch Intern Med 1922;30:563–77.

4. Mason RL, Hunt HM, Hurxthal L. Blood cholesterol values in hyperthyroidism and hypothyroidism-their significance. N Engl J Med 1930;203:1273–8.
5. Friedland IB. Investigations on the influence of thyroid preparations on experimental hypercholesterolemia and athereosclerosis. Zeitung Ges Exp Med 1933;87:683–9.
6. Loeb JN. Metabolic changes in hypothyroidism. In: Braverman LE, Utiger RD, editors. Werner and Ingbar's the thyroid. 7th edition. Philadelphia: Lippincott-Raven; 1996. p. 858–63.
7. Steinberg AD. Myxedema and coronary artery disease. A comparative autopsy study. Ann Intern Med 1968;68:338–44.
8. Tagami T, Kimura H, Ohtani S, et al. Multi-center study on the prevalence of hypothyroidism in patients with hypercholesterolemia. Endocr J 2001;58:449–57.
9. Walton KW, Scott PJ, Dykes PW, et al. The significance of alterations in serum lipids in thyroid dysfunction. II. Alterations of the metabolism and turnover of 131-I-low-density lipoproteins in hypothyroidism and thyrotoxicosis. Clin Sci 1965;29:217–38.
10. Riis AL, Gravholt CH. Elevated regional lipolysis in hyperthyroidism. J Clin Endocrinol Metab 2002;87:4747–53.
11. Duntas LH. Changes in lipid profile in overt and subclinical hypothyroidism. In: Derwahl KM, Duntas LH, Butz S, editors. The thyroid and cardiovascular risk. Stuttgart (Germany): Georg Thieme Verlag; 2005. p. 37–44.
12. Espenshade PJ, Hughes AL. Regulation of sterol synthesis in eukaryotes. Annu Rev Genet 2007;41:401–27.
13. Grifflin A, Zampelas A. Influence of dietary fatty acids on the atherogenic lipoprotein phenotype. Nutr Res Rev 1995;8:1–26.
14. Angles-Cano E, de la Pena Diaz A, Loyau S. Inhibition of fibrinolysis by lipoprotein (a). Ann N Y Acad Sci 2001;936:261–75.
15. Duntas L. Thyroid disease and lipids. Thyroid 2002;12:287–93.
16. Abrams JJ, Grundy SM. Cholesterol metabolism in hypothyroidism and hyperthyroidism in man. J Lipid Res 1981;22:323–38.
17. Chait A, Bierman EL, Albers J. Regulatory role of T_3 in the degradation of LDL by cultured human skin fibroblast. J Clin Endocrinol Metab 1979;48:887–9.
18. Staels B, Van Tol A, Chan L, et al. Alterations in thyroid status modulate apolipoprotein, hepatic triglyceride lipase, and low density lipoprotein receptor in rats. Endocrinology 1990;127:1144–52.
19. Salter AM, Hayashi R, al-Seeni M, et al. Effects of hypothyroidism and high-fat feeding on mRNA concentrations for the low-density-lipoprotein receptor and on acyl-CoA:cholesterol acyltransferase activities in rat liver. Biochem J 1991;276:825–32.
20. Weber LW, Boll M, Stampfl A. Maintaining cholesterol homeostasis: sterol regulatory element-binding proteins. World J Gastroenterol 2004;10:3081–7.
21. Bakker O, Hudig F, Meijssen S, et al. Effects of triiodothyronine and amiodarone on the promoter of the human LDL receptor gene. Biochem Biophys Res Commun 1998;249:517–22.
22. Ness G, Lopez D, Chambers C, et al. Effects of L-triiodothyronine and the thyromimetic L-94091 on serum lipoprotein levels and hepatic low density lipoprotein receptor, 3-hydroxy-3-methylglutaryl coenzyme A reductase, and apo A-I gene expression. Biochem Pharmacol 1998;56:121–9.
23. Choi J, Choi H. The regulatory effects of thyroid hormone on the activity of 3-hydroxy-3-methylglutaryl coenzyme A reductase. Endocr Res 2000;26:1–21.
24. Valdemarsson S, Nilsson-Ehle P. Hepatic lipase and the clearing reaction: studies in euthyroid and hypothyroid subjects. Horm Metab Res 1987;19:28–30.

25. Lithell H, Boberg J, Hellsing K, et al. Serum lipoprotein and apolipoprotein concentrations and tissue lipoprotein-lipase activity in overt and subclinical hypothyroidism: the effect of substitution therapy. Eur J Clin Invest 1981;11:3–10.

26. Kussi T, Taskinen MR, Nikkila EA. Lipoproteins, lipolytic enzymes, and hormonal status in hypothyroid women at different levels of substitution. J Clin Endocrinol Metab 1988;66:61–6.

27. Tan K, Shiu S, Kung A. Effect of thyroid dysfunction on high-density lipoprotein subfraction metabolism: roles of hepatic lipase and cholesteryl ester transfer protein. J Clin Endocrinol Metab 1998;83:2921–4.

28. Ridgway ND, Dolphin PJ. Serum activity and hepatic secretion of lecithin:cholesterol acyltransferase in experimental hypothyroidism and hypercholesterolemia. J Lipid Res 1985;26:1300–13.

29. Benvenga S, Robbins J. Altered thyroid hormone binding to plasma lipoproteins in hypothyroidism. Thyroid 1996;6:3377–8.

30. Shin DJ, Osborne TF. Thyroid hormone regulation and cholesterol metabolism are connected through sterol regulatory element-binding protein-2 (SREBP-2). J Biol Chem 2003;278:34114–8.

31. Johansson L, Puding M, Scanlan TS, et al. Selective thyroid receptor modulation by GC-1 reduces lipids and stimulates steps of reverse cholesterol transport in euthyroid mice. Proc Natl Acad Sci U S A 2005;102:10297–302.

32. Day R, Gebhard RL, Schwartz HL, et al. Time course of hepatic HMG-CoA reductase activity and mRNA, biliary lipid secretion, and hepatic cholesterol content in methimazole-treated hypothyroid and hypophysectomized rats after triiodothyronine administration: possible linkage of cholesterol synthesis to biliary secretion. Endocrinology 1989;125:459–68.

33. Ockenga J, Valentini L, Schuetz T, et al. Plasma bile acids are associated with energy expenditure and thyroid function in humans. J Clin Endocrinol Metab, in press.

34. Iizuka K, Horikawa Y. ChREBP: a glucose activated transcription factor. Endocr J 2008;55:617–24.

35. Hashimoto K, Ishida E, Matsumoto S, et al. Carbohydrate response element binding protein gene expression is positively regulated by thyroid hormone. Endocrinology 2009;150:3417–24.

36. Gauthier K, Billon C, Bissler M, et al. Thyroid hormone receptor beta (TRbeta) and liver X receptor (LXR) regulate carbohydrate-response element-binding protein (ChREBP) expression in a tissue-selective manner. J Biol Chem 2010;285: 28156–63.

37. Prieur X, Huby T, Coste H, et al. Thyroid hormone regulates the hypotriglyceridemic gene APOA5. J Biol Chem 2005;280:27533–43.

38. Verdugo C, Perrot L, Ponsin G, et al. Time-course of alterations of high density lipoproteins (HDL) during thyroxine administration to hypothyroid women. Eur J Clin Invest 1987;17:313–6.

39. O'Brien T, Dinneen SF, O'Brien PC, et al. Hyperlipidemia in patients with primary and secondary hypothyroidism. Mayo Clin Proc 1993;68:860–6.

40. Doi H, Kugiyama K, Oka H, et al. Remnant lipoproteins induce proatherothrombogenic molecules in endothelial cells through a redox-sensitive mechanism. Circulation 2000;102:670–6.

41. Duntas L, Mantzou E, Koutras DA. Circulating levels of oxidized low-density lipoprotein in overt and mild hypothyroidism. Thyroid 2002;12:1003–7.

42. Efrat M, Aviram M. Paraoxonase 1 interactions with HDL, antioxidants and macrophages regulate atherogenesis: a protective role for HDL phospholipids. Adv Exp Med Biol 2010;660:153–66.

43. Azizi F, Raiszadeh F, Solati M, et al. Serum paraoxonase 1 activity is decreased in thyroid dysfunction. J Endocrinol Invest 2003;26:703–9.
44. Abbas JM, Chakraborty J, Akanji AO, et al. Hypothyroidism results in small dense LDL independent of IRS and traits hypertriglyceridemia. Endocr J 2008; 55:381–9.
45. Roscini AR, Lupattelli G, Siepi D, et al. Low density lipoprotein size in primary hypothyroidism. Effects of hormone replacement therapy. Ann Nutr Metab 1999;43:374–9.
46. Pearce EN, Wilson PW, Yang Q, et al. Thyroid function and lipid subparticle in patients with short-term hypothyroidism and sizes a population-based cohort. J Clin Endocrinol Metab 2008;93:888–94.
47. Kim CS, Kang JG, Lee SJ, et al. Relationship of low-density lipoprotein (LDL) particle size to thyroid function status in Koreans. Clin Endocrinol (Oxf) 2009;71:130–6.
48. Rana JS, Boekholdt S, Kastelein JJ, et al. The role of non-HDL-cholesterol in risk stratification for coronary artery disease. Curr Atheroscler Rep, in press.
49. Ito M, Takamatsu J, Sasaki I, et al. Disturbed metabolism of remnant lipoproteins in patients with subclinical hypothyroidism. Am J Med 2004;117:696–9.
50. Ito M, Arishima T, Kudo T, et al. Effect of levothyroxine replacement on non-high density lipoprotein cholesterol in hypothyroid patients. J Clin Endocrinol Metab 2007;92:608–11.
51. Kutty KM, Bryant DG, Farid NR. Serum lipids in hypothyroidism – a re-evaluation. J Clin Endocrinol Metab 1978;46:55–6.
52. Ridgway EC, Cooper DS, Walker H, et al. Peripheral responses to thyroid hormone before and after l-thyroxine therapy in patients with subclinical hypothy-roidism. J Clin Endocrinol Metab 1981;53:1238–42.
53. Staub JJ, Althaus BU, Engler H, et al. Spectrum of subclinical and overt hypothy-roidism: effect on thyrotropin, prolactin, and thyroid reserve, and metabolic impact on peripheral target tissues. Am J Med 1992;92:631–42.
54. Pearce EN. Update in lipid alterations in subclinical hypothyroidism. J Clin Endo-crinol Metab, in press.
55. Canaris GJ, Manowitz NR, Mayor G, et al. The Colorado thyroid disease preva-lence study. Arch Intern Med 2000;160:526–34.
56. Vierhapper H, Nardi A, Grosser P, et al. Low-density lipoprotein cholesterol in subclinical hypothyroidism. Thyroid 2000;10:981–4.
57. Hueston WJ, Pearson W. Subclinical hypothyroidism and the risk of hypercholes-terolemia. Ann Fam Med 2004;2:351–5.
58. Bindels A, Westendorp R, Frolich M, et al. The prevalence of subclinical hypothy-roidism at different total plasma cholesterol levels in middle aged men and women: a need for case-finding? Clin Endocrinol 1999;50:217–20.
59. Leclère J, Cousty C, Schlienger JL, et al. Subclinical hypothyroidism and quality of life of women aged 50 or more with hypercholesterolemia: results of the HYOGA study. Presse Med 2008;37:1538–46.
60. Mueller B, Zulewski H, Huber P, et al. Impaired action of thyroid hormone asso-ciated with smoking in women with hypothyroidism. N Engl J Med 1995;333:964–9.
61. Bakker S, ter Maaten JC, Popp-Snijders C, et al. The relationship between thyro-tropin and low density lipoprotein cholesterol is modified by insulin sensitivity in healthy euthyroid subjects. J Clin Endocrinol Metab 2001;86:1206–11.
62. Chubb SA, Davis WA, Davis TM. Interactions among thyroid function, insulin sensitivity, and serum lipid concentrations: the fremantle diabetes study. J Clin Endocrinol Metab 2005;90:5317–20.

63. Brenta G, Berg G, Arias P, et al. Lipoprotein alterations, insulin sensitivity and hepatic lipase activity in Lipoprotein subclinical hypothyroidism (sH). Response to treatment with L-T4. Thyroid 2007;17:453–60.

64. Brenta G, Berg G, Arias P, et al. Proatherogenic mechanisms in subclinical hypothyroidism: hepatic lipase activity in relation to the VLDL remnant IDL. Thyroid 2008;18:1233–6.

65. Sigal GA, Medeiros-Neto G, Vinagre JC, et al. Lipid metabolism in subclinical hypothyroidism: plasma kinetics of triglyceride-rich lipoproteins and lipid transfers to high-density lipoprotein before and after levothyroxine treatment. Thyroid 2011;21:347–53.

66. Danese MD, Ladenson PW, Meinert CL, et al. Clinical review 115: effect of thyroxin therapy on serum lipoproteins in patients with mild thyroid failure: a quantitative review of the literature. J Clin Endocrinol Metab 2000;85:2993–3001.

67. Meier C, Straub JJ, Roth CB, et al. TSH-controlled L-thyroxine therapy reduces cholesterol level and clinical symptoms in subclinical hypothyroidism: a double-blind, placebo-controlled trial (Basel Thyroid Study). J Clin Endocrinol Metab 2001;86:4860–6.

68. Carraccio N, Ferrannini E, Monzani F. Lipoprotein profile in subclinical hypothyroidism: response to levothyroxine replacement a randomized placebo-controlled study. J Endocrinol Metab 2007;87:1533–8.

69. Taddei S, Caraccio N, Virdis A, et al. Impaired endothelium-dependent vasodilatation in subclinical hypothyroidism: beneficial effect of levothyroxine therapy. J Clin Endocrinol Metab 2003;88:3731–7.

70. Michalopoulou G, Alevizaki M, Piperingos G, et al. High serum cholesterol levels in persons with 'high-normal' TSH levels: should one extend the definition of subclinical hypothyroidism? Eur J Endocrinol 1998;138:141–5.

71. Iqbal A, Jorde R, Figenschau Y. Serum lipid levels in relation to serum thyroid-stimulating hormone and the effect of thyroxine treatment on serum lipid levels in subjects with subclinical hypothyroidism: the Tromsø Study. J Intern Med 2006;260:53–61.

72. Asvold BO, Vatten LJ, Nilsen TI, et al. The association between the TSH within the reference range and serum lipid concentrations in a population- based study: the HUNT study. Eur J Endocrinol 2007;156:181–6.

73. Razvi S, Ingoe L, Keeka G, et al. The beneficial effect of L-thyroxine on cardiovascular risk factors, endothelial function, and quality of life in subclinical hypothyroidism: randomized, crossover trial. J Clin Endocrinol Metab 2007;92:1715–23.

74. Teixeira PF, Reuters VS, Ferreira MM, et al. Treatment of subclinical hypothyroidism reduces atherogenic lipid levels in a placebo-controlled double-blind clinical trial. Horm Metab Res 2008;40:50–5.

75. Biondi B, Cooper DS. The clinical significance of subclinical thyroid dysfunction. Endocr Rev 2008;29:76–131.

76. Vanderpump MP, Tunbridge WM, French JM, et al. The development of ischemic heart disease in relation to autoimmune thyroid disease in a 20 year follow-up study of an English community. Thyroid 1996;6:155–60.

77. Hak AE, Pols HA, Visser TJ, et al. Subclinical hypothyroidism is an independent risk factor for atherosclerosis and myocardial infraction in elderly women: the Rotterdam Study. Ann Intern Med 2000;132:270–8.

78. Klein I, Ojamaa K. Thyroid hormone and the cardiovascular system. N Engl J Med 2001;344:501–9.

79. Cappola A, Ladenson P. Hypothyroidism and atherosclerosis. J Clin Endocrinol Metab 2003;88:2438–44.
80. Steinberg D, Parthasarathy S, Carew T, et al. Beyond cholesterol: modifications of low density lipoprotein that increase its atherogenicity. N Engl J Med 1989;320: 915–24.
81. Rizos CV, Elisaf MS, Liberopoulos EN. Effects of thyroid dysfunction on lipid profile. Open Cardiovasc Med J 2011;5:76–84.
82. Biondi B, Klein I. Hypothyroidism as a risk factor for cardiovascular disease. Endocrine 2004;24:1–13.
83. Rodondi N, Aujesky D, Vittinghoff E, et al. Subclinical hypothyroidism and the risk of coronary heart disease: a meta-analysis. Am J Med 2006;119:541–51.
84. Duntas LH, Wartofsky L. Cardiovascular risk and subclinical hypothyroidism: focus on lipids and new emerging risk factors. What is the evidence? Thyroid 2007;17:1075–84.
85. Rotondi N, den Elzen WP, Bauer DC, et al. Subclinical hypothyroidism and the risk of coronary heart disease and mortality. JAMA 2010;304:1365–74.
86. Raziel A, Rosenzweig B, Botvinic V, et al. The influence of thyroid function on serum lipid profile. Atherosclerosis 1982;41:321–6.
87. Heimberg M, Olubadewo JO, Wilcox HG. Plasma lipoproteins and regulation of hepatic metabolism of fatty acids in altered thyroid states. Endocr Rev 1985;6: 590–607.
88. Sundaram V, Hanna A, Koneru L, et al. Both hypothyroidism and hyperthyroidism enhance low density lipoprotein oxidation. J Clin Endocrinol Metab 1997;82: 3421–4.
89. Yavuz DG, Yüksel M, Deyneli O, et al. Association of serum paraoxonase activity with insulin sensitivity and oxidative stress in hyperthyroid and TSH-suppressed nodular goitre patients. Clin Endocrinol (Oxf) 2004;6:515–21.
90. Beylot M, Martin C, Laville M, et al. Lipolytic and ketogenic flux in hyperthyroidism. J Clin Endocrinol Metab 1991;73:42–9.
91. Hagenfeldt L, Wennlund A, Felig P, et al. Turnover and splanchnic metabolism of free fatty acids in hyperthyroid patients. J Clin Invest 1981;67:1672–7.
92. Cachefo A, Boucher P, Vidon C, et al. Hepatic lipogenesis and cholesterol synthesis in hyperthyroid patients. J Clin Endocrinol Metab 2001;86:5353–7.
93. Nishitani H, Okamura K, Noguchi S, et al. Serum lipid levels in thyroid dysfunction with special reference to transient elevation during treatment in hyperthyroid Graves' disease. Horm Metab Res 1990;22:490–3.
94. Diekman MJ, Anghelescu N, Endert E, et al. Changes in plasma low-density lipoprotein (LDL)-and high-density lipoprotein cholesterol in hypo- and hyperthyroid patients are related to changes in free thyroxine, not to polymorphisms in LDL receptor or cholesterol ester transfer protein genes. J Clin Endocrinol Metab 2000;85:1857–62.
95. Scanlan T. Thyroid hormone analogues: useful biological probes and potential therapeutic agents. Ann Endocrinol 2008;69:157–9.
96. Trancevski I, Eller P, Patsch JR, et al. The resurgence of thyromimetics as lipid-modifying agents. Curr Opin Investig Drugs 2009;10:912–8.
97. Trancevski I, Demetz E, Eller P. Sobetirome: a selective thyromimetic for the treatment of dyslipidemia. Recent Pat Cardiovasc Drug Discov 2011;6:16.
98. Ladenson PW, Kristensen JD, Ridgway EC, et al. Use of the thyroid hormone analogue eprotirome in statin-treated dyslipidemia. N Engl J Med 2010;362: 906–16.

The Effect of Medications on Thyroid Function Tests

Priya Kundra, MD[a,b,*], Kenneth D. Burman, MD[a,b]

KEYWORDS

• Thyroid function • Medication • Hormone • Euthyroid state

Abnormal results of thyroid function tests are possible effects of drugs and medications. The pathways of thyroid hormone synthesis, secretion, transport, metabolism, and absorption offer numerous targets for medication interactions (**Fig. 1**A, B). Normal thyroid secretion depends on thyroid-stimulating hormone (TSH), which is inhibited by thyroid hormones and stimulated by endogenous thyrotropin-releasing hormone (TRH). Circulating iodide is trapped by a specific iodide symporter protein in thyroid cells, after which it is oxidized and incorporated into tyrosine residues of thyroglobulin, which then couple to form thyroxine (T4) and triiodothyronine (T3). T4 and T3 are released from thyroglobulin and then secreted into the circulation. In the periphery, T4 is converted to T3 in the liver and other tissues by the action of 5′-T4 monodeiodinases. Type 1 5′-deiodinase predominates in the liver, kidneys, and thyroid; type 2 5′-deiodinase predominates in the brain, pituitary and skin. About 80% of T4 and T3 are metabolized by deiodination and 20% by other pathways that include conjugation with glucuronide and sulfate. T4 and T3 may be conjugated with glucuronide and sulfate in the liver, excreted in the bile, and partially hydrolyzed in the intestine; the T4 and T3 formed there may be reabsorbed in the gastrointestinal (GI) tract. In tissues, T3 and T4 are bound to nuclear receptor proteins that interact with regulatory regions of the genes, influencing their expression. In serum, most circulating T4 and T3 bind to proteins including thyroxine-binding globulin (TBG), transthyretin, and albumin. A small percentage (approximately 0.3% of T3 and 0.03% of T4) are unbound and available for binding to tissue T3 receptors. This article focuses on the groups of medications affecting production, regulation, secretion, transport, binding, metabolism, and absorption of T4 and T3. It also focuses on the medications that can clinically influence

[a] Endocrine Section, Washington Hospital Center, 110 Irving Street NW, Washington, DC 20010, USA
[b] Georgetown University Hospital, 3800 Reservoir Road NW, Washington, DC 20007, USA
* Corresponding author. Endocrine Section, Washington Hospital Center, 110 Irving Street NW, Washington, DC 20010.
E-mail address: Priya.Kundra@Medstar.net

Med Clin N Am 96 (2012) 283–295
doi:10.1016/j.mcna.2012.02.001
0025-7125/12/$ – see front matter © 2012 Elsevier Inc. All rights reserved.

medical.theclinics.com

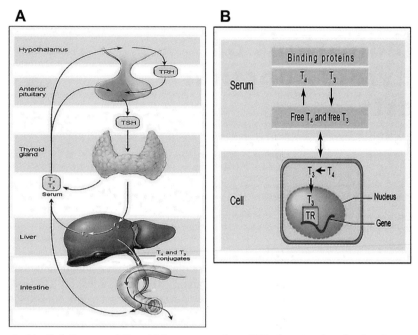

Fig. 1. (*A, B*) Pathways of thyroid hormone action. TRH, thyrotropin-releasing hormone; TSH, thyroid-stimulating hormone. (*Reprinted from* Surks MI, Sievert R. Drugs and thyroid function. N Engl J Med 1995;333:1689, published by The Massachusetts Medical Society; with permission.)

thyroid hormone homeostasis and on medications that we think are potentially significant or relevant. It does not include all possible medications that may influence thyroid function tests. **Box 1** provides a summary of the drugs involved with altered thyroid function tests discussed in this article.

TSH SUPPRESSION

Many agents can acutely suppress serum thyrotropin levels to subnormal levels, including dopamine, glucocorticoids, octreotide, and bexarotene. Dopamine infusions at greater than 1 μg/kg/min are known to block TSH release.[1,2] Glucocorticoids, particularly dexamethasone, at as low a dose as 0.5 mg/d and hydrocortisone at 100 mg/d, inhibit TSH secretion. However, clinically higher doses of dexamethasone (ie, >4 mg per day) inhibit extrathyroidal T3 production, leading to lower TSH values. Brabant and colleagues[3] showed that 4 mg of intravenous dexamethasone led to a rapid decrease in TSH concentrations and a decrease in TT3. Also, short-acting octreotide at 100 μg/d inhibits TSH release.[4] However, dopamine, glucocorticoids, and octreotide generally do not lower TSH concentrations to undetectable values (eg, less than 0.01 μU/mL). Bexarotene, a retinoid X receptor ligand, is known to suppress the pituitary TSH-β promoter, leading to central hypothyroidism. Sherman[5] showed that, in patients with T cell lymphoma receiving bexarotene, serum TSH levels decreased in proportion to the dose of bexarotene, with the greatest decrease for doses of more than 300 mg/m² with a mean TSH of 0.05 mU/L. Patients developed symptoms of hypothyroidism and thyroid hormone levels returned to normal following

Box 1
Drugs causing thyroid dysfunction

Decrease TSH secretion:

    Glucocorticoids: inhibit TSH release

    Dopamine: blocks TSH release

    Octreotide: inhibits TSH release

    Bexarotene: suppresses pituitary TSH-β promoter

Alter thyroid hormone secretion:

    Decrease thyroid hormone secretion: iodide, amiodarone, lithium

    Increase thyroid hormone secretion: iodide, amiodarone

Decrease T4 absorption:

    Cholesystramine, colestipol, sucralfate, ferrous sulfate, aluminum hydroxide, omeprazole

Alter T4 and T3 transport in serum:

    Increase serum TBG: estrogens, heroin, methadone, mitotane, fluorouracil

    Decrease serum TBG: androgens, anabolic steroids

    Displacement from protein-binding sites: furosemide, salicylates, meclofenamate, heparin

Alter T4 and T3 metabolism:

    Increase hepatic metabolism: phenobarbital and rifampin

    Increase hepatic metabolism and displace from binding proteins: phenytoin and carbamazepine

Cytokine mediated:

    Interferon (IFN) α

Immune reconstitution:

    Alemtuzumab

Hypothyroidism (tyrosine kinase inhibitors):

    Sunitinib: ? destructive thyroiditis,? blockade of iodine uptake,? inhibition of peroxidase activity

    Imatinib: ? induction of uridine diphosphate-glucuronosylotransferases (UGTs)

discontinuation of bexarotene. Smit and colleagues[6] also discovered that, in athyreotic subjects, bexarotene given for 6 weeks decreased free thyroxine (FT4) levels but the ratio of T4 sulfate/FT4 increased by 48%, possibly secondary to induction of T4 sulfation. There seemed to be a greater induction of the enzyme responsible for T4 conjugation with sulfate leading to an increased ratio of sulfated T4/FT4 (T4 sulfate/FT4) because more T4 was present in the sulfated form and less in the free form.

EFFECTS OF IODINE

Iodine has varied effects on the thyroid gland depending on the dose and duration of iodine exposure and on the underlying thyroid condition. Short-term iodine exposure (usually up to 7–10 days) can inhibit thyroid hormone secretion. This is called the Wolff-Chaikoff effect. However, with continued iodine exposure, there is an escape from this inhibition and hyperthyroidism can result (termed escape from the Wolff-Chaikoff effect or the Jod-Basedow phenomenon). Several agents can cause iodide-induced hyperthyroidism and many of these can also cause hypothyroidism. Iodide-induced hyperthyroidism generally develops in individuals with multinodular goiter (MNG) or hyperfunctioning thyroid adenoma secondary to the Jod-Basedow phenomenon, in which iodine serves as a substrate for thyroid hormone synthesis. Iodide-induced hypothyroidism generally develops secondary to a failure to escape from the Wolff-Chaikoff effect in chronic autoimmune thyroid disease, or Graves hyperthyroidism. Iodide inhibits thyroidal organification (Wolff-Chaikoff) but usually in up to 48 hours there is a decrease in sodium iodide symporter activity to allow restoration of organification (hence escape from Wolff-Chaikoff).

HYPOTHYROIDISM

The use of radiocontrast dyes and amiodarone are the most common medication-induced causes of hypothyroidism. Pharmacologic doses of iodine (up to 180 mg/d) can induce hypothyroidism in euthyroid patients with chronic thyroiditis.[7] In a large male cohort of more than 600 individuals, overt hypothyroidism (TSH >10 mU/L) developed in 5% of patients receiving amiodarone, but subclinical hypothyroidism (TSH 4.5–10 mU/L) developed in an additional 25%.[8] Hashimoto thyroiditis is the most common risk factor for the development of amiodarone-induced hypothyroidism (AIT).

AIT typically occurs between 6 and 12 months of treatment with amiodarone. If amiodarone cannot be discontinued, levothyroxine (L-T4) therapy can be initiated. Amiodarone administration to euthyroid subjects results in a decrease in serum T3 levels and an increase in serum T4, free T4, reverse T4, and TSH levels. These results are related to a decrease in intracellular T4 transport, inhibition of type 1 5′-deiodinase and pituitary type 2 5′-deiodinase, as well as antagonizing T3 binding to its nuclear receptor in the pituitary.[9] The dose of L-T4 needed to normalize TSH may be higher in patients treated with amiodarone as a result of the decreased intrapituitary T3 production caused by inhibition of pituitary type 2 5′-deiodinase. Basaria and Cooper[10] outlined surveillance and management of AIT (**Fig. 2**).

HYPERTHYROIDISM

Radiocontrast agents, which contain as much as 140 to 180 mg/mL of iodine, may cause hyperthyroidism within several weeks after exposure. Generally, pharmacologic doses of iodine (180 mg/d) can cause hyperthyroidism in patients with nontoxic nodular goiter, solitary autonomous goiter, or underlying Graves disease.[7] The frequency, timing, and duration of hyperthyroidism caused by various radiocontrast dyes may vary, in part depending on the underlying condition, but these issues have not been well studied. Amiodarone can cause hyperthyroidism by 2 mechanisms: iodine-induced hyperthyroidism or induction of thyroiditis. In the United States, 3% to 5% of patients treated with amiodarone become hyperthyroid, usually between 4 months and 3 years after the initiation of the drug.[8] There are 2 types of amiodarone-induced hyperthyroidism. Type 1 typically occurs in individuals with nontoxic MNG or Graves disease and type 2 is a drug-induced destructive thyroiditis. Many patients have an overlap syndrome between type 1 and type 2 disease. Basaria and Cooper[10] compared AIT type 1 and 2 (**Table 1**).

Traditionally, large doses of antithyroid drugs have been used to treat type 1 AIT, including methimazole 40 to 80 mg per day or propylthiouracil (PTU) 400 to 800 mg per day. For patients with type 2, prednisone is considered to be the treatment of choice. With daily prednisone at doses of 40 to 60 mg, there is rapid improvement

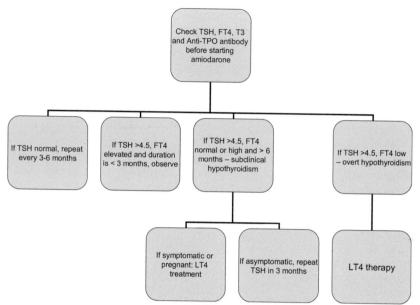

Fig. 2. Surveillance and management of amiodarone-induced hypothyroidism. TPO, thyroid peroxidase. (*Reprinted from* Basaria S, Cooper DS. Amiodarone and the thyroid. Am J Med 2005;118:709, published by Elsevier; with permission.)

in thyroid function in most patients. Basaria and Cooper[10] also comment on surveillance and management of amiodarone-induced hyperthyroidism (**Fig. 3**).

Our experience is that many patients may have an overlap between these 2 types of hyperthyroidism. Treatment approaches should be individualized and the patients monitored closely.

Table 1
AIT type 1 and 2

Factor	AIT Type 1	AIT Type 2
Preexisting thyroid disease	Yes (multinodular goiter or latent Graves)	No
Physical examination	Goiter, nodule(s)	Normal to slightly firm. Occasionally tender.
Duration of amiodarone	1–2 y	>2 y
Thyroid function tests	High FT4, T3 normal or high	High FT4, T3 normal or high
Thyroid autoantibodies	Absent (unless Graves)	Absent
Radioiodine uptake	Low	Very low
Thyroid ultrasound	Multinodular goiter or Graves	Heterogeneous
Color flow Doppler	Increased flow	Normal or decreased flow
Therapy	Stop amiodarone, if possible; high-dose antithyroid drugs	Prednisone
Subsequent hypothyroidism	No	Often

Reprinted from Basaria S, Cooper DS. Amiodarone and the thyroid. Am J Med 2005;118:711, published by Elsevier; with permission.

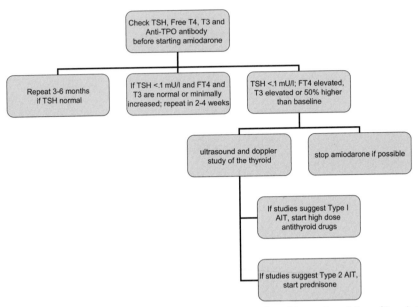

Fig. 3. Surveillance and management of amiodarone-induced hyperthyroidism. (*Reprinted from* Basaria S, Cooper DS. Amiodarone and the thyroid. Am J Med 2005;118:712, published by Elsevier; with permission.)

LITHIUM

Lithium can cause goiter, hypothyroidism, chronic autoimmune thyroiditis, and possibly hyperthyroidism. The mechanism by which lithium inhibits thyroid hormone secretion is not well understood. In vitro, lithium decreases colloid droplet formation within thyroid follicular cells, a reflection of decreased pinocytosis of colloid from the follicular lumen.[11] The efficiency of proteolytic digestion of thyroglobulin within phagolysosomes also may be impaired. The inhibition of thyroid hormone results in an increase in pituitary TSH and an enlarged thyroid gland. The prevalence of goiter may be as high as 50% and usually occurs within the first 2 years of treatment.[12] Hypothyroidism has been reported in 5% to 20% of patients treated with lithium, usually occurs within the first 2 years of therapy, and tends to be subclinical in nature. Lithium treatment usually need not be discontinued if levothyroxine replacement is initiated. It is likely that many patients who develop hypothyroidism during lithium treatment have underlying chronic autoimmune thyroiditis. In addition, lithium may induce autoimmune thyroid disease. Furthermore, Burman and colleagues[13] evaluated 7 patients who were euthyroid after treatment of Graves disease and showed that lithium administration in these patients resulted in lowering of T3, T4, and reverse T3 concentrations likely related to an inhibitory effect on thyroid hormone synthesis and release.

IFN

There are 3 different types of thyroid dysfunction associated with IFN α treatment: (1) autoimmune (often subclinical) hypothyroidism, (2) destructive thyroiditis, and (3) Graves-like hyperthyroidism. Hypothyroidism is more common than hyperthyroidism. Immune modulation may be a cause because IFN α is associated with development of antithyroid peroxidase antibodies in approximately 20% of patients. These abnormalities can occur as early as 4 weeks and as late as 23 months after initiation. In patients treated with IFN α, hypothyroidism occurs in 2.4% to 19%, with most patients having thyroid peroxidase (TPO) antibodies (87%).[14] Hypothyroidism can be transient, subsiding after discontinuation of IFN α. Koh and colleagues[15] showed that as many as 56% of patients had permanent hypothyroidism. In hypothyroidism, levothyroxine therapy is indicated without the need to withdraw IFN therapy. Destructive thyroiditis usually occurs in the first few weeks of IFN treatment in close temporal relationship with the appearance of thyroid autoantibodies, especially thyroglobulin antibodies. In addition, ribavarin along with IFN for the treatment of hepatitis C does not modify the thyroid autoantibody pattern, but is associated with a higher risk of hypothyroidism.[16] Thyrotoxicosis is frequently mild and transient without overt clinical manifestations and may be diagnosed only by obtaining frequent thyroid function tests. The duration of destructive thyroiditis is variable, ranging from a few weeks to a few months. IFN treatment may also cause hyperthyroidism, which may occur after a transient phase of destructive thyroiditis or following a period of hypothyroidism. Hyperthyroidism related to IFN is associated with thyroid-stimulating immunoglobulin (TSI) antibodies and increased uptake on technetium scintigraphy, but not with features of ophthalmopathy. TSH measurements should be performed every 8 to 12 weeks during IFN α treatment. When destructive thyroiditis is present, treatment with β-blockade is often useful to control the signs and symptoms of thyrotoxicosis. When IFN causes hyperthyroidism, antithyroid agents such as methimazole or propylthiouracil may be administered if clinically indicated in the setting of thyrotoxicosis.

ALEMTUZUMAB

Thyroid autoimmunity resulting from immune reconstitution from lymphocytopenia has been reported in the literature in patients receiving alemtuzumab, a humanized monoclonal antibody that targets CD52 on lymphocytes and monocytes. In 216 patients with multiple sclerosis treated with alemtuzumab, 32 developed hyperthyroidism and 15 developed hypothyroidism.[17] These events occurred with the presence of thyroid autoantibodies in 96% of affected patients and occurred up to 30 months after the last dose. Similarly, 4 patients with type 1 diabetes developed hyperthyroidism after immune suppressive therapy had been stopped 2 to 21 months earlier for a failing islet cell graft.[18] These 4 patients had a pretransplant positivity for TPO autoantibodies. It is hypothesized that drug-induced lymphopenia in patients with previously existing occult autoimmune thyroiditis predisposes to a reactivation of autoimmune mechanisms when T-lymphocytes are repopulated and thus to an aberrant immune reconstitution.

TBG

Medications may increase or decrease serum TBG concentrations, thereby causing changes in serum total, but not free, T4 and free T3 (FT3) concentrations. The most common cause of an increase in serum TBG concentration is the administration of estrogen (eg, birth control pills). Estrogens produce increased sialylation of TBG, which decreases its rate of clearance and raises its serum concentration. The increase in TBG in serum is dose dependent. In a study by Mandel and colleagues[19] of women with hypothyroidism who were receiving T4 and became pregnant, an increase of 45% in the dose was needed to maintain normal serum TSH concentrations because of estradiol-induced increases in TBG and 30% to 40% increase in plasma volume.[20]

In addition, in women with hypothyroidism treated with thyroxine, estrogen therapy may increase the need for thyroxine.[21]

Serum TBG concentrations are increased in about 50% of patients who use heroin or are treated with methadone.[22] There was a significant increase in the mean concentration of TT3, TT4, and TBG in the serum of 145 clinically euthyroid patients on maintenance methadone for approximately 6 weeks at doses of 15 to 45 mg/d compared with euthyroid controls not on methadone.[23] In contrast, free T4 and TSH levels were not different in the 2 groups. The increase in serum TBG, which can lead to increased TT4 and TT3 levels, may result from liver disease rather than from specific effects of these drugs. Mitotane and fluorouracil are also associated with increases in serum concentrations of total T4 and T3 and likely increase the serum concentration of TBG. Patients taking androgens or anabolic steroids have decreased serum TBG.[24]

At therapeutic concentrations, several drugs inhibit binding of T4 and T3 to TBG. Large doses of furosemide (>80 mg) result in a transient increase in serum-free T4 concentrations and a decrease in serum total T4 concentrations.[21] Several nonsteroidal antiinflammatory drugs have similar effects.[25] Salicylates (in doses of >2.0 g per day) and salsalate (in doses of 1.5–3 g per day) also inhibit the binding of T4 and T3 to TBG; salicylates inhibit binding to transthyretin as well.[26] Initially, the inhibition of binding to TBG results in transiently increased circulating thyroid hormone levels that cause transfer of T4 and T3 into intracellular sites, resulting in temporary TSH suppression and leading to a reduced thyroid hormone secretion. In particular, a study of 25 healthy adults receiving salsalate and aspirin at 1 g 4 times a day for 1 week showed an approximately 30% to 50% decrease in TT4, TT3, and TSH compared with time-adjusted baseline levels, but TSH remained within normal levels.[26] These thyroid function abnormalities are drug and dose dependent and can last several days after a large dose of salsalate. Serum-free T4 increases transiently after administration of heparin.[27] This increase is caused by in vitro inhibition of protein binding of T4 by free fatty acids generated as a result of the ability of heparin to activate lipoprotein lipase.[28]

MEDICATIONS THAT INTERFERE WITH T4 AND T3 METABOLISM

T4 and T3 are metabolized enzymatically mainly by deiodination but also by glucuronidation and sulfation. Phenobarbital and rifampin increase T4 and T3 metabolism by stimulating hepatic microsomal drug-metabolizing enzyme activity.[29,30] Patients with hypothyroidism who are treated with phenobarbital cannot augment thyroid hormone production and secretion, thereby exacerbating their hypothyroidism. Phenytoin and carbamazepine augment the rate of thyroid hormone metabolism and displace thyroid hormone from the serum binding proteins, principally TBG.[31] In 9 euthyroid patients treated with phenytoin at therapeutic levels, mean serum T4 decreased to 60% of that of the control group and mean T3 decreased to 78% of that of the control group.[31] In 10 euthyroid patients treated with carbamazepine at therapeutic levels, mean serum T4 decreased to 74% of that of the control group and mean T3 decreased to 83% of that of the control group. Serum FT4 concentrations remained unchanged by ultrafiltration and TSH levels remained within normal range in patients treated with phenytoin and carbamazepine. Hypothyroid patients treated with T4 may need a higher LT4 dose when treated with any of these agents.

MEDICATIONS THAT INTERFERE WITH GI ABSORPTION OF EXOGENOUS LEVOTHYROXINE

Multiple medications have been reported to impair the absorption of exogenous thyroxine and decrease its efficacy. Normally, about 80% of a usual dose of levothyroxine (eg, 50–150 µg per day) is absorbed, mostly in the jejunum and the upper part of the ileum.[32] The bile acid–binding resins, cholestyramine and colestipol, bind thyroid hormones and decrease their absorption. A decrease in serum T4 concentrations and an increase in serum TSH concentrations occurred when cholestyramine was administered to patients with hypothyroidism treated with T4.[33] Calcium carbonate reduces the absorption of exogenous T4. In a prospective cohort of 20 hypothyroid patients taking 1200 mg of elemental calcium (as calcium carbonate) for 3 months, the mean serum-free and total T4 concentrations decreased significantly during coadministration of calcium carbonate, by 8% and 7% respectively.[34] The mean serum TSH concentration increased by 69%, with 20% of patients having serum TSH concentrations greater than the normal range. These changes resolved after calcium carbonate was discontinued. Sucralfate, ferrous sulfate, and aluminum hydroxide also bind T4 in the gut, but their effect is smaller and also less consistent than those described earlier.[35–37] Normal gastric acid secretion seems to be necessary for normal thyroid hormone absorption. Centanni and colleagues[38] showed that, in 10 patients treated with omeprazole for multinodular goiter, a 37% increase in the dose of levothyroxine was required after 6 months to obtain similar TSH levels to those of patients treated without omeprazole. Italian coffee (espresso) has also been shown to interfere with T4 intestinal absorption. Benvenga and colleagues[39] reported 8 patients in whom coffee given with L-T4 compared with water lowered the average and peak incremental increases in serum T4. These changes are unrelated to change in intragastric pH and result from an interaction that makes L-T4 less available for absorption. It is unknown whether these effects are applicable more widely with varying types of coffee, and to what extent these findings apply clinically.

SUNITINIB

Sunitinib is an inhibitor of vascular endothelial growth factors (VEGF) tyrosine kinase and platelet-derived growth factor receptors used to treat renal cell cancer (RCC) and GI stromal tumors (GIST).[40] The potential mechanisms by which sunitinib might induce thyroid dysfunction include destructive thyroiditis, blockade of iodine uptake, and inhibition of peroxidase activity. Desai and colleagues[41] investigated 42 euthyroid patients receiving 50 mg of sunitinib for 2 to 4 weeks with 2 weeks of no therapy for 4 to 6 cycles. Hypothyroidism was developed by 15/42 patients after an average of 50 weeks. All patients normalized TSH values after receiving thyroxine. Two sonographic findings in hypothyroid patients showed atrophy of the thyroid gland, suggesting destructive thyroiditis as a cause. Rini and colleagues[42] investigated 66 patients with RCC treated with sunitinib (50 mg daily for first 28 days of a 42-day cycle). One or more thyroid function abnormalities of hypothyroidism were found in 56/66 at a median cycle of 2 with a range of 1 to 14. Rini and colleagues[42] suggested that sunitinib prevented binding of VEGF to normal thyroid cells and/or impaired thyroid blood flow resulting in thyroiditis. Grossmann and colleagues[43] studied 12/25 patients who developed thyroid dysfunction after receiving sunitinib 50 mg/d for 28 days for each 6-week cycle for metastatic renal cell carcinoma. Of these, 2 had a transiently reduced TSH with normal FT4 and FT3, 4 developed hypothyroidism without evidence of preceding hyperthyroidism, and 6 developed hyperthyroidism. Ultimately, 8 developed permanent hypothyroidism. It was postulated that, in the 6 patients who had thyrotoxicosis, thyroiditis was likely because of (1) rapid improvement in thyroid function tests with progression to hypothyroidism, (2) high thyroglobulin levels, (3) high FT4/FT3 ratio, and (4) decreased uptake on thyroid scan. Mannavola and colleagues[44] investigated 24 patients with GIST given 4 weeks of daily treatment with sunitinib at a dose of 50 mg orally and 2 weeks of withdrawal. After 1 to 6 cycles, 46% developed hypothyroidism. Thyroid sonographic abnormalities or variations in serum thyroglobulin and antithyroid antibodies were not found. ^{123}I was reduced, suggesting blockade of iodine uptake as a potential mechanism of hypothyroidism. Salem and colleagues[45] showed that FRTL-5 cells treated with 10 μM of sunitinib did not affect iodide efflux, but did increase influx at 24 hours in a dose-dependent manner. Wong and colleagues[46] discovered that 21/40 patients receiving sunitinib 50 mg daily for 4 weeks in a 6-week cycle (up to 48 months) developed hypothyroidism. Sunitinib inhibited peroxidase activity in the iodination and guaiacol assay. The antiperoxidase activity of sunitinib was 25% to 30% of that of PTU. In addition, Alexandrescu and colleagues[47] reported a case of sunitinib-associated lymphocytic thyroiditis without circulating antithyroid antibodies. There is a wide spectrum of thyroid alterations associated with sunitinib therapy, likely modulated by various molecular mediators. No prospective studies have evaluated the early treatment of subclinical hypothyroidism in patients treated with tyrosine kinase inhibitors. Systematic assessment of thyroid function at baseline and at the beginning of each treatment cycle is recommended. Treatment with levothyroxine should be based on clinical context and laboratory evaluation and may be considered, particularly if the TSH exceeds 10 mIU/L.[48] There are many other multikinase inhibitors being used clinically, but, in general, their likelihood of causing thyroid perturbations has not been adequately studied.

IMATINIB

Imatinib belongs to the 2-phenylaminopyridine class and targets BCR-ABL, platelet-derived growth factor receptor, and c-kit receptor tyrosine kinases. De Groot and colleagues[49] treated 11 patients (10 with medullary thyroid cancer and 1 with GIST) on levothyroxine and imatinib (400–800 mg) for an average of 6 months. TSH levels increased to 384% (±228%) of upper limits, whereas FT4 and FT3 decreased respectively to 59% (±17%) and 63% (±4%). De Groot and colleagues[49] suggested induction of UGTs involved in conjugation and T4/T3 clearance as a cause of hypothyroidism. In athyreotic patients, thyroidal compensation does not occur and the dose of levothyroxine sodium should be increased in a timely manner.

SUMMARY

In summary, drug-induced thyroid disorders are common in clinical practice. It is important to recognize the various drugs contributing to thyroid dysfunction for a timely intervention to help achieve a euthyroid state. **Box 1** provides a summary of the drugs involved with altered thyroid function tests.

REFERENCES

1. Brabant K, Prank C, Hoang-Vu RD, et al. Hypothalamic regulation of pulsatile thyrotropin secretion. J Clin Endocrinol Metab 1991;72(1):145–50.
2. Agner T, Hagen C, Anderson A, et al. Increased dopaminergic activity inhibits basal and metoclopramide-stimulated prolactin and thyrotropin secretion. J Clin Endocrinol Metab 1986;62(4):778–82.
3. Brabant G, Brabant U, Ranft K, et al. Circadian and pulsatile thyrotropin secretion in euthyroid man under the influence of thyroid hormone and glucocorticoid administration. J Clin Endocrinol Metab 1987;65(1):83–8.

4. Williams T, Kelijman M, Crelin W, et al. Differential effects of somatostatin (SRIH) and a SRIH analog, SMS 201-995, on the secretion of growth hormone and thyroid-stimulating hormone in man. J Clin Endocrinol Metab 1988;66(1):39–45.

5. Sherman SI. Etiology, diagnosis and treatment recommendations for central hypothyroidism associated with bexarotene therapy for cutaneous T cell lymphoma. Clin Lymphoma 2003;3(4):249–52.

6. Smit JW, Stokkel MP, Pereira AM, et al. Bexarotene induced hypothyroidism: bexarotene stimulates the peripheral metabolism of thyroid hormones. J Clin Endocrinol Metab 2007;92(7):2496–9.

7. Braverman L. Iodine induced thyroid disease. 3rd thyroid symposium, AMA.

8. Batcher EL, Tang XC, Singh BN, et al, SAFE-T Investigators. Thyroid function abnormalities during amiodarone therapy for persistent atrial fibrillation. Am J Med 2007;120(10):880–5.

9. Norman MF, Lavin TN. Antagonism of thyroid hormone action by amiodarone in rat pituitary tumor cells. J Clin Invest 1989;83:306–13.

10. Basaria S, Cooper DS. Amiodarone and the thyroid. Am J Med 2005;118:706–14.

11. Williams JA, Berens SC, Wolff J. Thyroid secretion in vitro: inhibition of TSH and dibutyryl cyclic-AMP stimulated ^{131}I release by Li$^+$. Endocrinology 1971;88:1385–8.

12. Lazarus JH, Richards AR, Addison GM, et al. Treatment of thyrotoxicosis with lithium carbonate. Lancet 1974;2:1160.

13. Burman KD, Dimond RC, Earll JM, et al. Wartofsky sensitivity to lithium in treated Grave's disease: effects on serum T4, T3 and reverse T3. J Clin Endocrinol Metab 1976;43(3):606–13.

14. Carella C, Mazziotti G, Amato G, et al. Interferon α related thyroid disease: pathophysiologic, epidemiologic, and clinical aspects. J Clin Endocrinol Metab 2004;89(8):3656–61.

15. Koh LK, Greenspan FS, Yeo PP. Interferon α induced thyroid dysfunction: three clinical presentations and a review of the literature. Thyroid 1997;7:891–6.

16. Carella C, Mazziotti G, Morisco F, et al. The addition if ribavirin to interferon-alpha therapy in patients with hepatitis C virus-related chronic hepatitis does not modify the thyroid autoantibody pattern but increases the risk of developing hypothyroidism. Eur J Endocrinol 2002;146:743–9.

17. CAMMS223 Trial Investigators, Coles AJ, Compston DA, et al. Alemtuzumab vs. interferon Beta-1a in early multiple sclerosis. N Engl J Med 2008;359:1786–801.

18. Gillard P, Huurman V, Van der Auwera B, et al. Graves' hyperthyroidism after stopping immune suppressive therapy in type I diabetic islet cell recipients with pretransplant TPO-autoantibodies. Diabetes Care 2009;32:1–8.

19. Mandel SJ, Larsen PR, Seely EW, et al. Increased need for thyroxine during pregnancy in women with primary hypothyroidism. N Engl J Med 1990;323:91–6.

20. Alexander EK. Timing and magnitude of increases in levothyroxine requirements during pregnancy in women with hypothyroidism. N Engl J Med 2004;351(3):241–9.

21. Arafah BM. Increased need for thyroxine in women with hypothyroidism during estrogen therapy. N Engl J Med 2001;344:1743–9.

22. Surks MI, Sievert R. Drugs and thyroid function. N Engl J Med 1995;333:1688–94.

23. English T, Ruxton D, Eastman C. Abnormalities in thyroid function associated with chronic therapy with methadone. Clin Chem 1988;34/11:2202–4.

24. Deyssig R, Weissel M. Ingestion of androgenic-anabolic steroids induces mild thyroidal impairment in male body builders. J Clin Endocrinol Metab 1993;76(4):1069–71.

25. Wang R, Nelson JC, Wilcox RB. Salsalate and salicylate binding to and their displacement of thyroxine from thyroxine-binding globulin, transthyrin, and albumin. Thyroid 1999;9(4):359–64.

26. Samuels MH, Pillote K, Asher D, et al. Variable effects of nonsteroidal anti-inflammatory agents on thyroid test results. J Clin Endocrinol Metab 2003; 88(12):5710.

27. Jain R, Uy HL. Increase in serum free thyrosine levels related to intravenous heparin treatment. Ann Intern Med 1996;124(1 Pt 1):74–5.

28. Jaume JC, Mendel CM, Frost PH, et al. Extremely low doses of heparin release lipase activity into the plasma and can thereby cause artifactual elevations in the serum-free thyroxine concentration as measured by equilibrium dialysis. Thyroid 1996;6:79.

29. Oppenheimer JH, Bernstein G, Surks MI. Increased thyroxine turnover and thyroidal function after stimulation of hepatocellular binding of thyroxine by phenobarbital. J Clin Invest 1968;47:1399.

30. Isley WL. Effect of rifampin therapy on thyroid function tests in a hypothyroid patient on replacement L-thyroxine. Ann Intern Med 1987;107:517.

31. Surks MI, DeFesi CR. Normal serum free thyroid hormone concentrations in patients treated with phenytoin or carbamezipine. JAMA 1996;275:1495–8.

32. Hays MT. Thyroid hormone and the gut. Endocr Res 1988;14(2-3):203–24.

33. Harmon SM, Siefert CF. Levothyroxine-cholestyramine interaction reemphasized. Ann Intern Med 1991;115:658.

34. Singh N, Singh PN, Hershman JM. Effect of calcium carbonate on the absorption of levothyroxine. JAMA 2000;283:2822.

35. Sherman SI, Tielens ET, Ladenson PW. Sucralfate causes malabsorption of L-thyroxine. Am J Med 1994;96(6):531–5.

36. Campbell NR, Hasinoff BB, Stalts H, et al. Ferrous sulfate reduces thyroxine efficacy in patients with hypothyroidism. Ann Intern Med 1992;117(12):1010–3.

37. Sperber AD, Liel Y. Evidence for interference with the intestinal absorption of levothyroxine sodium by aluminum hydroxide. Arch Intern Med 1992;152(1): 183–4.

38. Centanni M, Gargano L, Canettieri G, et al. Thyroxine in goiter, Helicobacter pylori infection, and chronic gastritis. N Engl J Med 2006;354:1787.

39. Benvenga S, Bartolone L, Pappalardo MA, et al. Altered intestinal absorption of L-thyroxine caused by coffee. Thyroid 2008;18(3):293–301.

40. Chow LQ, Eckhardt SG. Sunitinib: from rational design to clinical efficacy. J Clin Oncol 2007;25(7):884–96.

41. Desai J, Yassa L, Marqusee E, et al. Hypothyroidism after sunitinib treatment for patients with gastrointestinal tumors. Ann Intern Med 2006;145:660–4.

42. Rini BI, Tamaskar I, Shaheen P, et al. Hypothyroidism in patients with metastatic renal cell carcinoma treated with sunitinib. J Natl Cancer Inst 2007;99:81–3.

43. Grossmann M, Premaratne E, Desai J, et al. Thyrotoxicosis during sunitinib treatment for renal cell carcinoma. Clin Endocrinol 2008;69(4):669–72.

44. Mannavola D, Coco P, Vannachi G, et al. A novel tyrosine-kinase selective inhibitor, sunitinib, induces transient hypothyroidism by blocking iodine uptake. J Clin Endocrinol Metab 2007;92(9):3531–4.

45. Salem AK, Fenton MS, Marion KM, et al. Effect of sunitinib on growth and function of FRTL-5 thyroid cells. Thyroid 2008;18(6):631–5.

46. Wong E, Rosen LS, Mulay M, et al. Sunitinib induces hypothyroidism in advanced cancer patients and may inhibit thyroid peroxidase activity. Thyroid 2007;17(4): 351–5.

47. Alexandrescu DT, Popoveniuc G, Farzanmehr H, et al. Sunitinib-associated lymphocytic thyroiditis without circulating antithyroid antibodies. Thyroid 2008; 18(7):809–12.

48. Torino F, Corsello S, Longo R, et al. Is hypothyroidism a clinically relevant toxicity of tyrosine kinase inhibitors? Thyroid 2009;19(5):539–40.

49. De Groot JW, Zonnenberg BA, Plukker JT, et al. Imatinib induces hypothyroidism in patients receiving levothyroxine. Clin Pharmacol Ther 2005;78:433–8.

Approach to and Treatment of Thyroid Disorders in the Elderly

Maria Papaleontiou, MD[a], Megan R. Haymart, MD[b],*

KEYWORDS

- Older adults • Thyroid cancer • Longevity
- Thyroid function • Hyperthyroidism • Hypothyroidism
- Thyroid nodule • Age

Interpretation of thyroid function tests in older adults is difficult because of the age-dependent physiologic changes in thyroid function, coexistent chronic illness, and polypharmacy.[1–4] However, thyroid dysfunction is common in older adults and may be associated with significant morbidity if not treated. The classic symptoms of thyroid dysfunction are usually absent or may be overlooked in older patients, making the diagnosis and subsequent management challenging.

The management of thyroid disorders in older adults remains controversial. There has been conflicting literature regarding the approach. Despite the ongoing debate, current guidelines suggest considering treatment on an individual basis according to symptoms and possible treatment benefit.[5] However, in older patients the risk of harm from treatment complicates the decision-making process.

The objective of this article is to review the epidemiology, clinical presentation, risks and complications, and management of thyroid disorders in older adults, including hyperthyroidism, hypothyroidism, thyroid nodules and thyroid cancer.

THYROID FUNCTION IN OLDER ADULTS

Several studies have investigated the role of thyroid function in the aging process. Recent reports have shown increased levels of serum thyrotropin (TSH) with increasing age, independent of antithyroid antibody presence[1]; by contrast, others have demonstrated decreased serum TSH in older adults.[2,3] Populations in which

Disclosures: Drs Papaleontiou and Haymart have no commercial relationships to disclose.
[a] Division of Metabolism, Endocrinology and Diabetes, Department of Medicine, University of Michigan Health System, 24 Frank Lloyd Wright Drive, PO Box 451, Ann Arbor, MI 48105, USA
[b] Division of Metabolism, Endocrinology and Diabetes, and Hematology/Oncology, Department of Medicine, University of Michigan Health System, 300 North Ingalls Building, NI 3A17, Ann Arbor, MI 48109, USA
* Corresponding author.
E-mail address: meganhay@umich.edu

Med Clin N Am 96 (2012) 297–310
doi:10.1016/j.mcna.2012.01.013
0025-7125/12/$ – see front matter © 2012 Elsevier Inc. All rights reserved.

medical.theclinics.com

the dominant abnormality is thyroid deficiency secondary to Hashimoto thyroiditis display a trend for the upper limit of TSH to increase with age.[6,7] On the contrary, an inverse relationship between TSH and age is seen in iodine-deficient populations in which the dominant thyroid abnormality is nodularity and increasing thyroid autonomy with age.[8] Most studies have demonstrated an age-dependent decline in free triiodothyronine (T3) levels, whereas free thyroxine (T4) levels remain relatively unchanged[2,3] and reverse T3 (rT3) levels increase with increasing age. However, interpretation of thyroid function tests in older adults is often complicated by the presence of chronic illness (whereby free T3 can be low and rT3 high) and polypharmacy.[4] Furthermore, differences in iodine intake and the presence of autoimmune thyroid disease make the distinction between age-related and disease-related abnormalities in thyroid function even more challenging.[9]

There is convincing evidence that higher levels of TSH are associated with longevity. Atzmon and colleagues[10] concluded that serum TSH levels were significantly higher in centenarians (mean age 98 years) compared with controls ($P<.001$). Several other studies have also shown increased TSH levels (mean age 85 years) and low to low-normal free T4 levels (mean age 78 years) to be associated with a better survival in older adults.[11,12] It is hypothesized that the association of a higher TSH level with longevity may be due to a correlated lower bioactivity of thyroid hormone, which in turn leads to a lower basal metabolic rate and thus potentially may serve as an adaptive mechanism to prevent catabolism in older adults.[12] Moreover, the offspring of individuals with longevity were also shown to have higher TSH levels than those of age-matched controls without familial longevity (mean age 70 years), indicating a genetic predisposition.[13]

HYPERTHYROIDISM
Epidemiology and Clinical Presentation

The prevalence of hyperthyroidism in older adults is estimated to be 0.5% to 4%.[14] Although Graves' disease still remains the most common cause of hypothyroidism, the prevalence of multinodular goiter and toxic nodular adenomas tends to increase with age.[15,16] Two-thirds of older adults with hyperthyroidism have a similar presentation to younger patients. Symptoms are consistent with sympathetic overactivity and include tremors, anxiety, palpitations, weight loss, and heat intolerance. However, one-third of older adults present with apathetic hyperthyroidism.[17] The paucity of clinical signs of hyperthyroidism in older adults ($\geq$70 years) has been confirmed by several studies,[18,19] with weight loss, apathy, and tachycardia the most commonly occurring symptoms ($P<.001$). A large cross-sectional study by Boelaert and colleagues[20] (N = 3049) showed an increased prevalence of weight loss in older patients (>61 years) and identified shortness of breath as a symptom commonly reported in older adults ($P<.001$). This study also demonstrated a higher proportion of older adults reporting only 1 or 2 symptoms, versus 5 or more in the younger patients. The absence of classic symptoms and signs in older adults presents a diagnostic challenge, and may lead to a delay in treatment and worse outcome.[19,20]

More common than overt hyperthyroidism in older adults is subclinical hyperthyroidism, which is estimated to have a prevalence of 3% to 8%[21–23] and is more common in women than in men, especially in patients older than 70 years.[24] In a study of the natural history of subclinical hyperthyroidism in female patients 60 years or older (N = 102), Rosario[25] showed that progression to overt hyperthyroidism is infrequent, at 1% per year.

Risks, Complications, and Sequelae

Atrial fibrillation

It has been clearly demonstrated that age is independently associated with an increased risk of developing atrial fibrillation. Atrial fibrillation is estimated to be present in up to 20% to 35% of older patients suffering from hyperthyroidism,[19,26,27] and is especially common in those with hyperthyroidism secondary to toxic nodule(s).[19] Long-standing low serum TSH concentration in older patients is associated with a 3-fold increased risk of developing atrial fibrillation.[28] Because of the greater incidence of underlying cardiac disease, the risk of developing atrial fibrillation is increased in patients older than 60 years. Atrial fibrillation in older adults may sometimes be the only clinical sign of hyperthyroidism. However, the degeneration of the sinus node and fibrotic changes in the cardiac conduction system make the presence of palpitations less likely. In addition, frequent use of β-blockers or amiodarone in these patients can mask the arrhythmia. By contrast, younger hyperthyroid patients often present with sinus tachycardia.[20]

Cardiovascular mortality

Overt hyperthyroidism, and less often subclinical hyperthyroidism, can be accompanied by several cardiovascular changes including widened pulse pressure, exercise intolerance, increased risk for atrial fibrillation, and increased cardiac mass.[29] Several cross-sectional and case-control studies have found that decreased levels of serum TSH are associated with increased cardiovascular mortality in older adults.[30] In addition, subclinical hyperthyroidism has been shown to be associated with left ventricular hypertrophy, which is a predictor of cardiovascular mortality.[29]

Osteoporosis

Overt hyperthyroidism is a well-recognized risk factor leading to low bone mineral density and osteoporotic fractures, especially in older women.[31] Thyroid hormone acts on osteoblasts and osteoclasts to increase bone turnover, leading to net bone loss.[32] Of note, most studies investigating the relationship between thyroid dysfunction and fracture risk have been specific to women. Bauer and colleagues,[33] in a large prospective study of fractures (N = 686), reported that women older than 65 with a TSH level of 0.1 mIU/L or less had a 3-fold increased risk for hip fracture and a 4-fold increased risk for vertebral fracture compared with euthyroid counterparts. In a study of subclinical hyperthyroidism in older adults (mean age 72.8 years) with sex-specific analysis, men were found to have an increased incidence of hip fractures compared with women (13.8% vs 12%; $P<.01$).[34]

Ophthalmopathy

Contradicting studies exist regarding the association of symptoms and signs of ophthalmopathy in Graves' disease with increasing age. Most studies published on this subject have demonstrated a positive correlation between prevalence and severity of ophthalmopathy with increasing age.[19,35] However, one prospective cohort study found ophthalmopathy to be more frequent in younger patients than in older adults with Graves' disease (46% vs 6%; $P<.001$).[20]

Management

As in younger patients, the initial diagnostic test for suspected hyperthyroidism in older adults is a serum TSH test. However, hospitalized elderly patients who are acutely ill may demonstrate depressed TSH without actually being hyperthyroid.

When the clinical presentation of thyrotoxicosis is not diagnostic of Graves' disease, a radioactive iodine (RAI) uptake test should be performed to help determine the cause. A scan should be added if thyroid nodules are also identified.[5]

Symptomatic treatment of hyperthyroidism in older adults consists of β-adrenergic blockade. β-Adrenergic blockade decreases the heart rate and systolic blood pressure and can also improve tremor, irritability, emotional lability, and exercise intolerance. Anticoagulation may be indicated in patients who present with atrial fibrillation.

Treatment modalities that may be used for hyperthyroidism include RAI ablation therapy, antithyroid medications, and thyroidectomy.

RAI ablation is often used in older adults because of its efficacy, safety, and cost-effectiveness.[36] An appropriate dose is calculated from the previous thyroid-uptake scan. A drawback to this management approach is that hyperthyroidism is reversed gradually over months, and cardiac issues may need to be managed aggressively until the thyrotoxic state is reversed. More than 80% of these patients subsequently develop hypothyroidism and require thyroid hormone replacement therapy.[36]

Methimazole is the preferred antithyroid medication. However, older adults may be at greater risk of recurrence of hyperthyroidism after drug therapy and of side effects of medication.[36] Data suggest that older adults taking propylthiouracil or high doses of methimazole may be at greater risk for side effects. Agranulocytosis is the major adverse event in this population, occurring in 0.5% of those treated. Rash, arthralgias, and myalgias also occur more frequently.[36]

Depending on comorbidities, surgical approaches are less commonly used in older adults with hyperthyroidism, because of the increased risk of morbidity.[37] Surgery is reserved for large goiters with obstructive symptoms, or known or suspected malignancy.[38]

Regarding subclinical hyperthyroidism in older adults, guidelines advocate periodic clinical and biochemical assessment. Recent guidelines by the American Thyroid Association (ATA) and American Association of Clinical Endocrinologists recommend that patients older than 65 years be treated if their TSH level is less than 0.1 mIU/L and that treatment can be considered if their TSH level is between 0.1 and 0.5 mIU/L.[22,39]

HYPOTHYROIDISM
Epidemiology and Clinical Presentation

Estimates of the prevalence and incidence of hypothyroidism among older adults are variable, depending on populations studied and criteria used to define the condition.[40] A large screening study (N = 25,000) revealed that 10% of men and 16% of women aged 65 to 74 years had TSH levels above the upper limit of the reference range.[41] The most recent National Health and Nutrition Examination Survey (NHANES) reported that compared with men in the same age range, a significantly greater number of women aged 50 to 69 met criteria for subclinical and clinical hypothyroidism.[6] Moreover, a study evaluating geriatric patients under medical care demonstrated that 15% of the women and 17% of the men had previously undiagnosed hypothyroidism.[42]

The incidence of hypothyroidism steadily increases with advancing age, predominantly because of a rising incidence of autoimmune thyroiditis (Hashimoto).[43–45] In a survey by Reinhardt and Mann,[46] the reported incidence of Hashimoto thyroiditis was 67% in a patient population with a mean age of 73 years (N = 24). A survey of patients in the endocrinology clinic revealed that 47% of patients aged 55 years and older presenting with primary hypothyroidism carried a diagnosis of autoimmune thyroiditis, whereas 27% had postsurgical hypothyroidism and 10% had post-RAI hypothyroidism.[47]

A high index of suspicion is required for a diagnosis of hypothyroidism in older adults because symptoms and signs such as fatigue, weakness, constipation, dry skin, and cold intolerance may be attributed to other diseases common in older patients, medication side effects, or aging itself.[3,48] Psychiatric symptoms, such as depression, are also common in older adults with hypothyroidism. A prospective study by Doucet and colleagues[49] compared 24 clinical symptoms and signs of hypothyroidism between older (n = 67; mean age 79.3 years) and younger (n = 54; mean age 40.8 years) patients. It was concluded that the mean number of clinical signs in older adults was 6.6, compared with 9.3 in the younger population. Fatigue and weakness were the most common symptoms in older adults, with cold intolerance, paresthesia, weight gain, and abdominal cramps being less common.

Risks, Complications, and Sequelae

Cognitive impairment

Hypothyroidism in older adults has been associated with impairment of several cognitive domains including memory, attention and concentration, language, executive function, and perceptual and visuospatial function.[50,51] Severe hypothyroidism may mimic depression and dementia. Neuropsychiatric symptoms usually improve with treatment and restoration of a euthyroid state.[52]

The relationship between subclinical hypothyroidism and cognition is less clear. It is postulated that older adults may be more vulnerable to the effects of subclinical hypothyroidism, given age-related changes to the hypothalamic-pituitary-thyroid axis. However, several studies in older adults did not show a significant association between mildly elevated TSH and reduced cognitive performance.[53,54]

Cardiovascular effects

The cardiovascular consequences of hypothyroidism in older adults are thought to be due to a reduction in both stroke volume and heart rate.[55] Other contributing factors include increased risk of atherosclerosis, increased arterial stiffness, endothelial dysfunction, and altered coagulation parameters.[56] All of these abnormalities regress with levothyroxine replacement.

Myxedema coma

Myxedema coma occurs almost exclusively in older adults with long-standing primary hypothyroidism, and is usually precipitated by a concomitant medical illness. Patients may present with a rapid development of stupor, seizures, or coma along with respiratory depression. Hallmark signs of myxedema coma include localized neurologic signs, hypothermia, bradycardia, hyponatremia, and hypoglycemia.[55] Myxedema coma is a severe and life-threatening clinical state in older adults, with a mortality rate as high as 40%.[57–59]

Management

Despite the high prevalence of thyroid hormone use in this population, there are no concrete data on when and at what dose to initiate thyroid hormone replacement in older adults. Somwaru and colleagues[60] collected data on thyroid hormone medication from community-dwelling individuals aged 65 years and older (mean age 72.8 years) enrolled in the Cardiovascular Health Study (N = 5888) over a span of 16 years. It was concluded that thyroid hormone use is common in patients older than 65, with up to 20% being treated with levothyroxine. The incidence of thyroid hormone replacement in adults aged 85 years and older was more than twice as frequent as that in adults aged 65 to 89 years (hazard ratio 2.34; 95% confidence interval 1.43–3.85).[60]

Older patients often have lower dose requirements for levothyroxine, which may be related to several factors including declining metabolic clearance, slow progression of underlying thyroid failure, declining body mass, and interactions with other medications.[61] On average, older adults with primary hypothyroidism receive initial daily doses that are 20 μg lower and maintenance daily doses that are 40 μg lower than those prescribed for younger patients of comparable weight.[62–64] Thyroid hormone increases myocardial oxygen demand, which may induce cardiac arrhythmias, angina pectoris, or myocardial infarction in older patients. Once the cardiovascular tolerance of a starting dose has been assessed, a gradual increase by 12.5 to 25 μg every 4 to 6 weeks is recommended until adequate replacement is confirmed by serum TSH measurement.[65]

Physicians treating hypothyroidism in older adults should target a normal TSH range.[65] In a recent survey of ATA members, 39% of them recommended targeting a TSH range of 0.5 to 2.0 mIU/L when treating younger patients, whereas a comparable number reported being more liberal in their approach to older adults, targeting a TSH range of 1.0 to 4.0 mIU/L.[65] This approach avoids overtreatment with excessive doses of levothyroxine, which can be associated with increased risks of atrial fibrillation and progressive loss of bone mineral density in this population.[66]

Management of subclinical hypothyroidism in older adults is controversial, and guidelines have been published both for[67] and against[68,69] routine treatment in older adults. Several placebo-controlled randomized trials have failed to find a reduction in the symptoms of subclinical hypothyroidism with treatment,[70,71] suggesting there is no benefit to treatment.[72,73] Surks and colleagues[68] recommend against routine treatment of patients older than 58 years with TSH levels between 4.5 and 10 mIU/L because of the lack of evidence indicating adverse health outcomes in untreated patients in this group, excluding progression to overt hypothyroidism. Chu and Crapo[69] recommend levothyroxine replacement therapy in patients with a TSH level greater than 10 mIU/L on repeated measurements, clear symptoms or signs associated with thyroid failure, a family history of thyroid disease, or severe hyperlipidemia not previously diagnosed.

THYROID NODULES
Epidemiology and Clinical Presentation

It is known that the prevalence of thyroid nodules increases with age.[74] By the age of 65 years, nearly 50% of individuals in iodine-sufficient areas have thyroid nodules when evaluated with ultrasonography.[75] A survey by Cavaliere and colleagues[76] showed that the prevalence of multinodular goiter in older adults in an iodine-deficient area was 74% in patients aged 55 to 75 years and 54% in patients aged 76 to 84 years. Thyroid nodules may be benign adenomas, cysts, cancers, or inflammation.

Management

The approach to the management of a solitary thyroid nodule in an older adult is the same as that in a younger patient. With the discovery of a new thyroid nodule, a complete history and physical examination should be performed. Pertinent questions should include history of head and neck or whole-body irradiation, exposure to ionizing radiation, and family history of thyroid cancer or syndromes such as multiple endocrine neoplasia. Physical findings such as palpable cervical lymphadenopathy, hoarseness, or fixation of the nodule to surrounding tissue raise suspicion for malignancy.

As per recent ATA guidelines,[77] initial evaluation constitutes measurement of serum TSH. If the TSH is subnormal, the next step consists of a radionuclide thyroid scan using either technetium pertechnetate or RAI. A diagnostic thyroid ultrasonogram should be performed in all patients with known or suspected thyroid nodules when TSH is found to be normal or high. Ultrasonographic features associated with a higher likelihood of malignancy include hypoechogenicity, increased intranodular vascularity, presence of microcalcifications, absence of a halo, irregular borders, a nodule with a height greater than width, and presence of suspicious cervical lymphadenopathy. Ultrasound-guided fine-needle aspiration (FNA) is the subsequent specific diagnostic test, but this is not generally recommended for subcentimeter nodules.

THYROID CANCER
Epidemiology and Clinical Presentation

The prevalence of clinically apparent thyroid cancer in adults aged 50 to 70 years is estimated to be 0.1%.[78] As patients age, there is a greater incidence in poorly differentiated types of thyroid cancer.[79,80]

However, well-differentiated papillary thyroid cancer is still the most common thyroid cancer in older adults, with a presentation similar to that in younger patients. These tumors are slow growing, and most patients are asymptomatic or may present with a painless neck mass. More advanced disease may present with palpable cervical lymphadenopathy, hoarseness, dysphagia, and respiratory distress secondary to local invasion and compression. A retrospective study of data from the National Cancer Institute's Surveillance, Epidemiology, and End Results (SEER) registry reported that the incidence of papillary thyroid cancer is increasing disproportionally in patients older than 45 years, and the most commonly found tumor in this group is now a papillary thyroid microcarcinoma (<1 cm).[81] It is speculated that these increased rates are due to the increasing use of imaging studies and subsequent discovery of incidental thyroid nodules in older patients.

Follicular thyroid cancer is more common in areas of iodine deficiency, with the peak incidence in the sixth decade of life.[74,82] It commonly presents with an asymptomatic neck mass, which may be incidentally discovered on imaging studies.

Sporadic forms of medullary thyroid cancer are more common than familial forms in older patients.[83] Many patients present with a palpable neck mass. There may be local or systemic symptoms secondary to metastases. Symptoms of hormone hypersecretion include diarrhea, flushing, and bronchospasm.

Anaplastic thyroid cancer is aggressive and has a peak incidence in the seventh decade of life.[74] It often arises within a more differentiated thyroid cancer, and usually presents as a rapidly growing neck mass with metastases at the time of diagnosis. In a recent retrospective study, 26 anaplastic thyroid cancers were identified out of 1500 thyroid cancers over a span of 16 years. The average anaplastic tumor size at diagnosis was 7.35 cm, with lymph node involvement in 61.5% and distant metastases in 34.5% of cases.[84]

Risks, Complications, and Sequelae

Thyroid cancer is the only cancer for which age is included in the American Joint Committee on Cancer TNM staging system.[85–87] The mortality rates of patients with thyroid cancer increase starting at age 45 years.[88] A steady decline in survival rates has been reported with increasing age, regardless of the degree of differentiation of the thyroid cancer.[89,90] A large retrospective study (N = 53,856) demonstrated lower 10-year survival rates in patients older than 45 years with papillary (47%–85% vs 97%), follicular (57%–66% vs 98%), medullary (63%–80% vs 88%), and anaplastic (5-year survival rate: 13% vs 55%) thyroid cancer.[78] Extension of thyroid cancer outside the gland significantly worsened the prognosis in older patients, whereas it did not alter the favorable prognosis in younger patients.[91–94] In a study of the SEER database, the presence of lymph node metastases had no effect on survival in patients younger than 45 years. However, in patients 45 years or older, there was an associated 46% increased risk of death with lymph node positivity (P<.001).[95] Distant metastases are also a serious prognostic sign in older patients with thyroid cancer[91]; this may be related to thyroid cancer being less RAI-avid in older patients than in younger patients.[85,96]

Recurrence rates of thyroid cancer have also been shown to be influenced by age.[86] Cady and colleagues[91] demonstrated that women older than 50 years had a 32% risk of thyroid cancer recurrence compared with 10% in those younger than 50.

Management

The modalities used for the management of thyroid cancer in older adults are essentially the same as those used in younger patients. Frequently the surgical approach for a thyroid cancer larger than 1 cm is near-total or total thyroidectomy. Thyroid lobectomy alone may be sufficient for tumors smaller than 1 cm. Central neck dissection should accompany total thyroidectomy in patients with clinically involved central or lateral neck lymph nodes.[77] Even though older patients may exhibit a higher surgical risk because of comorbidities, age by itself is not a contraindication to thyroidectomy.

Postoperative RAI ablation of thyroid remnants is indicated for all patients with known iodine-avid distant metastases, gross extrathyroidal extension of the tumor regardless of tumor size, or primary tumor size greater than 4 cm, even in the absence of other risk factors.[77] Dosimetry-guided RAI ablation therapy may be preferable to fixed-dose RAI ablation treatment strategies in older patients with advanced thyroid cancer, as evidenced by a study showing that administered activities above 7.4 GBq (200 mCi) will exceed the maximal safe level in a substantial number of patients older than 70 years.[97] Older age, renal failure, and liver failure are associated with lower clearance of radioiodine.[97]

Unstimulated thyroglobulin should be periodically assessed. One year after RAI ablation, measurement of thyroglobulin under TSH stimulation is useful because it is more sensitive. If the stimulated level is greater than 2 ng/mL, diagnostic imaging studies should be performed for localization of persistent versus recurrent disease.

Thyroxine-suppression therapy is used for the treatment of differentiated thyroid cancers. Jonklaas and colleagues[98] showed that aggressive thyroid hormone–suppression therapy was independently associated with longer overall survival in high-risk patients, and that moderate thyroid hormone suppression led to improved overall survival in stage II patients. Because outcome is good regardless of intervention, survival was not altered in stage I patients. The TSH-suppressive doses of 2 to 2.2 μg/kg often required in younger patients with thyroid cancer may be excessive in older adults, as thyroxine degradation is reduced with age.[99] In the Framingham Heart Study, individuals older than 60 years with TSH values of 0.1 mIU/L or less had an adjusted relative risk of 3.8 for developing atrial fibrillation during a 10-year follow-up, and those with TSH values between 0.1 and 0.4 mIU/L had an adjusted relative risk of 1.6.[28] The beneficial effect of TSH suppression is a considerable reduction in recurrence rates of differentiated thyroid cancer, but this should be weighed against potential complications.

Indications for external beam radiation include the presence of aggressive and unresectable cancer, painful bone metastases, or risk of spinal cord compression.[77] Current clinical trials for novel therapies in thyroid cancer treatment, for example, tyrosine kinase inhibitors, are promising, and older age may not preclude participation.

Table 1
Unique features of the approach and management of thyroid disorders in older adults

Thyroid Disorder	Unique Features in Older Adults
Hyperthyroidism • Overt	• Less symptomatic with apathetic hyperthyroidism common • Greater likelihood of developing atrial fibrillation or osteoporosis • Antithyroid medications (propylthiouracil, methimazole): increased risk of side effects, especially agranulocytosis • Surgery: increased risk of morbidity, but not contraindicated. Primarily used if large, obstructive goiter or suspected malignancy
• Subclinical	• Treat if age >65 y with TSH persistently <0.1 mIU/L
Hypothyroidism • Overt	• Myxedema coma almost exclusively occurs in older adults • Age >50 y: initiate lower dose of levothyroxine, usually 25 μg orally daily and titrate to cardiovascular tolerance • Target a wider TSH range because overtreatment may lead to significant morbidity
• Subclinical	• Treat if TSH >10 mIU/L or clear symptoms/signs of thyroid failure
Thyroid nodules	• Prevalence increases with age
Thyroid cancer	• Greater risk of cancer recurrence and mortality with older age • Age is involved in cancer staging • Greater incidence of poorly differentiated thyroid cancer, including anaplastic, with increasing age • Surgery: higher surgical risk because of comorbidities • Postoperative radioactive iodine ablation: increased risk of empiric dosing exceeding maximum tolerated activity. Consider dosimetry in advanced disease • Thyroxine-suppression therapy for some well-differentiated cancers for a limited period: Lower doses required

SUMMARY

Thyroid gland dysfunction is prevalent in older adults and may be associated with significant morbidity if misdiagnosed and untreated. Factors contributing to misinterpretation of thyroid function tests in older adults include age-dependent physiologic changes, comorbidities, and polypharmacy. Moreover, clinical signs and symptoms of thyroid dysfunction may be subtle or absent, making diagnosis more difficult. As thyroid disorders are often amenable to effective treatments that can improve the quality of life of patients, a high index of clinical suspicion is warranted.

Treatment of hyperthyroidism in older adults is usually similar to that for younger adults, with antithyroid medications, RAI ablation, or surgery. Side effects of antithyroid medication occur more commonly in older adults, and surgery is less favorable because of the increased risk of morbidity and mortality.

There are no concrete guidelines as to when and at what dose to initiate levothyroxine replacement therapy in older adults with hypothyroidism. However, after assessing the cardiovascular tolerance of a starting dose, the dose should be gradually increased by 12.5 to 25 μg every 4 to 6 weeks until adequate replacement is confirmed by serum TSH measurement.

Thyroid nodules are more common in older adults and are managed with an initial measurement of TSH, followed by an ultrasonogram if TSH is normal or high. Depending on nodule size and ultrasonographic features, ultrasound-guided FNA may be performed.

With increasing age, the incidence of thyroid cancer shifts from well-differentiated to poorly differentiated types. Thyroid cancer is unique because age is included in the staging system. The modalities used for the management of thyroid cancer in older adults are in essence the same as those used in younger patients. These methods include surgery, and when appropriate, postoperative RAI ablation, serial thyroglobulin measurements, and thyroxine-suppression therapy (**Table 1**).

REFERENCES

1. Surks MI, Hollowell JG. Age-specific distribution of serum thyrotropin and antithyroid antibodies in the US population: implications for the prevalence of subclinical hypothyroidism. J Clin Endocrinol Metab 2007;92:4575–82.
2. Mariotti S, Franceschi C, Cossarizza A, et al. The aging thyroid. Endocr Rev 1995; 16:686–715.
3. Mariotti S, Barbesino G, Caturegli P, et al. Complex alteration of thyroid function in healthy centenarians. J Clin Endocrinol Metab 1993;77:1130–4.
4. Peeters RP, Debaveye Y, Fliers E, et al. Changes within the thyroid axis during critical illness. Crit Care Clin 2006;22:41–55.
5. Bahn RS, Burch HB, Cooper DS, et al. Hyperthyroidism and other causes of thyrotoxicosis: management guidelines of the American Thyroid Association and American Association of Clinical Endocrinologists. Endo Pract 2011;17(3): 456–520.
6. Hollowell JG, Staehling NW, Flanders WD, et al. Serum TSH, T(4), and thyroid antibodies in the United States population (1988 to 1994): National Health and Nutrition Examination Survey (NHANES III). J Clin Endocrinol Metab 2002;87(2):489–99.
7. Bjoro T, Holmen J, Kruger O, et al. Prevalence of thyroid disease, thyroid dysfunction and thyroid peroxidase antibodies in a large, unselected population. The Health Study of Nord-Trondelag (HUNT). Eur J Endocrinol 2000;143(5):639–47.
8. Volzke H, Alte D, Kohlmann T, et al. Reference intervals of serum thyroid function tests in a previously iodine-deficient area. Thyroid 2005;15(3):279–85.
9. Chiovato L, Mariotti S, Pinchera A. Thyroid diseases in the elderly [review]. Baillieres Clin Endocrinol Metab 1997;11(2):251–70.
10. Atzmon G, Barzilai N, Hollowell JG, et al. Extreme longevity is associated with increased serum thyrotropin. J Clin Endocrinol Metab 2009;94:1251–4.
11. Gussekloo J, van Exel E, de Craen AJ, et al. Thyroid function, activities of daily living and survival in extreme old age: the 'Leiden 85-plus Study'. Ned Tijdschr Geneeskd 2006;150(2):90–6.
12. Van Den Beld AW, Visser TJ, Feelders RA, et al. Thyroid hormone concentrations, disease, physical function and mortality in elderly men. J Clin Endocrinol Metab 2005;90(12):6403–9.
13. Atzmon G, Barzilai N, Surks MI, et al. Genetic predisposition to elevated serum thyrotropin is associated with exceptional longevity. J Clin Endocrinol Metab 2009;94:4768–75.
14. Bannister P, Barnes I. Use of sensitive thyrotropin measurements in an elderly population. Gerontology 1989;35:225–9.
15. Balles BK. Hyperthyroidism in elderly patients. AORN J 1999;69(1):254–8.
16. Thomas FB, Mazzaferri EL, Skillman TG. Apathetic thyrotoxicosis: a distinctive clinical and laboratory entity. Ann Intern Med 1970;72(5):679–85.
17. Diez JJ. Hyperthyroidism in patients older than 55 years: an analysis of the etiology and management. Gerontology 2003;49(5):316–23.
18. Nordyke RA, Gilbert FT Jr, Harada AS. Graves' disease, influence of age on clinical findings. Arch Intern Med 1988;148(3):626–31.
19. Trivalle C, Doucet J, Chassagne P, et al. Differences in the signs and symptoms of hyperthyroidism in older and younger patients. J Am Geriatr Soc 1996;44(1):50–3.

20. Boelaert K, Torlinska B, Holder RL, et al. Older subjects with hyperthyroidism present with a paucity of symptoms and signs: a large cross-sectional study. J Clin Endocrinol Metab 2010;95(6):2715–26.
21. Benseñor IM, Goulart AC, Lotufo PA, et al. Prevalence of thyroid disorders among older people: results from the São Paulo Ageing & Health Study. Cad Saude Publica 2011;27(1):155–61.
22. Samuels MH. Subclinical thyroid disease in the elderly. Thyroid 1998;8:803–13.
23. Ceresini G, Morganti S, Maggio M, et al. Subclinical thyroid disease in elderly subjects. Acta Biomed 2010;81(Suppl 1):31–6.
24. Morganti S, Ceda GP, Saccani M, et al. Thyroid disease in the elderly: sex-related differences in clinical expression. J Endocrinol Invest 2005;28(Suppl 11):101–4.
25. Rosario PW. Natural history of subclinical hyperthyroidism in elderly patients with TSH between 0.1 and 0.4 mIU/l: a prospective study. Clin Endocrinol 2010;72(5): 685–8.
26. Klein I, Ojamaa K. Thyroid hormone and the cardiovascular system. N Engl J Med 2001;344(7):501–9.
27. Cooper DS. Approach to the patient with subclinical hyperthyroidism. J Clin Endocrinol Metab 2007;92(1):3–9.
28. Sawin CT, Geller A, Wolf PA, et al. Low serum thyrotropin concentrations as a risk factor for atrial fibrillation in older persons. N Engl J Med 1994;331(19): 1249–52.
29. Dorr M, Wolff B, Robinson DM, et al. The association of thyroid function with cardiac mass and left ventricular hypertrophy. J Clin Endocrinol Metab 2005;90(2):673–7.
30. Rodondi N, Bauer DC, Cappola AR, et al. Subclinical thyroid dysfunction, cardiac function, and the risk of heart failure. The Cardiovascular Health study. J Am Coll Cardiol 2008;52(14):1152–9.
31. Cummings SR, Nevitt MC, Browner WS, et al. Study of osteoporotic fractures research group. Risk factors for hip fracture in white women. N Engl J Med 1995;332(12):767–73.
32. Bassett JH, Williams GR. The molecular actions of thyroid hormone in bone. Trends Endocrinol Metab 2003;14(8):356–64.
33. Bauer DC, Ettinger B, Nevitt MC, et al. Study of osteoporotic fractures research group. Risk for fracture in women with low serum levels of thyroid-stimulating hormone. Ann Intern Med 2001;134(7):561–8.
34. Schuit SC, van der Klift M, Weel AE, et al. Fracture incidence and association with bone mineral density in elderly men and women: the Rotterdam Study. Bone 2004;34(1):195–202.
35. Lin MC, Hsu FM, Bee YS, et al. Age influences the severity of Graves' ophthalmopathy. Kaohsiung J Med Sci 2008;24(6):283–8.
36. Shakaib U, Rehman MD, Dennis W, et al. Thyroid disorders in elderly patients: Hyperthyroidism. South Med J 2005;98(5):543–9.
37. Faggiano A, Del Prete M, Marciello F, et al. Thyroid diseases in elderly. Minerva Endocrinol 2011;36(3):211–31.
38. Mitrou P, Raptis SA, Dimitriadis G. Thyroid disease in older people. Maturitas 2011;70(1):5–9.
39. Baskin HJ, Cobin RH, Duick DS, et al. American Association of Clinical Endocrinologists. American Association of Clinical Endocrinologists medical guidelines for clinical practice for the evaluation and treatment of hyperthyroidism and hypothyroidism. Endocr Pract 2002;8(6):457–69.
40. Sawin CT, Castelli WP, Hershman JM, et al. The aging thyroid. Thyroid deficiency in the Framingham Study. Arch Intern Med 1985;145(8):1386–8.

41. Canaris GJ, Manowitz NR, Mayor G, et al. The Colorado thyroid disease prevalence study. Arch Intern Med 2000;160(4):526–34.
42. Bemben DA, Winn P, Hamm RM, et al. Thyroid disease in the elderly. Part 1. Prevalence of undiagnosed hypothyroidism. J Fam Pract 1994;38(6):577–82.
43. Dayan CM, Daniels GH. Chronic autoimmune thyroiditis. N Engl J Med 1996; 335(2):99–107.
44. Mariotti S, Chiovato L, Franseschi C, et al. Thyroid autoimmunity and aging. Exp Gerontol 1998;33(6):535–41.
45. Pinchera A, Mariotti S, Barbesino G, et al. Thyroid autoimmunity and ageing. Horm Res 1995;43(1–3):64–8.
46. Reinhardt W, Mann K. Incidence, clinical picture and treatment of hypothyroid coma. Results of a survey. Med Klin (Munich) 1997;92(9):521–4.
47. Diez JJ. Hypothyroidism in patients older than 55 years: an analysis of the etiology and assessment of the effectiveness of therapy. J Gerontol A Biol Sci Med Sci 2002;57(5):315–20.
48. Maselli M, Inelmen EM, Giantin V, et al. Hypothyroidism in the elderly: diagnostic pitfalls illustrated by a case report. Arch Gerontol Geriatr 2011. [Epub ahead of print].
49. Doucet J, Trivalle C, Chassagna P, et al. Does age play a role in clinical presentation of hypothyroidism? J Am Geriatr Soc 1994;42(9):984–6.
50. Kramer CK, von Muhlen D, Kritz-Silverstein D, et al. Treated hypothyroidism, cognitive function, and depressed mood in old age: the Rancho Bernardo Study. Eur J Endocrinol 2009;161(6):917–21.
51. Davis JD, Tremont G. Neuropsychiatric aspects of hypothyroidism and treatment reversibility. Minerva Endocrinol 2007;32(1):49–65.
52. Correia N, Mullally S, Cooke G, et al. Evidence for a specific defect in hippocampal memory in overt and subclinical hypothyroidism. J Clin Endocrinol Metab 2009;94(10):3789–97.
53. Jorde R, Waterloo K, Storhaug H, et al. Neuropsychological function and symptoms in subjects with subclinical hypothyroidism and the effect of thyroxine treatment. J Clin Endocrinol Metab 2006;91(1):145–53.
54. Roberts LM, Pattison H, Roalfe A, et al. Is subclinical thyroid dysfunction in the elderly associated with depression or cognitive dysfunction? Ann Intern Med 2006;145(8):573–81.
55. Li TM. Hypothyroidism in elderly people. Geriatr Nurs 2002;23(2):88–93.
56. Mariotti S, Cambuli VM. Cardiovascular risk in elderly hypothyroid patients. Thyroid 2007;17(11):1067–73.
57. Yamamoto T, Fukuyama J, Fujiyoshi A. Factors associated with mortality of myxedema coma: report of eight cases and literature survey. Thyroid 1999; 9(12):1167–74.
58. Nicoloff JT, LoPresti JS. Myxedema coma. A form of decompensated hypothyroidism. Endocrinol Metab Clin North Am 1993;22(2):279–90.
59. Jordan RM. Myxedema coma. Pathophysiology, therapy, and factors affecting prognosis. Med Clin North Am 1995;79(1):185–94.
60. Somwaru LL, Arnold AM, Cappola AR. Predictors of thyroid hormone initiation in older adults: results from the cardiovascular health study. J Gerontol A Biol Sci Med Sci 2011;66(7):809–14.
61. Laurberg P, Andersen S, Bulow Pedersen I, et al. Hypothyroidism in the elderly: pathophysiology, diagnosis and treatment. Drugs Aging 2005;22(1):23–38.
62. Rosenbaum RL, Barzel US. Levothyroxine replacement dose for primary hypothyroidism decreases with age. Ann Intern Med 1982;96(1):53–5.

63. Young RE, Jones SJ, Bewsher PD, et al. Age and the daily dose of thyroxine replacement therapy for hypothyroidism. Age Ageing 1984;13(5):293–303.

64. Sawin CT, Geller A, Hershman JM, et al. The aging thyroid. The use of thyroid hormone in older persons. JAMA 1989;261(18):2653–5.

65. McDermott MT, Haugen BR, Lezotte DC, et al. Management practices among primary care physicians and thyroid specialists in the care of hypothyroid patients. Thyroid 2001;11(8):757–64.

66. Koch L. Pharmacotherapy: levothyroxine in the elderly—finding the breaking point. Nat Rev Endocrinol 2011;7(8):435.

67. Gharib H, Tuttle RM, Baskin HJ, et al. Subclinical thyroid dysfunction: a joint statement on management from the American Association of Clinical Endocrinologists, the American Thyroid Association, and the Endocrine Society. J Clin Endocrinol Metab 2005;90(1):581–5.

68. Surks MI, Ortiz E, Daniels GH, et al. Subclinical thyroid disease: scientific review and guidelines for diagnosis and management. JAMA 2004;291(2):228–38.

69. Chu JW, Crapo LM. The treatment of subclinical hypothyroidism is seldom necessary. J Clin Endocrinol Metab 2001;86(10):4591–9.

70. Kong WM, Sheikh MH, Lumb PJ, et al. A 6-month randomized trial of thyroxine treatment in women with mild subclinical hypothyroidism. Am J Med 2002; 112(5):348–54.

71. Jaeschke R, Guyatt G, Gerstein H, et al. Does treatment with L-thyroxine influence health status in middle-aged and older adults with subclinical hypothyroidism? J Gen Intern Med 1998;11(12):733–9.

72. Nystrom E, Caldahl K, Fager G, et al. A double-blind cross-over 12-month study of L-thyroxine treatment of women with subclinical hypothyroidism. Clin Endocrinol (Oxf) 1988;29(1):63–75.

73. Ayala C, Cozar MV, Rodriguez JR, et al. Subclinical thyroid disease in institutionalized healthy geriatric population. Med Clin (Barc) 2001;117(14):534–5.

74. Gupta KL. Neoplasm of the thyroid gland. Clin Geriatr Med 1995;11:271–90.

75. Mazzaferri EL. Management of a solitary thyroid nodule. N Engl J Med 1993; 328(8):553–9.

76. Cavaliere R, Antonangeil L, Vitti P, et al. The aging thyroid in a mild to moderate iodine deficient area of Italy. J Endocrinol Invest 2002;25(Suppl 10):66–8.

77. Cooper DS, Doherty GM, Haugen BR, et al. Revised American Thyroid Association management guidelines for patients with thyroid nodules and differentiated thyroid cancer. Thyroid 2009;19(11):1167–214.

78. Castro MR, Gharib H. Continuing controversies in the management of thyroid nodules. Ann Intern Med 2005;142(11):926–31.

79. Hundahl SA, Fleming ID, Fremgen AM, et al. A National Cancer Data Base report on 53,856 cases of thyroid carcinoma treated in the U.S., 1985-1995. Cancer 1998;83(12):2638–48.

80. Aschebrook-Kilfoy B, Ward MH, Sabra MM, et al. Thyroid cancer incidence patterns in the United States by histologic type, 1992-2006. Thyroid 2011;21(2):125–34.

81. Hughes DT, Haymart MR, Miller BS, et al. The most commonly occurring papillary thyroid cancer in the United States in now a microcarcinoma in a patient older than 45 years. Thyroid 2011;21(3):231–6.

82. Woolner LB, Beahrs OH, Black BM, et al. Classification and prognosis of thyroid carcinoma. Am J Surg 1961;102:354–87.

83. Kebebew E, Ituarte PH, Siperstein AE, et al. Medullary thyroid carcinoma clinical characteristics, treatment, prognostic factors, and a comparison of staging systems. Cancer 2000;88:1139–47.

84. Roche B, Larroumets G, Dejax C, et al. Epidemiology, clinical presentation, treatment and prognosis of a regional series of 26 anaplastic thyroid carcinomas (ATC). Comparison with the literature. Ann Endocrinol (Paris) 2010;71(1):38–45.
85. Haymart MR. Understanding the relationship between age and thyroid cancer. Oncologist 2009;14:216–21.
86. Greene FL, Page DL, Fleming ID, et al, editors. Thyroid. In: American Joint Committee on Cancer: cancer staging manual. 6th edition. New York: Springer-Verlag; 2002. p. 77–87.
87. Dean DS, Hay ID. Prognostic indicators in differentiated thyroid carcinoma. Cancer Control 2000;7:229–39.
88. Mazzaferri EL, Kloos RT. Current approaches to primary therapy for papillary and follicular thyroid cancer. J Clin Endocrinol Metab 2001;86:1447–63.
89. Halnan KE. Influence of age and sex on incidence and prognosis of thyroid cancer. Three hundred forty-four cases followed for ten years. Cancer 1966; 19(11):1534–6.
90. Sautter-Bihl ML, Raub J, Hetzel-Sesterheim M, et al. Differentiated thyroid cancer: prognostic factors and influence of treatment on the outcome in 441 patients. Strahlenther Onkol 2001;177(3):125–31.
91. Cady B, Sedgwick CE, Meissner WA, et al. Risk factor analysis in differentiated thyroid cancer. Cancer 1979;43:810–20.
92. Brennan MD, Bergstralh EJ, Van Heerden JA, et al. Follicular thyroid cancer treated at the Mayo Clinic, 1946 through 1970: initial manifestations, pathologic findings, therapy, and outcome. Mayo Clin Proc 1991;66:11–22.
93. Ladurner D, Zechmann W, Hofstadter F. Prognosis of the follicular thyroid carcinoma in an endemic goiter area—results of a retrospective study. Acta Endocrinol Suppl 1983;252:28–9.
94. Crile G, Pontius KI, Hawk WA. Factors influencing the survival of patients with follicular carcinoma of the thyroid gland. Surg Gynecol Obstet 1985;160:409–13.
95. Zaydfudim V, Feurer ID, Griffin MR, et al. The impact of lymph node involvement on survival in patients with papillary and follicular thyroid carcinoma. Surgery 2008;144:1070–7.
96. Vini L, Hyer SL, Marshall J, et al. Long-term results in elderly patients with differentiated thyroid carcinoma. Cancer 2003;97:2736–42.
97. Tuttle RM, Leboeul R, Robbins RJ, et al. Empiric radioactive iodine dosing regimens frequently exceed maximum tolerated activity levels in elderly patients with thyroid cancer. J Nucl Med 2006;47:1587–91.
98. Jonklaas J, Sarlis NJ, Litofsky D, et al. Outcomes of patients with differentiated thyroid carcinoma following initial therapy. Thyroid 2006;16(12):1229–42.
99. Gregerman RI, Gaffney GW, Shock NW. Thyroxine turnover in euthyroid man with special reference to changes with age. J Clin Invest 1962;41:2065–74.

The Evaluation and Treatment of Graves Ophthalmopathy

Marius N. Stan, MD[a], James A. Garrity, MD[b],
Rebecca S. Bahn, MD[a],*

KEYWORDS

- Graves ophthalmopathy • Graves disease
- Thyrotropin receptor autoantibodies • Radioactive iodine

Graves ophthalmopathy (GO) is an inflammatory disorder of the orbit that occurs in association with autoimmune thyroid disease.[1] Although most patients with GO have a history of Graves disease (GD) with hyperthyroidism, some are euthyroid with no such history or have hypothyroidism primarily caused by Hashimoto thyroiditis.[2] A close temporal relationship exists between the onset of Graves hyperthyroidism and the onset of GO. Regardless of which condition occurs first, the other condition develops within 18 months in 80% of patients, although GO may occasionally precede or follow hyperthyroidism by many years.[3] The common manifestations of the disease vary considerably from patient to patient in expression, severity, and duration. Such signs include proptosis, upper eyelid retraction, and swelling with or without erythema of the periocular tissues, lids, and conjunctivae. The natural history of GO is characterized by fairly steady deterioration over 3 to 6 months, followed by a plateau phase of often between 1 and 3 years, then gradual improvement toward the baseline.[4] Whereas the inflammatory signs and symptoms generally resolve over time, proptosis, lid retraction, and extraocular dysfunction may persist. A cohort of patients with GO followed for a median of 12 months showed spontaneous improvement in ocular manifestations in approximately two-thirds, stability in 20%, and worsening in 14%.[5]

PATHOPHYSIOLOGY

As with hyperthyroidism of GD, GO likely evolves from an autoimmune process primarily directed against the thyrotropin receptor (TSHR).[6] However, rather than TSHR on thyroid follicular cells being the autoimmune target, this same receptor

[a] Division of Endocrinology, Metabolism and Nutrition, Mayo Clinic School of Medicine, Mayo Clinic, 200 First Street Southwest, Rochester, MN 55905, USA
[b] Department of Ophthalmology, Mayo Clinic School of Medicine, Mayo Clinic, 200 First Street Southwest, Rochester, MN 55905, USA
* Corresponding author.
E-mail address: Bahn.rebecca@mayo.edu

Med Clin N Am 96 (2012) 311–328
doi:10.1016/j.mcna.2012.01.014
0025-7125/12/$ – see front matter © 2012 Elsevier Inc. All rights reserved.

expressed on orbital fibroblasts is recognized by TSHR autoantibodies (TRAb) directed against this receptor (**Fig. 1**).[7] As a result, these cells are stimulated to produce hydrophilic hyaluronan,[8] and a subset differentiates into mature adipocytes.[9] This process leads to enlargement of the extraocular muscles and to expansion of the orbital adipose tissue. Many of the clinical manifestations of GO can be explained in a mechanical sense by this increase in tissue volume within the bony orbit that displaces the globe forward and hinders venous outflow. Cytokines and other mediators of inflammation, produced by infiltrating mononuclear cells and resident macrophages, accumulate within the orbit and contribute to the local inflammatory process.[10] No unique genetic associations have been identified that distinguish individuals with GO from those having GD without evident GO. However, environmental factors, including smoking, radioactive iodine (RAI) therapy for hyperthyroidism, and posttreatment hypothyroidism, may play an important role in disease development and progression.[11]

EPIDEMIOLOGY

The annual adjusted incidence rate of Graves hyperthyroidism is 0.50 per 1000 population,[12] with some 25% to 50% of these patients having clinical eye involvement.

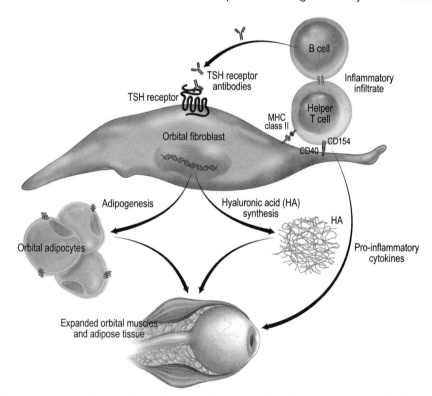

Fig. 1. Immunopathogenesis of Graves ophthalmopathy. Circulating autoantibodies directed against the thyrotropin receptor activate this receptor on orbital fibroblasts; this results in their increased secretion of hyaluronic acid, and the differentiation of a subset into mature adipocytes. In addition, activated T cells infiltrate the orbit, interact with autoreactive B cells, and secrete proinflammatory cytokines. These cellular changes lead to the extraocular muscle enlargement, orbital adipose tissue expansion, and orbital inflammation characteristic of the disease. XRT, radiotherapy.

Most patients with GO show mild signs and symptoms including corneal irritation, periocular swelling, eyelid retraction, conjunctival erythema/chemosis, and mild extraocular muscle dysfunction. A much smaller proportion of patients (approximately 5%) experience severe disease including significant inflammation/congestion, excessive proptosis, and sight-threatening corneal ulceration or optic neuropathy. Although GO is overall more frequent in women than in men, men are overly represented in severe forms of the disease, with a female-to-male ratio of 1:4.[13] Subclinical eye involvement is common, with approximately 70% of hyperthyroid patients showing evidence of GO on magnetic resonance imaging (MRI) or orbital computed tomography (CT) scanning.[14] The overall incidence of GO varies depending on the diagnostic criteria; the annual adjusted incidence rate of clinically significant GO in Olmsted County, Minnesota is 16 women and 3 men per 100,000 population.[15] A bimodal age distribution is followed, with peak incidence of GO in women occurring between age 40 to 44 years and 60 to 64 years, and in men between 45 to 49 years and 65 to 69 years. The other peripheral manifestations of GD, dermopathy and acropachy, occur with lower frequency and almost always develop in patients with more severe GO.[16]

DIAGNOSIS

There is no single clinical finding or laboratory test that is diagnostic of GO. A careful history and physical examination often allows for a firm diagnosis of GO to be made. Although the diagnosis is generally straightforward without the need for additional laboratory or imaging data in a thyrotoxic patient with bilateral proptosis, it can be more difficult in a euthyroid patient with unilateral proptosis. In this instance, CT scanning or MRI with special attention paid to the orbits is indicated, and may identify an orbital mass lesion, an infiltrative process, idiopathic orbital inflammation (pseudotumor), or other orbital abnormality. If the imaging is compatible with GO, the finding of elevated TRAb is helpful in making the diagnosis in a euthyroid patient.[2] Although the absence of elevated TRAb in this setting does not rule out the diagnosis of GO, it makes the diagnosis less likely and necessitates further evaluation and/or observation over time. The differential diagnosis of GO regarding particular findings on physical examination is outlined in **Table 1**.

CLINICAL EVALUATION

The clinical evaluation and management of GO, as well as any accompanying hyperthyroidism, is optimally performed in a multidisciplinary clinic having both endocrine and ophthalmologic expertise in the condition as well as access to ancillary specialties.[17] All patients with GO, except for the mildest cases, should be examined by both an ophthalmologist and an endocrinologist. Proper management of GO is based on accurate determination of both the severity of the disease, or extent of ocular dysfunction or involvement, and its clinical activity, or degree of active inflammation present. Although severity and activity may peak simultaneously, often the two are not congruent, with peak activity preceding the most significant clinical expressions of the disease.[18]

The degree of severity can be classified as mild, moderate to severe, or sight-threatening, following quantitative assessment of lid aperture width, proptosis measurement, diplopia score (1 = intermittent [ie, when tired or on awakening]; 2 = inconstant [ie, only at extremes of gaze]; 3 = constant), degrees of abduction in eye muscle movement, examination of the cornea for evidence of exposure keratitis or ulceration, and assessment of optic nerve function (**Table 2**).[17]

Table 1
Differential diagnosis

Primary Examination Feature	Differential Diagnosis	Symmetry	Prevalence[a]
Proptosis	Primary cancer	Unilateral	Uncommon
	Metastatic cancer	Unilateral	Uncommon
	Orbital meningioma	Unilateral	Common
	Orbital myositis	Uni-/bilateral	Common
	IgG$_4$ disease	Uni-/bilateral	Uncommon
	Sarcoidosis	Uni-/bilateral	Rare
	Wegener granulomatosis	Uni-/bilateral	Rare
	Carotid cavernous fistula	Unilateral	Uncommon
	Paranasal sinus mucocele	Unilateral	Uncommon
Periocular inflammation/ congestion/edema	Allergy	Bilateral	Common
	Nephrotic syndrome	Bilateral	Uncommon
	Facial cellulitis	Unilateral	Uncommon
Diplopia	Orbital myositis	Uni-/bilateral	Common
	Myasthenia gravis	Uni-/bilateral	Common
	Contralateral blowout fracture	Unilateral	Uncommon
Lid retraction	Midbrain disease	Unilateral	Uncommon
	Contralateral ptosis	Unilateral	Uncommon
	Sympathomimetic drugs	Bilateral	Common
	Thyrotoxicosis	Bilateral	Common

[a] Prevalence within all patients with primary examination feature.

The activity of GO can be graded using a clinical activity score (CAS) that ranges from 0 to 10 and predicts response to anti-inflammatory therapies.[18] The CAS is generated by the addition of 1 point for the presence of each the following features: chemosis, eyelid swelling, eyelid erythema, conjunctival erythema, caruncular swelling, pain in primary gaze, and pain with ocular movement. In addition, if the patient has been examined within the 3 months prior, additional points may be given for decreased visual acuity, worsened diplopia, and increased proptosis compared with that visit. GO is considered active in patients with a CAS of 3 or more out of 7 (if no previous assessment is available), or 4 out of 10 on the complete scale.

Dysthyroid optic neuropathy (DON) is a severe complication of GO that affects approximately 5% of GO patients, and may lead to loss of vision. The condition may present as unexplained deterioration in vision or change in intensity or quality of color vision.[19] Corneal breakdown with subsequent ulceration is another sight-threatening complication, and may be found in patients who experience corneal exposure in the setting of poor blinks, excessive upper lid retraction, and/or lagophthalmos (inability to fully close the eye), which can be exacerbated with greater amounts of proptosis. Globe subluxation is a form of partial displacement of the globe from the orbit whereby the eyelids are repositioned behind the protruding globe. It is typically seen with greater amounts of proptosis and lid retraction, and is associated with pain and risk of loss of vision caused by optic nerve compromise with repeated episodes As immediate treatment is essential for each of these conditions, patients in whom they occur or are suspected should be referred urgently to an ophthalmologist.

Clinical assessment of GO also includes evaluation of the impact of the disease on the patient's quality of life (QOL). The QOL has been shown to be impaired in GO, with both physical and mental health being adversely affected. Patients have poorer self-image, more sleep disturbance, and more impaired social and work functioning than controls.[20] Several QOL questionnaires have been developed and validated for

Table 2
GO severity assessment

Degree of Severity	Lid Retraction	Soft Tissue Involvement	Proptosis[a]	Diplopia	Corneal Exposure	Optic Nerve Status
Mild (≥1 of following)	<2 mm	Mild	<3 mm	Transient[b] or absent	Absent	Normal
Moderate to severe (≥1 of following)	≥2 mm	Moderate or severe	≥3 mm	Inconstant[b] or constant	Mild	Normal
Sight threatening (1 of last 2 categories)	Not contributory	Not contributory	Not contributory	Not contributory	Ulceration	Compromised

[a] Proptosis refers to the variation compared with the norm for each race or to the patient's baseline if available.
[b] Intermittent diplopia: present when the patient is fatigued; inconstant diplopia: present at extremes of gaze; constant diplopia: present in primary gaze.

use in patients with GO.[20–22] While being essential for treatment evaluation in clinical studies, such instruments may also be useful in clinical practice to aid in decisions regarding disease intervention.

RISK FACTORS FOR GO DEVELOPMENT OR PROGRESSION

Several risk factors have been identified that predispose to the development or progression of GO (**Table 3**). Among the most carefully studied factors in randomized trials have been the various treatment options for Graves hyperthyroidism. Risks in these studies ranged from 33% for radioactive iodine (RAI) compared with 10% for antithyroid drugs and 16% for surgery,[31] to 39% for RAI compared with 21% for anti-thyroid drugs.[32] In one large randomized study, patients were treated with RAI with or without concurrent corticosteroid (to determine whether this might be preventive), or methimazole.[37] Within 6 months of treatment, progression was seen in 15% of patients treated with RAI alone, in approximately 3% of patients treated with methima-zole, and in no patients treated with RAI plus corticosteroid. By 1 year most patients with progression had improved, with only 5% of the RAI group experiencing persistent worsening that required additional treatment. Overall, studies suggest that antithyroid drug therapy or thyroidectomy do not affect the course of GO, whereas there is a small but significant increased risk of worsening following RAI therapy in patients with active disease. By contrast, it appears that patients with inactive GO may be treated with RAI without increased risk.[17,38]

Smoking is the risk factor most strongly and consistently linked with the development or progression of GO and with poorer response to therapy.[32,39,40] Several studies suggest that smokers develop more severe GO, that the risk is proportional to the number of cigarettes smoked per day, and that former smokers have significantly lower risk than current smokers.[33,41] In a recent randomized trial of patients with newly diagnosed GD treated with either RAI or antithyroid drugs, smoking was found to be a more important risk factor for GO than was RAI.[32] Regardless of which

Table 3			
Risk factors for GO development or deterioration			
Risk Factor	**Relative Risk**	**Details**	**References**
Genetics	+	Complex genetic basis; similar to Graves disease	23
Ancestry	++	Caucasians > Asians	24
Gender	++	Frequency: women > men Severity: men > women	25,26
Thyroid dysfunction	+++	Both hypo- and hyperthyroidism increase risk	27–29
Mechanical factors	+	Narrower lateral orbital wall angle may affect progression	30
Thyroid hormone levels	+	Both high triiodothyronine and thyroxine levels increase risk (inconsistent results in the literature)	29,31,32
Smoking	++++	Active and passive smoking increases risk	33,34
TSH receptor antibody	++	High titer 5 months after diagnosis predicts worse course of disease	35,36
Radioactive iodine	++	RAI treatment increases risk primarily in smokers and patients with active GO	31,32,37

therapy they received, more than 40% of smokers either developed GO or experienced deterioration of their eye involvement. This rate was almost double that of nonsmokers. In another study wherein hyperthyroid patients with established GO were treated with RAI, smoking was found to add additional risk for GO over that conferred by RAI alone, and GO progression was prevented when RAI was combined with steroids in only 14.9% of smokers compared with 63.8% of nonsmokers.[42] Second-hand smoking has also been linked, albeit indirectly, with GO development.[34] Although no intervention trial of smoking cessation has been successfully undertaken, there is retrospective evidence that quitting is associated with a better outcome.[33] Counseling and aiding GO patients to stop smoking is the standard of care.[17,43]

The relationship between TRAb level and disease activity or progression has been studied by several groups. TRAb level was found in one study to be strongly correlated with the CAS or degree of proptosis in euthyroid patients with untreated GO of moderate severity.[36] In another study, 159 GO patients were followed for 1 to 2 years, with TRAb levels recorded every 3 months.[35] Using specific levels of TRAb as threshold points at various times following the diagnosis of GO, the prognosis of GO was predictable as being either mild or severe in 50% of patients. Both hyperthyroidism and hypothyroidism have also been shown in multiple reports to be associated with increased risk for development or deterioration of GO. When GO patients in a referral population were stratified into groups using a severity index, approximately twice as many patients with current thyroid dysfunction were identified in the groups having more severe GO than in the more mildly affected groups.[27] The impact on GO of early supplementation with levothyroxine (to avoid hypothyroidism following RAI therapy) was studied in a group of patients receiving levothyroxine beginning 2 weeks following RAI.[28] The investigators compared GO progression in these patients with a historical cohort of patients who did not receive levothyroxine until they were documented to be hypothyroid following RAI therapy (permissive hypothyroidism). The investigators found the relative risk of GO development or worsening in the permissive hypothyroidism group compared with the early treatment group to be 1.64 (95% confidence interval: 1.1–2.6), and additionally documented more severe GO in the former. The association between hypothyroidism following RAI therapy and progression of GO was later confirmed in a prospective cohort of 114 patients followed for 2 years.[29] Based on these studies, it has become widely accepted that hypothyroidism following treatment of Graves hyperthyroidism is a risk factor for GO, warranting active prevention.[43] The complication of DON has its own risk factors that include smoking, advanced age, and the presence of diabetes.[44]

INITIAL MANAGEMENT

Optimum management of GO requires a partnership between the endocrinologist and ophthalmologist, with the goal of preserving the patient's vision and restoring favorable self-perception and QOL. Although either partner may make the diagnosis, the initial steps in management are generally the purview of the endocrinologist, who evaluates and addresses the reversible risk factors associated with disease progression and severity.[13] Smokers should be offered participation in a structured smoking cessation program, and patients exposed to second-hand smoke should be identified and advised of its negative impact.[45] If the patient is hyperthyroid, prompt attention should be directed toward the restoration of euthyroidism. Whereas RAI therapy with or without concurrent corticosteroid treatment for GO prophylaxis may be considered in nonsmokers with mild active GO, smokers who choose this treatment option should receive oral corticosteroids. A common regimen consists of prednisone (0.4–0.5 mg/kg/d) started 1 to 3 days following RAI administration and continued for 1 month, with tapering over the 2 subsequent months.[17] However, a recent retrospective cohort study suggested that lower doses of prednisone (0.2 mg/kg/d) for 6 weeks may be equally effective.[46] RAI treatment in patients with active and moderate or severe GO should be avoided in favor of either antithyroid drug therapy or thyroidectomy.[45]

As described earlier, therapeutic decision making hinges on proper evaluation of the clinical activity of the disease and its severity, with particular attention paid to the possible presence of the sight-threatening complications of corneal ulceration and DON. While these elements are addressed by the endocrinologist, a complete evaluation by the ophthalmologist, especially in patients with moderate or severe disease, is essential for appropriate assessment. Generally mild disease is treated with local supportive measures. A patient having moderate or severe active disease may benefit from systemic medical therapy or external radiation therapy, whereas inactive disease of the same severity might be considered for rehabilitative surgery.

LOCAL THERAPY

In both active and inactive GO, the use of local measures can afford good symptomatic relief.[17] Ocular lubrication with artificial tears (administered 4–6 times per day) or gels (applied at nighttime) benefits the corneal symptoms of dryness, photophobia, and grittiness. The application of viscous gels or ointment at bedtime lengthens the duration of action and is useful for patients with nocturnal lagophthalmos, who typically have prominent symptoms on awakening. Cool compresses and sunglasses are also helpful with ocular irritation. Temporary relief from diplopia may be obtained from botulinum toxin A injected in the extraocular muscles, and symptomatic lid retraction may improve with injection into the levator palpebralis.[47] This effect is temporary, however, and in the authors' experience botulinum injections have not been as helpful as initially hoped.

Approximately two-thirds of patients with mild disease experience spontaneous improvement within about 6 months, and thus need no treatment beyond local measures.[5] In these patients, observation every few months is appropriate until the inactive stage is reached, and rehabilitative surgery can be performed if needed. However, in some patients with mild disease the QOL is significantly diminished and additional intervention may be warranted.[17]

ANTIOXIDANT THERAPY

Antioxidant therapy generally carries with it few side effects and may have a beneficial effect on GO outcome. An early intervention study consecutively assigned patients to allopurinol (300 mg daily) plus nicotinamide (300 mg daily) or placebo.[48] A promising result was noted in this nonrandomized study, with a total eye score index showing improvement in 82% of treated patients compared with 27% of those receiving placebo. Selenium was recently reported to improve mild GO in a trial conducted by the European Group on Graves Orbitopathy (EUGOGO) consortium.[49] Patients were randomized to receive selenium (100 μg twice daily), pentoxifylline, or placebo. Evaluation at 6 months, with confirmation at 12 months, documented an improvement not only in several ocular parameters but also in QOL, compared with placebo or pentoxifylline. The selenium-treated group did not experience any significant side effects, and in particular there was no increase in blood glucose levels, as has been noted in studies of selenium treatment in other diseases. An important caveat is that these subjects were from a population with marginally decreased selenium levels, leaving unanswered the question of selenium-related benefit in patients living in selenium-sufficient regions.

IMMUNOMODULATORY THERAPY

Oral glucocorticoids (GC) have long been used as treatment for GO (often in starting doses of between 40 and 100 mg/d with tapering over 10–24 weeks for a cumulative dose of 2–6 g), but more recent evidence suggests that the intravenous (IV) route is more effective. The two modes of GC administration have been assessed separately in several clinical trials and directly compared in 4.[50] In the largest trial, 70 patients with severe and active GO were randomized to receive either prednisolone (starting at 100 mg/d and tapered by 10 mg daily at weekly intervals for a total dose of 4.0 g) or IV methylprednisolone (500 mg weekly × 6 weeks then 250 mg weekly × 6 weeks for a total dose of 4.5 g).[51] After 3 months, the composite outcome (improvement in 3 or more of the following: proptosis, intraocular pressure, diplopia, muscle size, lid fissure width, visual acuity) was met in 77% of patients treated with IVGC and in 51% of those treated with oral GC. More importantly, the use of IVGC was associated with improved QOL and less need for subsequent surgery. Mild side effects were observed in 17% in the IVGC group and included palpitations (the most common), weight gain, gastrointestinal distress, and sleeplessness. By contrast, more significant side effects were reported with the use of oral GC and included cushingoid features, secondary adrenal insufficiency, weight gain, hypertension, myalgias, hirsutism, depression, hyperglycemia, and osteoporosis. Although similar efficacy and an equally favorable side-effect profile for IVGC were found in a comparable trial,[52] of concern is that fatal acute hepatotoxicity has been reported in 4 GO patients treated with IVGC.[53] Severe hepatotoxicity appears to be dose dependent, as it occurs only in patients receiving a cumulative dose of greater than 8 g of methylprednisolone.[54] Other severe complications of IVGC reported in a recent survey of members of the European Thyroid Association include cardiovascular or cerebrovascular events, autoimmune encephalitis, and liver test abnormalities (>4-fold upper limit of normal).[55] In light of these reports, it has been suggested that patients being considered for IVGC therapy be screened for chronic viral infections, underlying autoimmunity, and preexistent hepatic abnormalities, and that liver function be followed during therapy.[17,56] Retrobulbar injection of GCs was evaluated in a study of triamcinolone compared with placebo, with 25 patients in each arm.[57] The outcome was improved field of vision without diplopia and decreased muscle size on orbital CT in the triamcinolone group. However, because the effect was small and was associated with a risk of injury to the globe, retrobulbar GC injection is not a recommended therapy for GO.

Nonsteroidal immunomodulators have been studied in an attempt to identify agents that can supplant the need for high doses of GC or prevent GO remission after GC therapy is discontinued. Cyclosporine, the first of these agents to be investigated, showed an additive effect to oral steroids and extended the benefits of discontinued GC.[58] However, in a direct comparison with GC therapy, cyclosporine was less effective in reducing the total eye score (combination of extraocular muscle thickness, proptosis, and visual acuity), and the side-effect profile was significant (eg, pneumonia, renal failure, hepatitis, hypertension).[59] As the combination of cyclosporine with oral GC therapy was more effective than either agent alone, cyclosporine is sometimes used with benefit in oral GC–resistant patients or as a steroid-sparing agent. Azathioprine was compared with placebo in one study in which no benefit was identified.[60] By contrast, IV immunoglobulins (IVIg) have been found to be as effective as oral GC in patients with active GO. Studies have found the response rate to be between 62% (defined by an index of extraocular muscle area, proptosis, diplopia, and intraocular pressure) and 76% (assessed by a composite severity score).[61,62] The individual features that improved included soft tissue changes, diplopia, visual acuity, and proptosis. A low rate of side effects was seen, none of them serious. In these studies, IVIg were administered on 2 consecutive days every 3 weeks for 6 cycles in the former study, and daily for 5 days, repeated every 3 weeks for 3 cycles and then 1 dose every 3 weeks for an 9 additional cycles in the latter. Somatostatin analogues have been studied in 4 placebo-controlled trials which, in aggregate, demonstrated no clinically significant benefit and significant gastrointestinal side effects.[63–66]

Rituximab is an anti-CD20 chimeric monoclonal antibody that induces transient B-cell depletion, blocks early B-cell activation and differentiation, and inhibits cytokine secretion, antigen presentation, and T-cell activation.[67] This agent has been identified in case series to have a potentially beneficial effect on GD and GO.[68–71] In these case series with a total of 17 patients, rituximab treatment was associated with a decrease in the CAS of 3 to 4 points on average. However, as no randomized control trial of rituximab treatment in GO has yet been completed, its true efficacy is unknown. Given its side-effect profile (potential for infections, worsening hypertension, serum sickness, and so forth) and high cost, use of this agent in GO is currently best limited to centers performing randomized controlled trials.

Most randomized trials of orbital radiotherapy (OR) in GO have studied patients with moderate to severe disease and have shown a positive impact on ocular dysmotility, without improvement in disease progression.[72–76] The exception is a single trial using a somewhat different patient population, which failed to identify any clinically meaningful difference between OR and sham OR on the contralateral orbit.[77] Several studies addressed radiation dose and treatment duration to minimize exposure and side effects. One trial randomized patients to either 1 Gy/wk, 1 Gy/d, or 2 Gy/d, for a total dose of 20 Gy, and found 1 Gy/wk to be best tolerated and most effective in terms of regression in subjective signs and improvement in eye motility.[75] Another study found the lower total dose of 2.4 Gy to be as effective as higher doses.[78] A study of OR in patients with mild GO concluded that in these patients motility was improved, but that the treatment did not affect soft tissue swelling, proptosis, or QOL.[74] At present, several centers are using low cumulative-dose OR (<10 Gy) in selected active mild and moderate to severe GO, especially when significant diplopia or restricted motility is present. Several studies of OR used in conjunction with oral GC therapy have demonstrated the combination to be superior to oral GC used alone in expediting resolution of the active inflammatory phase of the disease.[76,79] A study of OR in which the therapy was used in conjunction with either oral GC or IVGC found IVGC to be better tolerated and somewhat more effective than oral GC in this regimen.[80] Whether IVGC therapy benefits from the addition of OR was examined in a nonrandomized study that suggested lack of additional benefit.[81] However, this finding has to be considered provisional until randomized clinical trials of IVGC with or without OR have been completed. The side-effect profile of OR includes retinopathy in 1% to 2% overall, with higher risk in patients with diabetes mellitus in whom the therapy is contraindicated owing to the lower threshold for radiation retinopathy in such patients.[82,83]

A caveat to the therapeutic trials discussed here is that although investigators studied various parameters or indices (proptosis, diplopia score, soft tissue features, QOL, CAS, and in many cases a composite score) to ascertain benefit, none is uniformly agreed to consistently represent "improvement" in GO. However, in summary it may be said that approximately 40% to 80% of GO patients treated with immunomodulatory therapy experience benefit, that patients with inactive disease are not likely to respond, and that IVGC therapy appears to be the most effective of the treatment options that have been well studied to date. Risks and benefits of these treatments should be carefully discussed with the patient who is best fully involved in the therapeutic decision-making process.

THYROIDECTOMY AND THYROID ABLATION

Interest in the potential benefit of eliminating the thyroid as a source of pathogenic antigen has increased as autoantibodies directed against the thyrotropin receptor have become more clearly implicated in the pathogenesis of GO.[1,7] A retrospective study of patients who were treated with IVGC and surgery compared those who underwent near-total thyroidectomy with patients receiving total thyroidectomy plus RAI for thyroid remnant ablation. Using a composite outcome (proptosis, CAS, eyelid fissure, diplopia) at 9 months following surgery, results showed a higher proportion of patients in the latter group with improved GO.[84] By contrast, another study comparing GO outcome in patients with moderate disease undergoing either subtotal (2 g thyroid remnant) or total thyroidectomy found no difference between groups and a higher surgical complication rate in the latter.[85] Recent guidelines recommend against RAI therapy for the management of hyperthyroidism in patients with moderate to severe active GO, extrapolating from its known deleterious impact on mild active disease.[43] Because no study to date has compared the therapeutic alternatives for hyperthyroidism therapy in these patients regarding GO progression, the choice between thyroidectomy and antithyroid medication is best based on clinical factors including degree of thyrotoxicosis, goiter size, comorbidities, and the preference of the patient. Given the paucity of evidence that thyroidectomy or thyroid remnant ablation in euthyroid GO patients is of value, neither practice is recommended.

THERAPY FOR SIGHT-THREATENING GO

Corneal ulceration, globe subluxation, and DON are sight-threatening disorders that require emergent therapy. DON is multifactorial in etiology, and generally occurs when the optic nerve is compressed by enlarged extraocular muscles at the orbital apex.[86] Response to therapy is not well studied because of the rarity of this condition (3%–5% of GO patients) and the lack of a uniformly accepted definition.[87] Therapy for DON consists of IVGC, orbital decompression surgery, or both modalities.[88] A direct comparison between the 2 modalities showed that 83% of patients needed additional therapy with IVGC following decompressive surgery, whereas only 56% of patients needed further therapy for DON (decompression surgery or OR) following IVGC therapy.[89] Although both approaches suffered from a significant failure rate, DON ultimately resolved in all cases as patients failing one approach responded to the other. Mainly based on these data showing overall excellent results, the EUGOGO consensus statement advises starting with IVGC therapy and observing the response over a 2- to 3-week period.[17] A commonly followed regimen is the administration of 1.0 g methylprednisolone for 3 consecutive days, repeated 1 week later.[90] If no improvement is seen or deterioration is noted, patients should be referred promptly for orbital decompression surgery. Surgery may be indicated as first-line therapy if the corneal exposure from proptosis is significant, if congestive features are prominent, or if side effects of steroids are to be avoided. Sight-threatening corneal breakdown or ulceration typically results from one or a combination of the following: excessive proptosis, excessive eyelid retraction, incomplete blinks, or incomplete eyelid closure.

Initial treatment includes the frequent use of topical lubricants, intensive topical anti-biotics where appropriate, moisture chambers, and surgical procedures to temporarily cover the globe until healing has taken place. Occasionally orbital decompression, eyelid surgery or even corneal grafting is required.[17]

REHABILITATIVE TREATMENT

After the eye disease has been inactive for 3 to 6 months, a patient may be evaluated for rehabilitative surgery, which can have a positive impact on both ocular function and QOL. Intervening earlier before a stable baseline is reached may increase the likeli-hood that additional surgery will be needed in future. The surgical sequence is gener-ally orbital decompression (if needed), followed by extraocular muscle surgery (if needed), with eyelid procedures (if needed) performed last. Thus, changes induced by one intervention can be addressed in a subsequent step. Indications for orbital decompression include excessive proptosis, orbital congestion, corneal exposure, side effects of steroids, deep orbital pain, and enhanced cosmesis. Patients with DON, or those who have shown intolerance or insufficient response to immunosup-pressive therapy or who have debilitating retrobulbar or periorbital pain, may also benefit from this surgery. Decompressive surgery involves removal of one or more orbital walls, retrobulbar fat, or both, to expand the retrobulbar space, decrease orbital pressure, and allow the globe to recede. The extent of the surgery generally depends on the degree and distribution of extraocular muscle involvement; the improvement in proptosis is directly related to the number of orbital walls removed.[91,92] Following decompression surgery, preexisting diplopia may worsen or new diplopia develop in 10% to 50% of patients.[93,94] If diplopia is mild, the use of prisms inserted in the eyeglass lens may suffice. The goal of extraocular muscle surgery (strabismus surgery) is single vision in primary gaze and the reading position; diplopia with deviant gaze may persist after surgery. Multiple surgeries over an extended period are

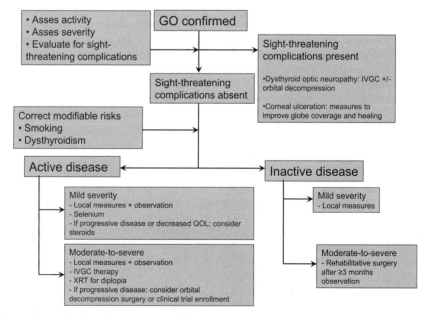

Fig. 2. Algorithm for the treatment of Graves ophthalmopathy.

sometimes needed to address limited extraocular muscle mobility. Eyelid surgery is generally performed to address symptomatic eyelid retraction or asymmetric lid position, its functional role being to ensure adequate corneal coverage. Upper lid retraction is relieved by weakening (recessing) the levator and/or Müller muscles. Lower lid retraction may be treated by recessing the lower lid retractors or, more typically, by inserting a spacer of some material, usually cartilage or a hard palate graft. Additional reconstructive procedures that may be performed include lateral tarsorrhaphy or blepharoplasty to remove excessive eyelid skin and eyelid fat. Removal of skin should be done with caution, as eyelid closure may be impaired if too much skin is removed.

SUMMARY

Optimum care of the patient with GO is achieved through teamwork between the endocrinologist and ophthalmologist, with input from ancillary specialists as needed. If no sight-threatening complications of the disease are initially identified, an accurate determination of disease activity and severity narrows the available treatment options to those most likely to benefit the patient (**Fig. 2**). Smoking and possible dysthyroidism constitute important modifiable risk factors for disease progression that should be addressed on diagnosis. Of importance is early assessment of the impact of disease on patients' QOL, and their priorities and expectations regarding management. Once this information has been gathered, careful discussion between patients and physicians can define the initial management plan, which includes the timing of the next visit and general parameters for a future change in course.

REFERENCES

1. Bahn RS. Graves' ophthalmopathy. N Engl J Med 2010;362:726–38.
2. Khoo DH, Eng PH, Ho SC, et al. Graves' ophthalmopathy in the absence of elevated free thyroxine and triiodothyronine levels: prevalence, natural history, and thyrotropin receptor antibody levels. Thyroid 2000;10:1093–100.
3. Wiersinga WM, Smit T, van der Gaag R, et al. Temporal relationship between onset of Graves' ophthalmopathy and onset of thyroidal Graves' disease. J Endocrinol Invest 1988;11:615–9.
4. Rundle FF, Wilson CW. Development and course of exophthalmos and ophthalmoplegia in Graves' disease with special reference to the effect of thyroidectomy. Clin Sci 1945;5:177–94.
5. Perros P, Crombie AL, Kendall-Taylor P. Natural history of thyroid associated ophthalmopathy. Clin Endocrinol 1995;42:45–50.
6. Bahn RS. Pathophysiology of Graves' ophthalmopathy: the cycle of disease. J Clin Endocrinol Metab 2003;88:1939–46.
7. Wiersinga WM. Autoimmunity in Graves' ophthalmopathy: the result of an unfortunate marriage between TSH receptors and IGF-1 receptors? J Clin Endocrinol Metab 2011;96:2386–94.
8. van Zeijl CJ, Fliers E, van Koppen CJ, et al. Thyrotropin receptor-stimulating Graves' disease immunoglobulins induce hyaluronan synthesis by differentiated orbital fibroblasts from patients with Graves' ophthalmopathy not only via cyclic adenosine monophosphate signaling pathways. Thyroid 2011;21:169–76.
9. Kumar S, Nadeem S, Stan MN, et al. A stimulatory TSH receptor antibody enhances adipogenesis via phosphoinositide 3-kinase activation in orbital preadipocytes from patients with Graves' ophthalmopathy. J Mol Endocrinol 2011;46:155–63.

10. Rapoport B, Alsabeh R, Aftergood D, et al. Elephantiasic pretibial myxedema: insight into and a hypothesis regarding the pathogenesis of the extrathyroidal manifestations of Graves' disease. Thyroid 2000;10:685–92.
11. Stan MN, Bahn RS. Risk factors for development or deterioration of Graves' ophthalmopathy. Thyroid 2010;20:777–83.
12. Tunbridge WM, Evered DC, Hall R, et al. The spectrum of thyroid disease in a community: the Whickham survey. Clin Endocrinol 1977;7:481–93.
13. Wiersinga WM, Bartalena L. Epidemiology and prevention of Graves' ophthalmopathy. Thyroid 2002;12:855–60.
14. Enzmann DR, Donaldson SS, Kriss JP. Appearance of Graves' disease on orbital computed tomography. J Comput Assist Tomogr 1979;3:815–9.
15. Bartley GB. The epidemiologic characteristics and clinical course of ophthalmopathy associated with autoimmune thyroid disease in Olmsted County, Minnesota. Trans Am Ophthalmol Soc 1994;92:477–588.
16. Fatourechi V. Pretibial myxedema: pathophysiology and treatment options. Am J Clin Dermatol 2005;6:295–309.
17. Bartalena L, Baldeschi L, Dickinson AJ, et al. Consensus statement of the European Group on Graves' Orbitopathy (EUGOGO) on management of Graves' orbitopathy. Thyroid 2008;18:333–46.
18. Mourits MP, Prummel MF, Wiersinga WM, et al. Clinical activity score as a guide in the management of patients with Graves' ophthalmopathy. Clin Endocrinol 1997; 47:9–14.
19. Wiersinga WM, Perros P, Kahaly GJ, et al. Clinical assessment of patients with Graves' orbitopathy: the European Group on Graves' Orbitopathy recommendations to generalists, specialists and clinical researchers. Eur J Endocrinol 2006; 155:387–9.
20. Yeatts RP. Quality of life in patients with Graves ophthalmopathy. Trans Am Ophthalmol Soc 2005;103:368–411.
21. Terwee CB, Gerding MN, Dekker FW, et al. Development of a disease specific quality of life questionnaire for patients with Graves' ophthalmopathy: the GO-QOL. Br J Ophthalmol 1998;82:773–9.
22. Terwee CB, Dekker FW, Mourits MP, et al. Interpretation and validity of changes in scores on the Graves' ophthalmopathy quality of life questionnaire (GO-QOL) after different treatments. Clin Endocrinol 2001;54:391–8.
23. Jacobson EM, Tomer Y. The CD40, CTLA-4, thyroglobulin, TSH receptor, and PTPN22 gene quintet and its contribution to thyroid autoimmunity: back to the future. J Autoimmun 2007;28:85–98.
24. Tsai CC, Kau HC, Kao SC, et al. Exophthalmos of patients with Graves' disease in Chinese of Taiwan. Eye 2006;20:569–73.
25. Burch HB, Wartofsky L. Graves' ophthalmopathy: current concepts regarding pathogenesis and management. Endocr Rev 1993;14:747–93.
26. Davies TF, Kendler DL. Mechanisms of human autoimmune thyroid disease. Monogr Pathol 1993;(35):103–17.
27. Prummel MF, Wiersinga WM, Mourits MP, et al. Effect of abnormal thyroid function on the severity of Graves' ophthalmopathy. Arch Intern Med 1990;150:1098–101.
28. Tallstedt L, Lundell G, Blomgren H, et al. Does early administration of thyroxine reduce the development of Graves' ophthalmopathy after radioiodine treatment? Eur J Endocrinol 1994;130:494–7.
29. Kung AW, Yau CC, Cheng A. The incidence of ophthalmopathy after radioiodine therapy for Graves' disease: prognostic factors and the role of methimazole. J Clin Endocrinol Metab 1994;79:542–6.

30. Baujat B, Krastinova D, Bach CA, et al. Orbital morphology in exophthalmos and exorbitism. Plast Reconstr Surg 2006;117:542–50 [discussion: 551–2].
31. Tallstedt L, Lundell G, Torring O, et al. Occurrence of ophthalmopathy after treatment for Graves' hyperthyroidism. The Thyroid Study Group [see comment]. N Engl J Med 1992;326:1733–8.
32. Traisk F, Tallstedt L, Abraham-Nordling M, et al. Thyroid-associated ophthalmopathy after treatment for Graves' hyperthyroidism with antithyroid drugs or iodine-131. J Clin Endocrinol Metab 2009;94:3700–7.
33. Pfeilschifter J, Ziegler R. Smoking and endocrine ophthalmopathy: impact of smoking severity and current vs lifetime cigarette consumption. Clin Endocrinol 1996;45:477–81.
34. Krassas GE, Segni M, Wiersinga WM. Childhood Graves' ophthalmopathy: results of a European questionnaire study. Eur J Endocrinol 2005;153:515–20.
35. Eckstein AK, Plicht M, Lax H, et al. Thyrotropin receptor autoantibodies are independent risk factors for Graves' ophthalmopathy and help to predict severity and outcome of the disease. J Clin Endocrinol Metab 2006;91:3464–70.
36. Gerding MN, van der Meer JW, Broenink M, et al. Association of thyrotrophin receptor antibodies with the clinical features of Graves' ophthalmopathy. Clin Endocrinol 2000;52:267–71.
37. Bartalena L, Marcocci C, Bogazzi F, et al. Relation between therapy for hyperthyroidism and the course of Graves' ophthalmopathy. N Engl J Med 1998;338:73–8.
38. Perros P, Kendall-Taylor P, Neoh C, et al. A prospective study of the effects of radioiodine therapy for hyperthyroidism in patients with minimally active graves' ophthalmopathy. J Clin Endocrinol Metab 2005;90:5321–3.
39. Eckstein A, Quadbeck B, Mueller G, et al. Impact of smoking on the response to treatment of thyroid associated ophthalmopathy. Br J Ophthalmol 2003;87:773–6.
40. Bartalena L, Marcocci C, Tanda ML, et al. Cigarette smoking and treatment outcomes in Graves ophthalmopathy. Ann Intern Med 1998;129:632–5.
41. Prummel MF, Wiersinga WM. Smoking and risk of Graves' disease. JAMA 1993;269:479–82.
42. Bartalena L, Marcocci C, Bogazzi F, et al. Use of corticosteroids to prevent progression of Graves' ophthalmopathy after radioiodine therapy for hyperthyroidism. N Engl J Med 1989;321:1349–52.
43. Bahn RS, Burch HB, Cooper DS, et al. Hyperthyroidism and other causes of thyrotoxicosis: management guidelines of the American Thyroid Association and American Association of Clinical Endocrinologists. Thyroid 2011;20:593–646.
44. Baldeschi L, Wakelkamp IM, Lindeboom R, et al. Early versus late orbital decompression in Graves' orbitopathy: a retrospective study in 125 patients. Ophthalmology 2006;113:874–8.
45. Bahn RS, Burch HB, Cooper DS, et al. Hyperthyroidism and other causes of thyrotoxicosis: management guidelines of the American Thyroid Association and American Association of Clinical Endocrinologists. Endocr Pract 2011;17:456–520.
46. Lai A, Sassi L, Compri E, et al. Lower dose prednisone prevents radioiodine-associated exacerbation of initially mild or absent graves' orbitopathy: a retrospective cohort study. J Clin Endocrinol Metab 2010;95:1333–7.
47. Uddin JM, Davies PD. Treatment of upper eyelid retraction associated with thyroid eye disease with subconjunctival botulinum toxin injection. Ophthalmology 2002;109:1183–7.
48. Bouzas EA, Karadimas P, Mastorakos G, et al. Antioxidant agents in the treatment of Graves' ophthalmopathy. Am J Ophthalmol 2000;129:618–22.

49. Marcocci C, Kahaly GJ, Krassas GE, et al. Selenium and the course of mild Graves' orbitopathy. N Engl J Med 2011;364:1920–31.
50. Zang S, Ponto KA, Kahaly GJ. Clinical review: intravenous glucocorticoids for Graves' orbitopathy: efficacy and morbidity. J Clin Endocrinol Metab 2011;96: 320–32.
51. Kahaly GJ, Pitz S, Hommel G, et al. Randomized, single blind trial of intravenous versus oral steroid monotherapy in Graves' orbitopathy. J Clin Endocrinol Metab 2005;90:5234–40.
52. Macchia PE, Bagattini M, Lupoli G, et al. High-dose intravenous corticosteroid therapy for Graves' ophthalmopathy. J Endocrinol Invest 2001;24:152–8.
53. Le Moli R, Baldeschi L, Saeed P, et al. Determinants of liver damage associated with intravenous methylprednisolone pulse therapy in Graves' ophthalmopathy. Thyroid 2007;17:357–62.
54. Marino M, Morabito E, Brunetto MR, et al. Acute and severe liver damage associated with intravenous glucocorticoid pulse therapy in patients with Graves' ophthalmopathy. Thyroid 2004;14:403–6.
55. Marcocci C, Watt T, Altea MA, et al. Fatal and non-fatal adverse events of glucocorticoid therapy for Graves' orbitopathy: a questionnaire survey among members of the European Thyroid Association. Eur J Endocrinol 2012;166(2):247–53.
56. Bahn R. High-dose intravenous glucocorticoid therapy for Graves' ophthalmopathy: where are we now? Thyroid 2012;22:1–2.
57. Ebner R, Devoto MH, Weil D, et al. Treatment of thyroid associated ophthalmopathy with periocular injections of triamcinolone. Br J Ophthalmol 2004;88:1380–6.
58. Kahaly G, Schrezenmeir J, Krause U, et al. Cyclosporin and prednisone versus prednisone in treatment of Graves' ophthalmopathy: a controlled, randomized and prospective study. Eur J Clin Invest 1986;16:415–22.
59. Prummel MF, Mourits MP, Berghout A, et al. Prednisone and cyclosporine in the treatment of severe Graves' ophthalmopathy. N Engl J Med 1989;321:1353–9.
60. Perros P, Weightman DR, Crombie AL, et al. Azathioprine in the treatment of thyroid-associated ophthalmopathy. Acta Endocrinol 1990;122:8–12.
61. Kahaly G, Pitz S, Muller-Forell W, et al. Randomized trial of intravenous immunoglobulins versus prednisolone in Graves' ophthalmopathy. Clin Exp Immunol 1996;106:197–202.
62. Baschieri L, Antonelli A, Nardi S, et al. Intravenous immunoglobulin versus corticosteroid in treatment of Graves' ophthalmopathy. Thyroid 1997;7:579–85.
63. Dickinson AJ, Vaidya B, Miller M, et al. Double-blind, placebo-controlled trial of octreotide long-acting repeatable (LAR) in thyroid-associated ophthalmopathy. J Clin Endocrinol Metab 2004;89:5910–5.
64. Wemeau JL, Caron P, Beckers A, et al. Octreotide (long-acting release formulation) treatment in patients with Graves' orbitopathy: clinical results of a four-month, randomized, placebo-controlled, double-blind study. J Clin Endocrinol Metab 2005;90:841–8.
65. Chang TC, Liao SL. Slow-release lanreotide in Graves' ophthalmopathy: a double-blind randomized, placebo-controlled clinical trial. J Endocrinol Invest 2006;29:413–22.
66. Stan MN, Garrity JA, Bradley EA, et al. Randomized, double-blind, placebo-controlled trial of long-acting release octreotide for treatment of Graves' ophthalmopathy. J Clin Endocrinol Metab 2006;91:4817–24.
67. El Fassi D, Banga JP, Gilbert JA, et al. Treatment of Graves' disease with rituximab specifically reduces the production of thyroid stimulating autoantibodies. Clin Immunol 2009;130:252–8.

68. Salvi M, Vannucchi G, Campi I, et al. Efficacy of rituximab treatment for thyroid-associated ophthalmopathy as a result of intraorbital B-cell depletion in one patient unresponsive to steroid immunosuppression. Eur J Endocrinol 2006;154:511–7.
69. El Fassi D, Nielsen CH, Hasselbalch HC, et al. Treatment-resistant severe, active Graves' ophthalmopathy successfully treated with B lymphocyte depletion. Thyroid 2006;16:709–10.
70. Khanna D, Chong KK, Afifiyan NF, et al. Rituximab treatment of patients with severe, corticosteroid-resistant thyroid-associated ophthalmopathy. Ophthalmology 2010;117:133–9, e132.
71. Heemstra KA, Toes RE, Sepers J, et al. Rituximab in relapsing Graves' disease, a phase II study. Eur J Endocrinol 2008;159:609–15.
72. Bradley EA, Gower EW, Bradley DJ, et al. Orbital radiation for Graves ophthalmopathy: a report by the American Academy of Ophthalmology. Ophthalmology 2008;115:398–409.
73. Prummel MF, Mourits MP, Blank L, et al. Randomized double-blind trial of prednisone versus radiotherapy in Graves' ophthalmopathy. Lancet 1993;342:949–54.
74. Prummel MF, Terwee CB, Gerding MN, et al. A randomized controlled trial of orbital radiotherapy versus sham irradiation in patients with mild Graves' ophthalmopathy. J Clin Endocrinol Metab 2004;89:15–20.
75. Kahaly GJ, Rosler HP, Pitz S, et al. Low- versus high-dose radiotherapy for Graves' ophthalmopathy: a randomized, single blind trial [see comment]. J Clin Endocrinol Metab 2000;85:102–8.
76. Marcocci C, Bartalena L, Bogazzi F, et al. Orbital radiotherapy combined with high dose systemic glucocorticoids for Graves' ophthalmopathy is more effective than radiotherapy alone: results of a prospective randomized study. J Endocrinol Invest 1991;14:853–60.
77. Gorman CA, Garrity JA, Fatourechi V, et al. A prospective, randomized, double-blind, placebo-controlled study of orbital radiotherapy for Graves' ophthalmopathy [see comment]. Ophthalmology 2001;108:1523–34 [erratum appears in Ophthalmology 2004;111(7):1306].
78. Gerling J, Kommerell G, Henne K, et al. Retrobulbar irradiation for thyroid-associated orbitopathy: double-blind comparison between 2.4 and 16 Gy. Int J Radiat Oncol Biol Phys 2003;55:182–9.
79. Bartalena L, Marcocci C, Chiovato L, et al. Orbital cobalt irradiation combined with systemic corticosteroids for Graves' ophthalmopathy: comparison with systemic corticosteroids alone. J Clin Endocrinol Metab 1983;56:1139–44.
80. Marcocci C, Bartalena L, Tanda ML, et al. Comparison of the effectiveness and tolerability of intravenous or oral glucocorticoids associated with orbital radiotherapy in the management of severe Graves' ophthalmopathy: results of a prospective, single-blind, randomized study. J Clin Endocrinol Metab 2001; 86:3562–7.
81. Ohtsuka K, Sato A, Kawaguchi S, et al. Effect of steroid pulse therapy with and without orbital radiotherapy on Graves' ophthalmopathy. Am J Ophthalmol 2003;135:285–90.
82. Marcocci C, Bartalena L, Rocchi R, et al. Long-term safety of orbital radiotherapy for Graves' ophthalmopathy. J Clin Endocrinol Metab 2003;88:3561–6.
83. Wakelkamp IM, Tan H, Saeed P, et al. Orbital irradiation for Graves' ophthalmopathy: is it safe? A long-term follow-up study. Ophthalmology 2004;111:1557–62.
84. Menconi F, Marino M, Pinchera A, et al. Effects of total thyroid ablation versus near-total thyroidectomy alone on mild to moderate Graves' orbitopathy treated with intravenous glucocorticoids. J Clin Endocrinol Metab 2007;92:1653–8.

85. Jarhult J, Rudberg C, Larsson E, et al. Graves' disease with moderate-severe endocrine ophthalmopathy-long term results of a prospective, randomized study of total or subtotal thyroid resection. Thyroid 2005;15:1157–64.

86. Feldon SE, Muramatsu S, Weiner JM. Clinical classification of Graves' ophthalmopathy. Identification of risk factors for optic neuropathy. Arch Ophthalmol 1984; 102:1469–72.

87. Wiersinga WM, Prummel MF. Graves' ophthalmopathy: a rational approach to treatment. Trends Endocrinol Metab 2002;13:280–7.

88. Soares-Welch CV, Fatourechi V, Bartley GB, et al. Optic neuropathy of Graves disease: results of transantral orbital decompression and long-term follow-up in 215 patients. Am J Ophthalmol 2003;136:433–41.

89. Wakelkamp IM, Baldeschi L, Saeed P, et al. Surgical or medical decompression as a first-line treatment of optic neuropathy in Graves' ophthalmopathy? A randomized controlled trial. Clin Endocrinol 2005;63:323–8.

90. Wiersinga WM. Management of Graves' ophthalmopathy. Nat Clin Pract Endocrinol Metab 2007;3:396–404.

91. Baldeschi L, MacAndie K, Hintschich C, et al. The removal of the deep lateral wall in orbital decompression: its contribution to exophthalmos reduction and influence on consecutive diplopia. Am J Ophthalmol 2005;140:642–7.

92. Cansiz H, Yilmaz S, Karaman E, et al. Three-wall orbital decompression superiority to 2-wall orbital decompression in thyroid-associated ophthalmopathy. J Oral Maxillofac Surg 2006;64:763–9.

93. Mourits MP, Koornneef L, Wiersinga WM, et al. Orbital decompression for Graves' ophthalmopathy by inferomedial, by inferomedial plus lateral, and by coronal approach. Ophthalmology 1990;97:636–41.

94. Boulos PR, Hardy I. Thyroid-associated orbitopathy: a clinicopathologic and therapeutic review. Curr Opin Ophthalmol 2004;15:389–400.

Thyroid Nodules

Geanina Popoveniuc, MD[a,b], Jacqueline Jonklaas, MD, PhD[a,*]

KEYWORDS

- Thyroid nodule • TSH • Ultrasonography • FNA biopsy
- Elastography • Molecular markers • Indeterminate cytology
- Malignancy

INTRODUCTION

Thyroid nodules are common entities, frequently discovered in clinical practice, either during physical examination, but also incidentally, during various imaging procedures. They are clinically important primarily due to their malignant potential. For this reason the initial evaluation should always include a history and physical examination focusing on features suggestive of malignancy. Serum thyrotropin (TSH) and thyroid ultrasonography (US) are pivotal in the evaluation of thyroid nodules, as they provide important information regarding thyroid nodule functionality and the presence of features suspicious for malignancy, respectively. Fine needle aspiration (FNA) biopsy is the most accurate and reliable tool for diagnosing thyroid malignancy and selecting candidates for surgery, particularly if performed under ultrasound guidance. The cytology findings from FNA biopsies will fall into an indeterminate category in approximately 25% of the cases, in which case malignancy cannot be safely excluded. The recent use of panels of gene mutations and molecular markers, when combined with the cytologic diagnosis, show promising results in improving the preoperative diagnosis of indeterminate thyroid nodules, thus reducing the number of unnecessary surgeries. Other tools for predicting the malignant potential of thyroid nodules still under investigation include elastography and 18F-fluorodeoxyglucose positron emission tomography (18FDG-PET) scanning. An approach to the initial evaluation and management of single nodules, functioning nodules, multinodular glands, incidental nodules, and cysts are discussed. Therapeutic interventions for benign nodules, when needed, may include surgery, radioiodine (131-I) therapy, or percutaneous

J.J. is supported by grant 1UL1RR031975 from the National Center for Research Resources, National Institutes of Health. Funding for publication of the figures in this article was provided by the Graduate Medical Education office at Washington Hospital Center.
Disclosure Summary: The authors have nothing to disclose.
a Division of Endocrinology, Georgetown University Medical Center, 4000 Reservoir Road, NW, Washington, DC 20007, USA
b Section of Endocrinology, Washington Hospital Center, 110 Irving Street, NW, Washington, DC 20010, USA
* Corresponding author. Division of Endocrinology, Georgetown University Medical Center, Suite 230, Building D, 4000 Reservoir Road, NW, Washington, DC 20007.
E-mail address: jonklaaj@georgetown.edu

Med Clin N Am 96 (2012) 329–349
doi:10.1016/j.mcna.2012.02.002
0025-7125/12/$ – see front matter © 2012 Elsevier Inc. All rights reserved.

ethanol injection (PEI), as indicated. Levothyroxine (T4) suppressive therapy is currently controversial and usually not recommended. The evaluation of thyroid nodules discovered during pregnancy is generally the same as for non-pregnant patients, except for the contraindication to radionuclide scanning. Thyroid cancer discovered during pregnancy may be safely managed by thyroidectomy after delivery in most of the cases, but if aggressive features are present, surgery should be ideally performed during the second trimester.

DEFINITION, CLINICAL IMPORTANCE, EPIDEMIOLOGY

- *Thyroid nodules are most common in women and older populations*
- *The purpose of thyroid nodule evaluation is to determine which nodules are malignant or require surgical attention*

Thyroid nodules have been defined by the American Thyroid Association (ATA) as "discrete lesions within the thyroid gland, radiologically distinct from surrounding thyroid parenchyma."[1] They may be discovered by palpation during a general physical examination or with radiographic studies performed for medical evaluations, such as carotid duplex ultrasound (US), computed tomography (CT) scans, magnetic resonance imaging (MRI) studies, or 18FDG-PET scanning. The latter entities are called "thyroid incidentalomas" and they generally do not correspond to palpable thyroid lesions. Conversely, clinicians may identify palpable thyroid lesions that do not correspond to distinct radiological entities, and therefore would not be defined as thyroid nodules.[2]

Thyroid nodules are common, their prevalence being largely dependent on the identification method. The estimated prevalence by palpation alone ranges from 4% to 7%,[3,4] whereas US detects nodules in 20% to 76% of the adult population,[4–6] particularly with the current use of high-resolution US techniques.[7] The reported frequencies detected by US correlate with the prevalence reported at surgery and autopsy with ranges between 50% and 65%.[8]

The estimated annual incidence of thyroid nodules in the United States is approximately 0.1% per year, conferring a 10% lifetime probability for developing a thyroid nodule.[6] Thyroid nodules are 4 times more common in women than men and their frequency increases with age and low iodine intake.[4] The gender disparity is perhaps explained by the hormonal influences of both estrogen and progesterone, as increasing nodule size and new nodule development have been demonstrated to be related to pregnancy and multiparity.[9,10] Exposure to ionizing radiation, either during childhood, or as an occupational exposure, will cause a rate of development of thyroid nodules of 2% per year, reaching a peak incidence in 15 to 25 years.[11,12]

Thyroid nodules are clinically important for several reasons. They may cause thyroid dysfunction and, rarely, compressive symptoms, but they are primarily important because of the need to exclude thyroid cancer. The reported prevalence of malignancy in thyroid nodules evaluated by biopsy ranges from 4.0% to 6.5% and is largely independent of the nodule size.[13,14] Despite this, papillary microcarcinomas (smaller than 1 cm) incidentally found at the time of surgery are much more common (up to 36%),[15,16] but it is controversial whether or not a survival benefit exists with the diagnosis and treatment of such entities, given their generally benign course.[17,18] Importantly, the incidence of thyroid nodules discovered incidentally during 18FDG-PET imaging is small (1%–2%), but the risk of malignancy may be as high as 27%, thus such nodules require immediate evaluation.[19]

HISTORY AND PHYSICAL EXAMINATION

- *History and physical examination should focus on detecting features particularly suggestive of malignancy*

The spectrum of disorders associated with thyroid nodules ranges from benign etiologies to malignant conditions that may either have an indolent course or a very aggressive behavior (**Box 1**). Therefore, clinical evaluation is best tailored to identification of clues suggestive of malignant disease. A careful history and physical examination should include information regarding previous radiation treatment of the head and neck area; growth of a neck mass; location, size, and consistency of the thyroid nodule; cervical lymphadenopathy; associated local symptoms such as pain, hoarseness, dysphagia, dysphonia, and dyspnea; and symptoms of hypothyroidism or hyperthyroidism.

Family history of thyroid disorders should always be investigated. Rare but important familial thyroid syndromes include familial medullary thyroid cancer (MTC), derived from calcitonin-producing C-cell tumors, and familial nonmedullary thyroid cancer, which is derived from follicular cells. History of papillary thyroid cancer (PTC) in a parent or sibling increases the patient's risk of developing PTC by threefold and sixfold, respectively.[20] Familial MTC may be a component of multiple endocrine neoplasia (MEN) IIA (pheochromocytoma, MTC, and primary hyperparathyroidism) and IIB (pheochromocytoma, MTC, marfanoid habitus, and mucosal and digestive neurofibromatosis), or may occur as the sole component. Follicular cell–derived familial thyroid cancer has been described in several syndromes, such as Cowden disease, Carney complex, Werner

---

Box 1
Etiology of thyroid nodules

Benign etiology

Follicular adenoma

Hurthle cell adenoma

Colloid cyst

Simple or hemorrhagic cyst

Lymphocytic thyroiditis

Granulomatous thyroiditis

Infectious processes

Malignant etiology

Malignancy of follicular or C-cell origin

    Papillary carcinoma

    Follicular carcinoma

    Hurthle cell carcinoma

    Medullary thyroid carcinoma

    Anaplastic carcinoma

Malignancy of other origin

    Thyroid lymphoma

    Malignancy metastatic to the thyroid

syndrome, and familial polyposis, as well as occurring in isolation. Cowden disease is an autosomal dominant condition, resulting from a mutation in the PTEN gene, and is characterized by hamartomatous neoplasms of the skin, oral mucosa, gastrointestinal tract, central nervous and genitourinary systems, with breast and thyroid cancers being the most commonly encountered malignancies.[21,22] Carney complex, another autosomal dominant condition, is characterized by cardiac and cutaneous myxomas, spotty skin pigmentation, various endocrinopathies, and malignancies of endocrine and nonendocrine origin.[23] Less commonly, thyroid cancer can be encountered in patients with Werner syndrome, of which the main characteristic is premature aging, and familial polyposis, which is primarily associated with colon cancer.

A personal history of head and neck irradiation, particularly as a child, young age (<20 years), or advanced age (>70 years), and male sex are demographic features associated with increased likelihood of malignancy in a patient with a thyroid nodule. **Table 1** summarizes clinical features that should alert the clinician to the possibility of thyroid carcinoma in a patient with a thyroid nodule.[13] It is important to know that symptoms, such as hoarseness, dysphagia, and cough, are rarely related to thyroid conditions, and a thorough workup should be pursued to exclude other, more common etiologies related to gastrointestinal and respiratory systems.

DIAGNOSTIC STUDIES

A spectrum of diagnostic studies is available to aid in the evaluation of a thyroid nodule (**Fig. 1**). These include serum markers, such as serum thyrotropin (TSH) and calcitonin. Fine-needle aspiration (FNA) cytology is the cornerstone of thyroid nodule evaluation. Genetic markers of thyroid cancer risk, such as the BRAF mutation, can also be determined using cytology samples. In addition, immunohistochemical markers, such as galectin-3, cyclooxygenase 2, and cyclin D2, may have potential use. Ultrasonography plays a pivotal role in the evaluation of thyroid nodules, and elastography may prove to

Table 1
Features suggestive of increased potential for thyroid carcinoma in a patient with thyroid nodule

Patient History or Characteristics	Findings on Physical Examination	Findings Seen on Imaging
Family history of MEN, MTC, and PTC	Firm nodule	Suspicious ultrasound features
History of head and neck irradiation	Nodule fixed to adjacent structures	Lymphadenopathy
History of Hodgkin and non-Hodgkin lymphoma	Growth of nodule, especially during therapy to suppress serum TSH	
Age <20	Abnormal cervical lymphadenopathy	
Age >70	Paralysis of the vocal cords	
Male sex		
Symptoms of compression: hoarseness, dysphagia, dysphonia, dyspnea, cough		

Abbreviations: MEN, multiple endocrine neoplasia; MTC, medullary thyroid cancer; PTC, papillary thyroid cancer; TSH, serum thyrotropin.

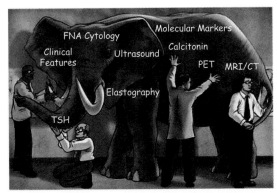

Fig. 1. Diagnostic studies available for evaluating thyroid nodules. (*Modified from* figure provided by Dr BR Haugen, University of Colorado at Denver and Health Sciences Center, Aurora, CO; with permission.)

be a valuable addition. Other imaging studies, including MRI, CT, and 18FDG-PET scans may be helpful in certain circumstances.

Serum Markers

- *The risk of malignancy in thyroid nodules increases as the serum TSH increases*

TSH measurement should be part of the initial workup in every patient with a thyroid nodule and be used as a guide for further management (**Fig. 2**).[1,24,25] A normal or high TSH level should raise concerns for possible malignant potential of a nodule, whereas a low TSH is an indicator of benignity in most cases. Therefore, the next step in the evaluation of a patient with a low TSH would be an iodine-123 (123-I) or pertechnetate scintigraphy scan, to explore the possibility of an autonomously functioning nodule. Hyperfunctioning thyroid nodules are almost always benign and generally do not require further cytologic investigation,[26,27] but a nonfunctioning or "cold" nodule in a patient with low TSH may indicate malignant potential. Recent studies have investigated the relationship between serum TSH concentration and thyroid cancer. TSH was found to be an independent predictor of malignancy in thyroid nodules.[28] The risk of malignancy rises in parallel with serum TSH, even within the normal range, and higher TSH levels were found to be associated with advanced-stage thyroid cancer.[26,29–31]

Calcitonin is a sensitive marker for detection of C-cell hyperplasia and MTC, as well as for surveillance and prognosis of MTC.[32] Calcitonin levels of more than 10 pg/mL were found to have high sensitivity for the detection of MTC,[33] with the specificity being enhanced by pentagastrin stimulation, when calcitonin levels exceed 100 pg/mL. Even though calcitonin screening was proved to be cost-effective and a useful tool in the evaluation algorithm for thyroid nodules,[34] it is not widely recognized in US,[1] partly because of the low prevalence of medullary thyroid cancer and lack of pentagastrin availability.

Serum thyroglobulin measurement is neither sensitive nor specific for the diagnosis of thyroid cancer in nodular thyroid disease, being more influenced by iodine intake and thyroid gland size.[35] Therefore, it is not recommended to be routinely measured in the initial evaluation of a thyroid nodule.[1]

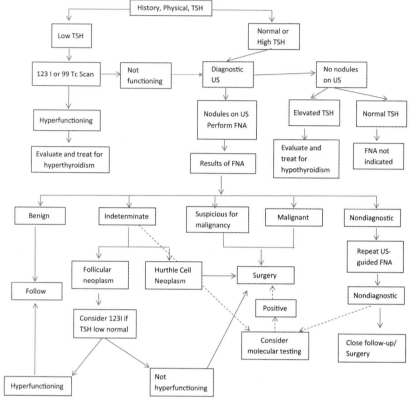

Fig. 2. Algorithm for initial evaluation of a patient with thyroid nodule. (*Modified from* Cooper DS. Revised American Thyroid Association management guidelines for patients with thyroid nodules and differentiated thyroid cancer. Thyroid 2009;19(11):1167–214; with permission.)

Thyroid Ultrasonography

- *Thyroid US allows targeting of nodules with suspicious appearance for biopsy*

Thyroid US is an important technique widely used in the detection and evaluation of thyroid nodules. It is a noninvasive, inexpensive procedure that provides information with regard to nodule dimensions, structure, and thyroid parenchymal changes. Nowadays, the use of brightness-mode US and high-frequency transducers may detect lesions as small as 2 to 3 mm, which raises the question of which thyroid nodules are clinically relevant for further evaluation.

Previous studies have investigated the ability of thyroid US to differentiate between benign and malignant lesions to avoid the unnecessary use of invasive procedures.[36–39] As a result, several US features have been found to be indicative of malignant potential. Microcalcifications (**Fig. 3**), irregular or microlobulated margins, hypoechogenicity, taller-than-wide shape, and increased intranodular vascularity (**Fig. 4**) were found to be independent risk factors for malignancy.[38,40,41] Even though these suspicious features are characterized by high specificity, their positive predictive value is lowered by their relatively low sensitivity (**Table 2**). It is important to know that none of these US features alone is sufficient to differentiate benign from

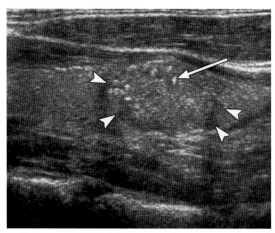

Fig. 3. US image of a thyroid nodule (*arrowheads*) containing multiple fine punctuate echogenicities (*arrow*) with no comet-tail artifact, indicating high suspicion for malignancy. FNA and surgery confirmed PTC. (*Reproduced from* Frates MC. Management of thyroid nodules detected at US: Society of Radiologists in Ultrasound consensus conference statement. Radiology 2005;237:794–800; with permission.)

malignant tumors, but a combination of at least 2 of them better succeeds in pointing out a subset of lesions at high risk for malignancy.[42,43] Papini and colleagues[38] demonstrated that nodules with a hypoechoic appearance and one of the other suspicious US characteristics successfully identifies thyroid lesions that need to undergo further cytologic examination. For example, a predominantly solid nodule with microcalcifications has a 31.6% likelihood of malignancy, whereas a predominantly cystic

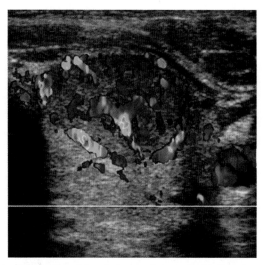

Fig. 4. Color Doppler US of a thyroid nodule showing marked internal vascularity, indicating increased likelihood of malignancy. Histology demonstrated PTC. (*Reproduced from* Frates MC. Management of thyroid nodules detected at US: Society of Radiologists in Ultrasound consensus conference statement. Radiology 2005;237:794–800; with permission.)

Table 2
Ultrasound characteristics of thyroid nodules predictive of malignancy

Ultrasound Feature	Sensitivity, %	Specificity, %	Positive Predictive Value, %	Negative Predictive Value, %
Microcalcifications	26.1–59.1	85.8–95.0	24.3–70.7	41.8–94.2
Hypoechogenicity	26.5–87.1	43.4–94.3	11.4–68.4	73.5–93.8
Irregular margins or no halo	17.4–77.5	38.9–85.0	9.3–60.0	38.9–97.8
Solid	69.0–75.0	52.5–55.9	15.6–27.0	88.0–92.1
Intranodule vascularity	54.3–74.2	78.6–80.8	24.0–41.9	85.7–97.4
More tall than wide	32.7	92.5	66.7	74.8

Reproduced from Frates MC. Management of thyroid nodules detected at US: Society of Radiologists in Ultrasound consensus conference statement. Radiology 2005;237(3):794–800; with permission.

lesion (**Fig. 5**) with no microcalcifications lowers the probability for being cancer to 1.0%.[44] US findings such as isoechogenicity and spongiform appearance (defined as aggregations of multiple microcysts in more than 50% of the nodule) are features highly suggestive of benignity.[41]

The number of nodules and their size are not predictive of malignancy, as a nodule smaller than 1 cm is as likely as a larger nodule to harbor neoplastic cells in the presence of suspicious US features.[44,45] Choosing an arbitrary size as cutoff for the likelihood of cancer or stratifying the risk in a multinodular goiter based on the "dominant" nodule has fallen into disfavor.[38]

US identification of cervical lymph nodes demonstrating microcalcifications, increased vascularity, cystic changes, and rounded shape, along with coexisting ipsilateral thyroid nodules, are also very important clues for malignant etiology.[42] Evidence of extracapsular growth, which may range from invasion of the thyroid capsule to perithyroidal muscle infiltration and recurrent laryngeal nerve extension, is another strong indicator of malignancy.[42,43]

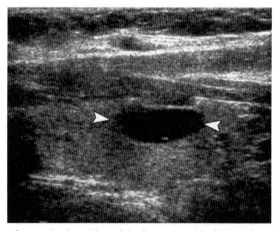

Fig. 5. US image of a cystic thyroid nodule (*arrowheads*). (*Reproduced from* Frates MC. Management of thyroid nodules detected at US: Society of Radiologists in Ultrasound consensus conference statement. Radiology 2005;237:794–800; with permission.)

Screening for thyroid nodules by US, or by any other types of imaging studies, is not recommended in the general population because of the minimal aggressiveness and indolent course of most of the thyroid cancers. Current ATA guidelines[1] recommend diagnostic thyroid sonography to be performed only in patients with known or suspected thyroid nodules, or in the presence of risk factors.[24,46]

Other diagnostic imaging techniques, such as MRI and CT scans, are not indicated for routine thyroid nodule evaluation, but they may be helpful for the assessment of nodule size, substernal extension of a nodular goiter, and airway compression.[25]

Elastography

- *Elastography is a promising tool for predicting the malignant potential of thyroid nodules*

A recent advancement in the diagnosis of thyroid nodules has been brought by the use of elastography. This is a dynamic technique that assesses the hardness of the tissue as an indicator of malignancy.[47] This technique was demonstrated to be highly specific (96%–100%) and sensitive (82%–97%) in the diagnostic evaluation of thyroid nodules, independent of nodule size, or location within the thyroid gland.[48,49] It was also found to be reliable in the diagnostic evaluation of indeterminate/follicular lesions, but this aspect of its use still needs to be confirmed.[50] The diagnostic yield of elastography is impaired in nodules with a calcified shell, cystic lesions, and multinodular goiter with coalescent nodules, because the margins need to be well demarcated for proper interpretation.[51] It is not suitable for diagnosis of follicular carcinoma and its use is restricted to high-end US devices. Although more data from larger prospective studies is needed to establish the accuracy of this diagnostic technique, it remains a promising tool in selecting nodules for FNA.

FNA Biopsy

- *FNA, in conjunction with US, forms the cornerstone of thyroid nodule evaluation*

Thyroid FNA biopsy is the most reliable, safe, and cost-effective diagnostic tool used in the evaluation of thyroid nodules.[52,53] FNA under US guidance is preferred over the palpation-guided approach because of lower rates of false-negative and nondiagnostic cytology.[54] This is particularly true for nodules that are nonpalpable, located deeply in the thyroid bed, or have a predominantly cystic component.[1]

The decision to pursue FNA sampling should be based on a risk-stratifying approach that includes history, US characteristics, and nodule size (**Table 3**). Subcentimeter nodules should be biopsied only if there is more than 1 suspicious US characteristic, extracapsular growth, abnormal cervical lymph nodes, or high-risk history (see **Table 1**). Otherwise, a cutoff size of 1 cm can be used for solid nodules that have only 1 suspicious sonographic feature, such as microcalcifications or hypoechoic appearance. Mixed cystic-solid nodules should undergo biopsy if they are more than 1.5 cm in size and the solid component should be targeted for biopsy. Purely cystic and spongiform lesions are considered to have low risk for malignancy; therefore, they could be either monitored or biopsied if larger than 2 cm (see **Table 3**).

Cytologic diagnosis

- *FNA based on an adequate sample is 95% accurate for diagnosing thyroid cancer*

Almost 20% of FNA results are nondiagnostic, because of sampling error or poor preparation technique.[55] In such cases, it is recommended that a repeat FNA be

Table 3
Sonographic and clinical features of thyroid nodules and recommendations for FNA

Nodule Sonographic or Clinical Features	Recommended[a] Nodule Threshold Size for FNA	
High-risk history		
Nodule with suspicious sonographic features	>5 mm	Recommendation A
Nodule without suspicious sonographic features	>5 mm	Recommendation I
Abnormal cervical lymph nodes	All	Recommendation A
Microcalcifications present in nodule	≥1 cm	Recommendation B
Solid nodule		
And hypoechoic	>1 cm	Recommendation B
And iso- or hyperechoic	≥1–1.5 cm	Recommendation C
Mixed cystic-solid nodule		
With any suspicious ultrasound features	≥1.5–2.0 cm	Recommendation B
Without suspicious ultrasound features	≥2.0 cm	Recommendation C
Spongiform nodule	≥2.0 cm[b]	Recommendation C
Purely cystic nodule	FNA not indicated[c]	Recommendation E

Abbreviation: FNA, fine-needle aspiration.

[a] Explanation of Recommendations: A, strongly recommends based on good evidence; B, recommends, based on fair evidence; C, recommends based on expert opinion; E, recommends against based on fair evidence; I, recommends neither for nor against, evidence insufficient.

[b] Sonographic monitoring without biopsy may be an acceptable alternative.

[c] Unless indicated as therapeutic modality.

Modified from Cooper D. Revised American Thyroid Association management guidelines for patients with thyroid nodules and differentiated thyroid cancer. Thyroid 2009;19(11):1167–214; with permission.

performed under US guidance, and if available, on-site cytologic examination for better cytologic adequacy.[56,57] Approximately 7% of the nodules will still yield unsatisfactory cytologic results on repeated biopsies. In this situation, surgery is strongly recommended for solid nodules and close observation or surgery for partially cystic lesions, as they may harbor neoplastic potential.[1,58]

Diagnostic FNA results are divided into 5 categories, based on the recent Bethesda System for Reporting Thyroid Cytopathology[59]: benign (70%), malignant (5%), suspicious for malignancy, follicular or Hurthle cell neoplasm, and follicular lesions of undetermined significance or atypia. The last 3 cytologic diagnoses, which represent 25% of the total cases, have been previously classified as indeterminate lesions. They have a predicted probability for cancer of 50% to 75%, 20% to 30%, and 5% to 10%, respectively.[59]

The most common benign lesions include colloid nodule, macrofollicular adenoma, and lymphocytic thyroiditis, among others.[24] The most prevalent malignant lesions by far are represented by PTC, followed by follicular thyroid cancer (FTC), MTC, anaplastic carcinoma, and high-grade metastatic neoplasms.[60] Suspicious lesions may represent PTC that lacks definitive diagnostic criteria, follicular neoplasm, Hurthle cell neoplasm, lymphoma, or PTC-follicular variant.

Surgery, with lobectomy or total thyroidectomy is the treatment of choice for malignant and suspicious lesions.[1] The same is true for follicular lesions, unless the nodule is found to be autonomous on a 123-I scan in the setting of low-normal TSH.[1] Thyroid nodules larger than 3 cm with mixed cystic/solid components should be strongly considered for surgery for diagnostic purposes, as FNA yields a high rate of false-negative results in these lesions.[61]

Indeterminate cytology

- *The cytology findings from some FNA biopsies fall into an indeterminate category in which malignancy cannot reliably be excluded*
- *Panels of gene mutations may serve as markers of which patients with cytologically indeterminate nodules may safely avoid surgery*

Current management for most patients with indeterminate cytology at FNA biopsy consists of diagnostic surgery to establish a histopathological diagnosis. However, only 10–40% of these cases will turn out to be malignant,[59,62] leading to more than 60% of surgeries being unnecessary, with their associated risks and costs. The evaluation of genetic markers associated with thyroid carcinoma (PTC: BRAF, RAS, RET/PTC; FTC: PAX8/PPARγ1) in the cytology specimen has been shown to improve preoperative diagnosis of thyroid nodules in large prospective studies, particularly when used in combination with cytologic features.[63,64] For example, in a Korean population, the combination of both cytology and BRAF mutation status increased the specificity of testing from 36% to 95% compared with FNA cytology alone.[65] The use of molecular markers, in the form of a panel of gene mutations, in patients with indeterminate cytology on FNA samples has been shown to increase the probability of cancer from 24% to 89% if any mutation is identified, whereas the lack of any mutation decreases the risk to 11%.[66] Cost-effectiveness analysis using a molecular panel of gene markers, coupled with classical cytologic findings, to increase the predictive power of diagnostic interpretations shows promising results when compared with the surgical approach, and is likely to be used in the future in clinical practice.[67]

Currently, there are 2 commercially available assays that provide molecular testing of the thyroid cytologic specimens from FNA biopsy. Veracyte Afirma Gene Expression Classifier, promoted by Genzyme (Cambridge, MA, USA), evaluates messenger RNA (mRNA) expression levels for 142 genes. It has a negative predictive value of 96% when evaluated in samples with indeterminate cytology, thus helping patients with benign lesions to avoid unnecessary surgeries.[68] The recent cost-effectiveness analysis by Li and colleagues[67] predicts that routine application of the gene expression classifier lowers the rate of surgeries for benign nodules from 57% (with current practice) to 14%. miRInform Thyroid is another commercially available assay provided by Asuragen (Austin, TX, USA), which analyzes a panel of 7 molecular markers most commonly encountered in thyroid cancers (BRAF, KRAS, HRAS, NRAS, RET/PTC1, RET/PTC3, PAX8/PPARγ). In contrast to the Veracyte product, it is thus designed to improve the preoperative cytologic diagnosis of indeterminate thyroid nodules by predicting which nodules are most likely to be malignant. Its clinical validation still needs to be determined, but the analytical specificity was found to be 99%, and the sensitivity 95%.

In addition to genetic markers, immunohistochemical staining of cytology specimens and other novel serum markers may be of use. With respect to immunohistochemical markers, galectin-3 is a protein marker that was also shown to improve preoperative diagnosis in indeterminate follicular lesions when used in combination with conventional cytomorphological diagnostic procedures.[69,70] However, recent data have shown that galectin-3 is more useful for diagnosing PTC than FTC.[71] Measurement of serum TSH receptor mRNA, which serves as an indicator of circulating thyroid cancer cells, may be useful for helping determine which nodules with indeterminate cytology are malignant. TSH receptor mRNA concentrations greater than 1 ng/μg had a positive predictive value of greater than 90% for carcinoma.[72]

The use of 18FDG-PET scan in the preoperative diagnosis of thyroid nodules with indeterminate cytology has high sensitivity, but histologic diagnosis is still required to distinguish benign from malignant etiology in 18FDG-PET–positive nodules.[73–76]

However, the use of 18FDG-PET could potentially reduce the number of unnecessary thyroidectomies by 39% to 46%.[73,74] It has limited value in selecting candidates for surgery among patients with the cytologic diagnosis of follicular neoplasm, as the glucose metabolic activity is similar in benign and malignant nodules with follicular pattern cytology.[45]

INITIAL EVALUATION OF SINGLE NODULES, FUNCTIONING NODULES, MULTINODULAR GLANDS, INCIDENTAL NODULES, AND CYSTS

- *A patient with a multinodular thyroid has the same risk of having a malignancy as a patient with a single thyroid nodule*

An algorithm for the initial evaluation of a thyroid nodule is shown in **Fig. 2**. Tests that direct the evaluation along different pathways depending on their results include TSH values, US findings, FNA results, scintigraphy findings, and results of molecular testing. Most nodules will be found to be benign based on cytology. Such nodules do not require immediate further diagnostic evaluation or treatment,[1] but can simply be monitored.

With respect to TSH values, a scintigraphy scan (123-I or technetium 99mTc pertechnetate) should be performed in patients with thyroid nodules and serologic evidence of low or low-normal TSH concentration for further evaluation of nodule functionality. Nodules that are interpreted as "hot" on scintigraphy represent hyperfunctioning nodules and should not be considered for FNA biopsy because they are very rarely malignant.[25] The isofunctioning or nonfunctioning nodules, also named "cold" nodules, have a risk for cancer between 5% and 15%, and therefore should be aspirated for further evaluation. The ability to assess nodular functioning with radioisotope scanning is generally limited in lesions smaller than 1 cm.[35]

US examination, in addition to providing information about the appearance and size of nodules, will also document the number of nodules. Of note, the prevalence of thyroid cancer in patients with a multinodular goiter is the same as in patients with a solitary nodule and is independent of the number of nodules. However, the likelihood of malignancy per nodule decreases as the number of nodules increases.[77] If 2 or more nodules larger than 1 cm are present, the selection of nodules for FNA biopsy should be made on the basis of the previously described suspicious US characteristics. Otherwise, the largest nodule should be targeted for biopsy.[1]

Thyroid incidentalomas discovered by CT or MRI should initially undergo US evaluation, with further management being guided based on the sonographic characteristics, as mentioned previously. In contradistinction, incidentalomas detected by 18FDG-PET examination have a high risk of malignancy, and US evaluation, along with FNA biopsy, should be performed.[25]

Totally cystic lesions are generally considered benign and, unless a solid component is present, further diagnostic investigation is not required (see **Table 3**).

TREATMENT FOR BENIGN NODULES

- *Surgical treatment is recommended for nodules causing compressive symptoms, and can be considered for toxic nodular disease and thyroid cysts*
- *T4 suppressive therapy is controversial: it is associated with the risks of iatrogenic hyperthyroidism, but may prevent new nodule formation*

Most benign thyroid nodules do not require any specific intervention, unless there are local compressive symptoms from significant enlargement, such as dysphagia, choking, shortness of breath, hoarseness, or pain, in which case thyroidectomy should be performed.

Other indications for surgery in benign nodules include the presence of a single toxic nodule, or a toxic multinodular goiter. Radioiodine (131-I) therapy is another option for treatment of toxic nodular goiters, but they are usually more radioresistant than toxic diffuse goiter and radioiodine is not the first-line therapy if compressive symptoms are present. Treatment with 131-I for larger nodules is not preferred either, as such nodules require high doses of 131-I with its associated side effects. Radioiodine therapy needs to be approached with caution in individuals with uncontrolled thyrotoxicosis. However, the only absolute contraindications to 131-I therapy are pregnancy and lactation.[78]

Aspiration is the treatment of choice in thyroid cysts, but the recurrence rates are high (60%–90% of patients), particularly with repeated aspirations and large-volume cysts.[79,80] Percutaneous ethanol injection (PEI) has been studied in several large randomized controlled studies, with reported success in 82–85% of the cases after an average of 2 sessions, with a volume reduction of more than 85% from baseline size.[79,80] PEI may also be considered for hyperfunctioning nodules, particularly if a large fluid component is present. It has a success rate ranging from 64% to 95%,[81–83] with a mean volume reduction of 66%,[81] but recurrences are more common and the number of sessions required to achieve good response is higher (about 4 sessions per patient). PEI is a safe procedure, with the most common reported adverse effects being local pain, dysphonia, flushing, dizziness, and, rarely, recurrent laryngeal nerve damage.[79,80,84] Surgery, in addition to serving as a suitable option for treatment of single toxic nodules and toxic multinodular goiter, is also a reasonable therapy for cystic lesions, as an alternative to the previously mentioned procedures.

Levothyroxine (T4) therapy for benign thyroid nodules has been proposed with the aim of achieving nodule shrinkage and preventing further appearance of new nodules through TSH suppression. Although several randomized control trials and meta-analyses have demonstrated nodule shrinkage in patients from areas of iodine deficiency,[85–88] a clinically significant decrease in nodule volume is achieved only in a minority of patients with sufficient iodine intake.[85,88,89] Other predictive features of good response to T4 treatment are recent diagnosis, small nodule size, and colloid appearance at FNA.[90]

T4 suppressive therapy is not devoid of adverse effects, such as decreased bone density, particularly in postmenopausal women, atrial fibrillation, and increased overall morbidity and mortality from cardiovascular diseases.[91] Current guidelines[1] do not recommend routine use of T4 suppressive treatment in patients with benign thyroid nodules from areas with iodine sufficiency. A recent study conducted in Italy in individuals with nontoxic goiter. However, a recent study conducted in Italy in individuals with non-toxic goiter showed decreased goiter growth, decreased formation of new nodules, and decreased risk of developing PTC in a population receiving T4, compared with an untreated population.[92] Thus, this management technique may have some utility.

FOLLOW-UP

- *A 50% increase in the volume of a previously biopsied thyroid nodule is a reasonable trigger for repeating an FNA*

Benign thyroid nodules require further long-term follow-up because of the risk of false-negative results after initial FNA, which is about 5%.[93] Serial US at 6 to 18 months from the initial FNA is the recommended investigation for the follow-up examination of thyroid nodules to accurately detect significant changes in size[94] or discover changes in appearance (**Fig. 6**).

There is no consensus definition for nodule growth and threshold size to repeat an FNA. However, many investigators propose a cutoff value of 50% for nodule volume growth, or more than 20% increase in at least 2 dimensions of a solid nodule, or the solid portion of a mixed cystic-solid nodule to be reasonable and safe.[95] An online calculator to determine the change in volume of a thyroid nodule from its serial dimensions is available on the ATA Web site (http://www.thyroid.org/professionals/calculators/CINV.php). Although nodule growth is an indication for repeat biopsy,[1] growth is not pathognomonic for malignancy.[96] Repeated FNA biopsy is recommended to be performed under US guidance, as false-negative rates are higher with palpation-guided FNA, compared with US-guided FNA.[54] A recent retrospective analysis of value of repeated FNAs of benign thyroid nodules demonstrated high accuracy (98%) of the initial diagnosis.[97]

If no significant nodule growth is observed at repeated US, a follow-up interval of 3 to 5 years may be reasonable (see **Fig. 6**).[1]

THYROID NODULES IN PREGNANCY

- *If a diagnosis of thyroid cancer is made during pregnancy, surgery usually may be delayed until after delivery*

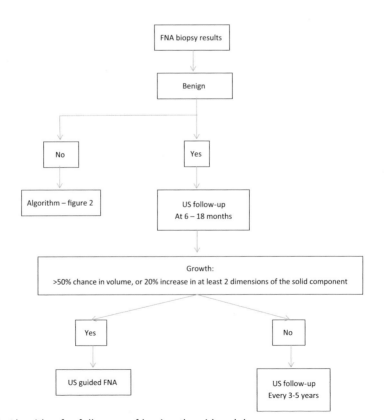

Fig. 6. Algorithm for follow-up of benign thyroid nodules.

- *In the case of aggressive or rapidly growing thyroid cancer, surgery during the second trimester is safest*

The etiology and behavior of thyroid nodules discovered during pregnancy as compared with the general population is unknown.[98] As a consequence, the evaluation should be similar to that for nonpregnant patients, except for the contraindication to radionuclide scanning. If a patient is found to have persistently suppressed serum TSH levels after the first trimester, the radionuclide scan and possible subsequent FNA can be safely postponed until after delivery and cessation of lactation.[1] In euthyroid or hypothyroid pregnant women with thyroid nodules, consensus guidelines recommend that an FNA biopsy should be performed.[1] An argument can be made, however, for deferring the FNA until after delivery unless there are worrisome clinical features that would perhaps lead to a recommendation for a thyroidectomy during pregnancy. If a diagnosis of malignancy results from the FNA, but postponement of thyroidectomy until the patient is post partum is the intended plan before the FNA, this simply exposes the patient to anxiety regarding a diagnosis about which she can take no action.

Previous studies have demonstrated similar cancer behavior in pregnant patients diagnosed with PTC when compared with the general population,[99,100] with no differences in survival rates or recurrences in pregnant women operated for PTC during or after delivery.[100] Rates of complications after thyroid surgery are higher in pregnant women than their nonpregnant counterparts, however.[101] Because additional retrospective data suggest that delaying surgery for less than 1 year from the time of the differentiated thyroid cancer diagnosis has no impact on patient outcome,[102] postponing the surgery until after delivery seems a reasonable approach. If more advanced or aggressive disease is present at the time of diagnosis, or a decision is made to pursue thyroidectomy for thyroid cancer discovered early in pregnancy, surgery should be ideally performed in the second trimester of pregnancy,[103] as this may decrease the risk of early miscarriage and premature delivery.

T4 suppressive therapy to maintain a serum TSH level between 0.1 and 1.0 mU/L is a reasonable approach in pregnant patients diagnosed with thyroid cancer on the basis of an FNA and who are awaiting thyroidectomy.[104]

REFERENCES

1. Cooper DS. Revised American Thyroid Association management guidelines for patients with thyroid nodules and differentiated thyroid cancer. Thyroid 2009; 19(11):1167–214.
2. Marqusee E, Benson CB, Frates MC, et al. Usefulness of ultrasonography in the management of nodular thyroid disease. Ann Intern Med 2000;133(9): 696–700.
3. Singer PA, Cooper DS, Daniels GH, et al. Treatment guidelines for patients with thyroid nodules and well-differentiated thyroid cancer. American Thyroid Association. Arch Intern Med 1996;156(19):2165–72.
4. Mazzaferri EL. Management of a solitary thyroid nodule. N Engl J Med 1993; 328(8):553–9.
5. Ezzat S, Sarti DA, Cain DR, et al. Thyroid incidentalomas. Prevalence by palpation and ultrasonography. Arch Intern Med 1994;154(16):1838–40.
6. Tan GH, Gharib H. Thyroid incidentalomas: management approaches to non-palpable nodules discovered incidentally on thyroid imaging. Ann Intern Med 1997;126(3):226–31.

7. Guth S, Theune U, Aberle J, et al. Very high prevalence of thyroid nodules detected by high frequency (13 MHz) ultrasound examination. Eur J Clin Invest 2009;39(8):699–706.

8. Mortensen JD, Woolner LB, Bennett WA. Gross and microscopic findings in clinically normal thyroid glands. J Clin Endocrinol Metab 1955;15(10):1270–80.

9. Kung AW, Chau MT, Lao TT, et al. The effect of pregnancy on thyroid nodule formation. J Clin Endocrinol Metab 2002;87(3):1010–4.

10. Struve CW, Haupt S, Ohlen S. Influence of frequency of previous pregnancies on the prevalence of thyroid nodules in women without clinical evidence of thyroid disease. Thyroid 1993;3(1):7–9.

11. DeGroot LJ. Clinical review 2: diagnostic approach and management of patients exposed to irradiation to the thyroid. J Clin Endocrinol Metab 1989;69(5):925–8.

12. Antonelli A, Silvano G, Bianchi F, et al. Risk of thyroid nodules in subjects occupationally exposed to radiation: a cross sectional study. Occup Environ Med 1995;52(8):500–4.

13. Hegedus L. Clinical practice. The thyroid nodule. N Engl J Med 2004;351(17):1764–71.

14. Lin JD, Chao TC, Huang BY, et al. Thyroid cancer in the thyroid nodules evaluated by ultrasonography and fine-needle aspiration cytology. Thyroid 2005;15(7):708–17.

15. de Matos PS, Ferreira AP, Ward LS. Prevalence of papillary microcarcinoma of the thyroid in Brazilian autopsy and surgical series. Endocr Pathol 2006;17(2):165–73.

16. Kovács GL, Gonda G, Vadász G, et al. Epidemiology of thyroid microcarcinoma found in autopsy series conducted in areas of different iodine intake. Thyroid 2005;15(2):152–7.

17. Pazaitou-Panayiotou K, Capezzone M, Pacini F. Clinical features and therapeutic implication of papillary thyroid microcarcinoma. Thyroid 2007;17(11):1085–92.

18. Sugitani I, Toda K, Yamada K, et al. Three distinctly different kinds of papillary thyroid microcarcinoma should be recognized: our treatment strategies and outcomes. World J Surg 2010;34(6):1222–31.

19. Kang KW, Kim SK, Kang HS, et al. Prevalence and risk of cancer of focal thyroid incidentaloma identified by 18F-fluorodeoxyglucose positron emission tomography for metastasis evaluation and cancer screening in healthy subjects. J Clin Endocrinol Metab 2003;88(9):4100–4.

20. Hemminki K, Eng C, Chen B. Familial risks for nonmedullary thyroid cancer. J Clin Endocrinol Metab 2005;90(10):5747–53.

21. Lloyd KM 2nd, Dennis M. Cowden's disease. A possible new symptom complex with multiple system involvement. Ann Intern Med 1963;58:136–42.

22. Liaw D, Marsh DJ, Li J, et al. Germline mutations of the PTEN gene in Cowden disease, an inherited breast and thyroid cancer syndrome. Nat Genet 1997;16(1):64–7.

23. Carney JA, Gordon H, Carpenter PC, et al. The complex of myxomas, spotty pigmentation, and endocrine overactivity. Medicine (Baltimore) 1985;64(4):270–83.

24. Gharib H, Papini E, Valcavi R, et al. American Association of Clinical Endocrinologists and Associazione Medici Endocrinologi medical guidelines for clinical practice for the diagnosis and management of thyroid nodules. Endocr Pract 2006;12(1):63–102.

25. Gharib H, Papini E, Paschke R, et al. American Association of Clinical Endocrinologists, Associazione Medici Endocrinologi, and European Thyroid Association

medical guidelines for clinical practice for the diagnosis and management of thyroid nodules: executive summary of recommendations. J Endocrinol Invest 2010;33(Suppl 5):51–6.

26. Fiore E, Rago T, Provenzale MA, et al. Lower levels of TSH are associated with a lower risk of papillary thyroid cancer in patients with thyroid nodular disease: thyroid autonomy may play a protective role. Endocr Relat Cancer 2009;16(4): 1251–60.

27. Meller J, Becker W. The continuing importance of thyroid scintigraphy in the era of high-resolution ultrasound. Eur J Nucl Med Mol Imaging 2002;29(Suppl 2): S425–38.

28. Boelaert K, Horacek J, Holder RL, et al. Serum thyrotropin concentration as a novel predictor of malignancy in thyroid nodules investigated by fine-needle aspiration. J Clin Endocrinol Metab 2006;91(11):4295–301.

29. Haymart MR, Glinberg SL, Liu J, et al. Higher serum TSH in thyroid cancer patients occurs independent of age and correlates with extrathyroidal extension. Clin Endocrinol (Oxf) 2009;71(3):434–9.

30. Haymart MR, Repplinger DJ, Leverson GE, et al. Higher serum thyroid stimulating hormone level in thyroid nodule patients is associated with greater risks of differentiated thyroid cancer and advanced tumor stage. J Clin Endocrinol Metab 2008;93(3):809–14.

31. Jonklaas J, Nsouli-Maktabi H, Soldin SJ. Endogenous thyrotropin and triiodothyronine concentrations in individuals with thyroid cancer. Thyroid 2008;18(9):943–52.

32. Jimenez C, Hu MI, Gagel RF. Management of medullary thyroid carcinoma. Endocrinol Metab Clin North Am 2008;37(2):481–96, x–xi.

33. Hahm JR, Lee MS, Min YK, et al. Routine measurement of serum calcitonin is useful for early detection of medullary thyroid carcinoma in patients with nodular thyroid diseases. Thyroid 2001;11(1):73–80.

34. Cheung K, Roman SA, Wang TS, et al. Calcitonin measurement in the evaluation of thyroid nodules in the United States: a cost-effectiveness and decision analysis. J Clin Endocrinol Metab 2008;93(6):2173–80.

35. Gharib H, Papini E. Thyroid nodules: clinical importance, assessment, and treatment. Endocrinol Metab Clin North Am 2007;36(3):707–35, vi.

36. Frates MC, Benson CB, Charboneau JW, et al. Management of thyroid nodules detected at US: Society of Radiologists in Ultrasound consensus conference statement. Radiology 2005;237(3):794–800.

37. Mandel SJ. Diagnostic use of ultrasonography in patients with nodular thyroid disease. Endocr Pract 2004;10(3):246–52.

38. Papini E, Guglielmi R, Bianchini A, et al. Risk of malignancy in nonpalpable thyroid nodules: predictive value of ultrasound and color-Doppler features. J Clin Endocrinol Metab 2002;87(5):1941–6.

39. Rago T, Vitti P, Chiovato L, et al. Role of conventional ultrasonography and color flow-Doppler sonography in predicting malignancy in 'cold' thyroid nodules. Eur J Endocrinol 1998;138(1):41–6.

40. Hong YJ, Son EJ, Kim EK, et al. Positive predictive values of sonographic features of solid thyroid nodule. Clin Imaging 2010;34(2):127–33.

41. Moon WJ, Jung SL, Lee JH, et al. Benign and malignant thyroid nodules: US differentiation—multicenter retrospective study. Radiology 2008;247(3):762–70.

42. Frasoldati A, Valcavi R. Challenges in neck ultrasonography: lymphadenopathy and parathyroid glands. Endocr Pract 2004;10(3):261–8.

43. Papini E. The dilemma of non-palpable thyroid nodules. J Endocrinol Invest 2003;26(1):3–4.

44. Frates MC, Benson CB, Doubilet PM, et al. Likelihood of thyroid cancer based on sonographic assessment of nodule size and composition [abstract]. In: Radiological Society of North America Scientific Assembly and Annual Meeting Program. Oak Brook (IL): Radiological Society of North America; 2004. p. 395.

45. Kim EK, Park CS, Chung WY, et al. New sonographic criteria for recommending fine-needle aspiration biopsy of nonpalpable solid nodules of the thyroid. AJR Am J Roentgenol 2002;178(3):687–91.

46. Baskin HJ. Thyroid ultrasound and ultrasound-guided FNA biopsy. In: Baskin HJ, editor. Ultrasound of thyroid nodules. Boston: Kluwer Academic Publishers; 2000. p. 71–86.

47. Ueno E, Ito A. Diagnosis of breast cancer by elasticity imaging. Eizo Joho Medical 2004;36:2–6.

48. Rago T, Santini F, Scutari M, et al. Elastography: new developments in ultrasound for predicting malignancy in thyroid nodules. J Clin Endocrinol Metab 2007;92(8):2917–22.

49. Bojunga J, Herrmann E, Meyer G, et al. Real-time elastography for the differentiation of benign and malignant thyroid nodules: a meta-analysis. Thyroid 2010; 20(10):1145–50.

50. Rago T, Scutari M, Santini F, et al. Real-time elastosonography: useful tool for refining the presurgical diagnosis in thyroid nodules with indeterminate or nondiagnostic cytology. J Clin Endocrinol Metab 2010;95(12):5274–80.

51. Rago T, Vitti P. Role of thyroid ultrasound in the diagnostic evaluation of thyroid nodules. Best Pract Res Clin Endocrinol Metab 2008;22(6):913–28.

52. Castro MR, Gharib H. Thyroid fine-needle aspiration biopsy: progress, practice, and pitfalls. Endocr Pract 2003;9(2):128–36.

53. Gharib H, Goellner JR. Fine-needle aspiration biopsy of the thyroid: an appraisal. Ann Intern Med 1993;118(4):282–9.

54. Danese D, Sciacchitano S, Farsetti A, et al. Diagnostic accuracy of conventional versus sonography-guided fine-needle aspiration biopsy of thyroid nodules. Thyroid 1998;8(1):15–21.

55. Fraker DL. Thyroid tumors. In: HS De Vita Jr V, Rosenberg S, editors. Cancer: principles and practice of oncology. Philadelphia: Lippincott-Raven; 1997. p. 1629–52.

56. Baloch ZW, Tam D, Langer J, et al. Ultrasound-guided fine-needle aspiration biopsy of the thyroid: role of on-site assessment and multiple cytologic preparations. Diagn Cytopathol 2000;23(6):425–9.

57. Braga M, Cavalcanti TC, Collaço LM, et al. Efficacy of ultrasound-guided fine-needle aspiration biopsy in the diagnosis of complex thyroid nodules. J Clin Endocrinol Metab 2001;86(9):4089–91.

58. Yeh MW, Demircan O, Ituarte P, et al. False-negative fine-needle aspiration cytology results delay treatment and adversely affect outcome in patients with thyroid carcinoma. Thyroid 2004;14(3):207–15.

59. Baloch ZW, LiVolsi VA, Asa SL, et al. Diagnostic terminology and morphologic criteria for cytologic diagnosis of thyroid lesions: a synopsis of the National Cancer Institute Thyroid Fine-Needle Aspiration State of the Science Conference. Diagn Cytopathol 2008;36(6):425–37.

60. Gharib H, Goellner JR. Fine-needle aspiration biopsy of thyroid nodules. Endocr Pract 1995;1(6):410–7.

61. Meko JB, Norton JA. Large cystic/solid thyroid nodules: a potential false-negative fine-needle aspiration. Surgery 1995;118(6):996–1003 [discussion: 1003–4].

62. Baloch ZW, Fleisher S, LiVolsi VA, et al. Diagnosis of "follicular neoplasm": a gray zone in thyroid fine-needle aspiration cytology. Diagn Cytopathol 2002; 26(1):41–4.
63. Nikiforov YE, Steward DL, Robinson-Smith TM, et al. Molecular testing for mutations in improving the fine-needle aspiration diagnosis of thyroid nodules. J Clin Endocrinol Metab 2009;94(6):2092–8.
64. Franco C, Martínez V, Allamand JP, et al. Molecular markers in thyroid fine-needle aspiration biopsy: a prospective study. Appl Immunohistochem Mol Morphol 2009;17(3):211–5.
65. Kim SK, Hwang TS, Yoo YB, et al. Surgical results of thyroid nodules according to a management guideline based on the BRAF(V600E) mutation status. J Clin Endocrinol Metab 2011;96(3):658–64.
66. Nikiforov YE, Ohori NP, Hodak SP, et al. Impact of mutational testing on the diagnosis and management of patients with cytologically indeterminate thyroid nodules: a prospective analysis of 1056 FNA samples. J Clin Endocrinol Metab 2011;96(11):3390–7.
67. Li H, Robinson KA, Anton B, et al. Cost-effectiveness of a novel molecular test for cytologically indeterminate thyroid nodules. J Clin Endocrinol Metab 2011; 96(11):E1719–26.
68. Chudova D, Wilde JI, Wang ET, et al. Molecular classification of thyroid nodules using high-dimensionality genomic data. J Clin Endocrinol Metab 2010;95(12): 5296–304.
69. Bartolazzi A, Gasbarri A, Papotti M, et al. Application of an immunodiagnostic method for improving preoperative diagnosis of nodular thyroid lesions. Lancet 2001;357(9269):1644–50.
70. Bartolazzi A, Orlandi F, Saggiorato E, et al. Galectin-3-expression analysis in the surgical selection of follicular thyroid nodules with indeterminate fine-needle aspiration cytology: a prospective multicentre study. Lancet Oncol 2008;9(6): 543–9.
71. Weber KB, Shroyer KR, Heinz DE, et al. The use of a combination of galectin-3 and thyroid peroxidase for the diagnosis and prognosis of thyroid cancer. Am J Clin Pathol 2004;122(4):524–31.
72. Milas M, Shin J, Gupta M, et al. Circulating thyrotropin receptor mRNA as a novel marker of thyroid cancer: clinical applications learned from 1758 samples. Ann Surg 2010;252(4):643–51.
73. Giovanella L, Suriano S, Maffioli M, et al. 18FDG-positron emission tomography/computed tomography (PET/CT) scanning in thyroid nodules with nondiagnostic cytology. Clin Endocrinol (Oxf) 2011;74(5):644–8.
74. Sebastianes FM, Cerci JJ, Zanoni PH, et al. Role of 18F-fluorodeoxyglucose positron emission tomography in preoperative assessment of cytologically indeterminate thyroid nodules. J Clin Endocrinol Metab 2007;92(11):4485–8.
75. de Geus-Oei LF, Pieters GF, Bonenkamp JJ, et al. 18F-FDG PET reduces unnecessary hemithyroidectomies for thyroid nodules with inconclusive cytologic results. J Nucl Med 2006;47(5):770–5.
76. Kresnik E, Gallowitsch HJ, Mikosch P, et al. Fluorine-18-fluorodeoxyglucose positron emission tomography in the preoperative assessment of thyroid nodules in an endemic goiter area. Surgery 2003;133(3):294–9.
77. Frates MC, Benson CB, Doubilet PM, et al. Prevalence and distribution of carcinoma in patients with solitary and multiple thyroid nodules on sonography. J Clin Endocrinol Metab 2006;91(9):3411–7.

78. Lazarus JH. Guidelines for the use of radioiodine in the management of hyperthyroidism: a summary. Prepared by the Radioiodine Audit Subcommittee of the Royal College of Physicians Committee on Diabetes and Endocrinology, and the Research Unit of the Royal College of Physicians. J R Coll Physicians Lond 1995;29(6):464–9.

79. Bennedbaek FN, Hegedus L. Treatment of recurrent thyroid cysts with ethanol: a randomized double-blind controlled trial. J Clin Endocrinol Metab 2003; 88(12):5773–7.

80. Valcavi R, Frasoldati A. Ultrasound-guided percutaneous ethanol injection therapy in thyroid cystic nodules. Endocr Pract 2004;10(3):269–75.

81. Tarantino L, Francica G, Sordelli I, et al. Percutaneous ethanol injection of hyperfunctioning thyroid nodules: long-term follow-up in 125 patients. AJR Am J Roentgenol 2008;190(3):800–8.

82. Papini E, Panunzi C, Pacella CM, et al. Percutaneous ultrasound-guided ethanol injection: a new treatment of toxic autonomously functioning thyroid nodules? J Clin Endocrinol Metab 1993;76(2):411–6.

83. Lippi F, Manetti L, Rago T. Percutaneous ultrasound-guided ethanol injection for treatment of autonomous thyroid nodules: results of a multicentric study [abstract]. J Endocrinol Invest 1994;17(Suppl 2):71.

84. Verde G, Papini E, Pacella CM, et al. Ultrasound guided percutaneous ethanol injection in the treatment of cystic thyroid nodules. Clin Endocrinol (Oxf) 1994; 41(6):719–24.

85. Castro MR, Caraballo PJ, Morris JC. Effectiveness of thyroid hormone suppressive therapy in benign solitary thyroid nodules: a meta-analysis. J Clin Endocrinol Metab 2002;87(9):4154–9.

86. Papini E, Bacci V, Panunzi C, et al. A prospective randomized trial of levothyroxine suppressive therapy for solitary thyroid nodules. Clin Endocrinol (Oxf) 1993; 38(5):507–13.

87. Papini E, Petrucci L, Guglielmi R, et al. Long-term changes in nodular goiter: a 5-year prospective randomized trial of levothyroxine suppressive therapy for benign cold thyroid nodules. J Clin Endocrinol Metab 1998;83(3):780–3.

88. Wemeau JL, Caron P, Schvartz C, et al. Effects of thyroid-stimulating hormone suppression with levothyroxine in reducing the volume of solitary thyroid nodules and improving extranodular nonpalpable changes: a randomized, double-blind, placebo-controlled trial by the French Thyroid Research Group. J Clin Endocrinol Metab 2002;87(11):4928–34.

89. Zelmanovitz F, Genro S, Gross JL. Suppressive therapy with levothyroxine for solitary thyroid nodules: a double-blind controlled clinical study and cumulative meta-analyses. J Clin Endocrinol Metab 1998;83(11):3881–5.

90. La Rosa GL, Ippolito AM, Lupo L, et al. Cold thyroid nodule reduction with L-thyroxine can be predicted by initial nodule volume and cytological characteristics. J Clin Endocrinol Metab 1996;81(12):4385–7.

91. Parle JV, Maisonneuve P, Sheppard MC, et al. Prediction of all-cause and cardiovascular mortality in elderly people from one low serum thyrotropin result: a 10-year cohort study. Lancet 2001;358(9285):861–5.

92. Fiore E, Rago T, Provenzale MA, et al. L-thyroxine-treated patients with nodular goiter have lower serum TSH and lower frequency of papillary thyroid cancer: results of a cross-sectional study on 27 914 patients. Endocr Relat Cancer 2010;17(1):231–9.

93. Carmeci C, Jeffrey RB, McDougall IR, et al. Ultrasound-guided fine-needle aspiration biopsy of thyroid masses. Thyroid 1998;8(4):283–9.

94. Tan GH, Gharib H, Reading CC. Solitary thyroid nodule. Comparison between palpation and ultrasonography. Arch Intern Med 1995;155(22):2418–23.

95. Brauer VF, Eder P, Miehle K, et al. Interobserver variation for ultrasound determination of thyroid nodule volumes. Thyroid 2005;15(10):1169–75.

96. Asanuma K, Kobayashi S, Shingu K, et al. The rate of tumour growth does not distinguish between malignant and benign thyroid nodules. Eur J Surg 2001; 167(2):102–5.

97. Oertel YC, Miyahara-Felipe L, Mendoza MG, et al. Value of repeated fine needle aspirations of the thyroid: an analysis of over ten thousand FNAs. Thyroid 2007; 17(11):1061–6.

98. Tan GH, Gharib H, Goellner JR, et al. Management of thyroid nodules in pregnancy. Arch Intern Med 1996;156(20):2317–20.

99. Morris DM, Herzon FS, Segal MN, et al. Coexistent thyroid cancer and pregnancy. Arch Otolaryngol Head Neck Surg 1994;120(11):1191–3.

100. Moosa M, Mazzaferri EL. Outcome of differentiated thyroid cancer diagnosed in pregnant women. J Clin Endocrinol Metab 1997;82(9):2862–6.

101. Kuy S, Roman SA, Desai R, et al. Outcomes following thyroid and parathyroid surgery in pregnant women. Arch Surg 2009;144(5):399–406 [discussion: 406].

102. Mazzaferri EL, Jhiang SM. Long-term impact of initial surgical and medical therapy on papillary and follicular thyroid cancer. Am J Med 1994;97(5):418–28.

103. Mestman JH, Goodwin TM, Montoro MM. Thyroid disorders of pregnancy. Endocrinol Metab Clin North Am 1995;24(1):41–71.

104. Rosen IB, Korman M, Walfish PG. Thyroid nodular disease in pregnancy: current diagnosis and management. Clin Obstet Gynecol 1997;40(1):81–9.

Approach to and Treatment of Goiters

Geraldo Medeiros-Neto, MD, MACP[a],*,
Rosalinda Y. Camargo, MD, PhD[b], Eduardo K. Tomimori, MD, PhD[c]

KEYWORDS

- Simple goiter • Multinodular goiter • Sonography • Surgery
- L-thyroxine therapy • Radioiodine ablation

Simple and nodular goiters are common and geographically widespread conditions. Since remote times, goiter has been described as an enlargement of the neck, and a pictorial description of this anomaly has been present in several cultures and civilizations.[1] The Chinese identified goiter in people living in the countryside and empirically treated them successfully with extracts of dry sea sponges. The traditional Chinese medical doctors were not aware of the iodine-rich content of dry sea sponges and they must have discovered the efficacy of this treatment by trial and error. When Roman armies were crossing the Alps to conquer the Celtic tribes, it was noted that most of the villagers had goiters (*Quis tumidum guttur miratur in Alpibus?*: Do not be surprised to observe goitrous [people] in the Alps). The Latin *guttur* may be the obvious root for the French, English, and Italian words for the enlargement of the neck (*goiter*, goiter, and *gozzo*). During medieval and Renaissance periods, many sculptures, paintings, and works of folk art depicted goitrous people; most of them were villagers from the Alps and other mountainous regions of Europe. Goiter was common in Switzerland, as indicated by medical reports.[1] In South America, goiter was observed after the Spanish and Portuguese conquerors started the process of colonization. It is debatable if the indigenous civilizations in the Andes mountains had a goiter or not, but after the miscegenation of the local population, goiter became common in the Andes. In the Alps, the Andes, and the Himalayas as well as in China, Brazil, Indonesia, Thailand, Vietnam, and other countries, goiter was the visible

This article was partially supported by a grant from Instituto da Tiróide-São Paulo, Brazil- www.indatir.org.br.

The authors declare that they have nothing to disclosure.

[a] Division of Endocrinology, Department of Medicine, University of Sao Paulo Medical School, Rua Artur Ramos, 96 – 5A, 01454-903 Sao Paulo, Brazil

[b] Thyroid Unit, Division of Endocrinology, University of Sao Paulo Medical School, Rua Mirassol, 216 – apartment 82, 04044-010 São Paulo, Brazil

[c] Section of Ultrasonography at the Hospital das Clínicas, University of São Paulo Medical School, Rua Artur Ramos, 241 - Room 63, 01454-011 São Paulo, Brazil

* Corresponding author.

E-mail address: medneto@uol.com.br

consequence of chronic iodine deficiency, but this was clearly shown only at the beginning of the nineteenth century, when iodine was discovered. Later, iodine drops were used to cure goiters in Geneva, Switzerland, but a few cases of excessive thyroid function and dramatic cardiac arrhythmias were detected with deaths from the excessive iodine administered to goitrous elderly people.[2] Iodine started to be widely distributed to afflicted populations in the mountainous regions of Europe late in the nineteenth century. The first attempt at an epidemiologic approach to prevent endemic goiter was made in France and Switzerland in the early twentieth century. In the United States, Marine and Taylor[1] reported on clinical and pathologic aspects of multinodular goiters, and general prophylaxis with iodine administration was suggested. Later, several countries started their own programs to distribute iodine to their populations. Most of the studies of the prevalence of goiters were based on physical examination of schoolchildren. If more than 5% of all schoolchildren had thyroid enlargement, supplementation of iodine through salt was recommended. In 1986, the International Council for Control of Iodine Deficiency Disorders started a new period of globalization in the permanent fight against iodine-deficiency disorders, including goiter. Almost 2 billion people are still at risk of iodine deficiency and its consequences, mostly pregnant women and their babies, as well as children of school age.[3]

Iodine deficiency was and still is a major cause for goiter in schoolchildren, young adults, and elderly people. As discussed in the following sections, goiter may have a familial incidence and a strong genetic predisposition. Other causes of goiter may relate to smoking, natural goitrogens, autoimmune disorders, dyshormonogenesis, certain iodine-rich drugs, and environmental agents. The approach to a patient with a goiter should consider and evaluate many and multiple factors that induce an abnormal growth of the thyroid gland.

WHAT IS A GOITER?

Simple diffuse goiter (SDG) is an enlargement of the thyroid volume occurring in an iodine-sufficient area or, more frequently, in young individuals living in mild to moderate iodine-deficiency areas. The goiters should not have signs and symptoms related to autoimmune thyroid disorders or neoplasia. SDG volume has been clinically evaluated by palpation, which is considered inaccurate. More recently, ultrasonography of the thyroid gland conducted in schoolchildren[4] has provided a more accurate measurement of thyroid volume. If more than 5% of the schoolchildren have more than the reference volume value for their age, the geographic area is considered to be less than a low iodine intake (**Fig. 1**); measurement of urinary iodine excretion confirms this assumption.[3]

Multinodular goiter (MNG) is a clinically recognizable enlargement of the thyroid gland characterized by excessive growth of more than 1 nodule, which undergoes a structural and functional transformation within the normal thyroid tissue. Simple nodular goiter or MNG occurs both endemically (low iodine intake; more than 5% of population has this condition) and sporadically (<5% of the population has SDG and MNG).

Both MNG and SDG may be familial, when several members of the family have a diffuse or nodular enlargement of the thyroid. In familial clustering, a simple mode of transmission has been recognized. Both endemic and sporadic goiter belong to the group of diseases referred to as complex diseases; they commonly vary in their severity and are multifactorial, with the clinical phenotype representing contributions from both genetic and environmental factors.[4]

Prevalence of goiter [*]

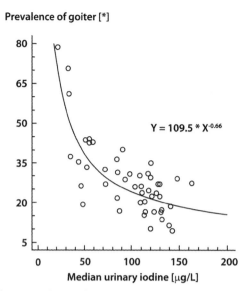

$$Y = 109.5 * X^{-0.66}$$

Median urinary iodine [μg/L]

Fig. 1. Relationship between the median urinary iodine concentration and the prevalence of goiter (measuring volume by echography) at 57 locations in 12 European countries. (*From* Delange F, Benker G, Caron P, et al. Thyroid volume and urinary iodine in European schoolchildren; standardization values for assessment of iodine deficiency. Eur J Endocrinol 1997;136:182; with permission.)

EPIDEMIOLOGY

Studies on the epidemiology of SDG and MNG in a given population have been hampered by selection criteria, influence of environmental factors, methodology for measuring size, and morphology, as well as methods for evaluating thyroid function.[5,6]

Survey of a representative sample of the adult population from a geographic area of the United Kingdom[7] indicated that 15.5% of the individuals had a palpable goiter, with a female/male ratio of 4.5:1. No relation to iodine excretion was found. In the Framingham, United States, study[8] the iodine intake was high (urinary iodine 246 μg iodine/L), and MNG was found by palpation in only 1% of individuals between 30 and 50 years of age. MNG is a frequent clinical entity in countries with a history of chronic iodine deficiency. After correction of the iodine deficiency most schoolchildren, young adults, and middle-aged individuals do not present with an SDG. However, older individuals who have suffered from lack of proper iodine nutrition since childhood may have a clinically visible and palpable MNG. It is estimated that about 6% of elderly individuals in a given population, previously suspected to have iodine deficiency, may have visible MNG.[9]

EVOLUTION OF SDG AND MNG

The evolution of SDG (either endemic or sporadic) is limited to primary and secondary factors.[6] Primary factors are functional heterogeneity of normal follicular cells, caused by genetics, and acquisition of new inheritable qualities by replicating epithelial cells. An important primary factor is gender (females are affected more than males). Later, with the evolution of SDG and MNG, several functional and structural anomalies in growing goiters emerge (**Fig. 2**).

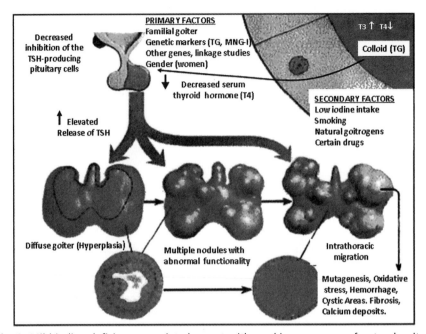

Fig. 2. Mild iodine deficiency associated or not with smoking, presence of natural goitrogenic drugs, familial goiter, genetic markers, and gender (female) decreases the inhibition of serum T_4 on the pituitary thyrotrophs. Increased TSH production causes diffuse goiter followed by nodule formation. After decades of life, a large MNG is present with cystic areas, hemorrhage, fibrosis, and calcium deposits. (*From* Medeiros-Neto G, Henneman G. Multinodular goiter. 2010. Available at: http://www.thyroidmanager.org. Accessed November 7, 2011; with permission.)

Secondary factors are mostly linked to persistent increased levels of serum thyroid-stimulating hormone (TSH) (induced by iodine deficiency), presence of natural goitrogens, dyshormonogenesis, nutritional deficiencies, oxidative stress, smoking, and environmental and endocrine disruptors.

The secondary factors discussed later stimulate thyroid cell growth or function, and, because of presumed differences in cellular responsiveness, aggravate the expression of heterogeneity, which leads to further growth and focal autonomic function of the thyroid gland. Local necrosis and cyst formation (sometimes with bleeding and fibrosis) may be the anatomic end stage of such processes (see **Fig. 2**).

Iodine Deficiency

Stimulation of new follicle generation seems to be necessary in the formation of simple goiter (see **Fig. 2**). Evidence accumulated from many studies indicates that iodine deficiency negatively modifies the iodine metabolism in the thyroid gland, and this may be an important mechanism leading to increases in TSH secretion.[10–13] Because in experimental animals the level of iodine per se may modulate the response of thyroid cells to TSH, this is an additional mechanism by which small increases in serum TSH level cause substantial effects on thyroid growth in iodine-deficient areas.[12,14] The thyroidal iodine clearance of patients with nontoxic nodular goiter was, on average, higher than that in normal persons. When data published from various major cities in Western Europe regarding thyroid volume and iodine excretion are put together,[4] an inverse relation is found between urinary iodine excretion and thyroid volume (see **Fig. 1**). Physiologic stresses, such as pregnancy, may increase the need for iodine and require thyroid hypertrophy to increase iodine uptake. Moreover, increased renal clearance of iodine occurs during normal pregnancy.[10] Increased need for thyroxine (T_4) during pregnancy may also lead to significant transfer of thyroid hormone from the mother to the fetus. Mutations in the thyroglobulin gene may impair the efficiency of thyroid hormone synthesis and release, leading to a decrease inhibition of TSH at the pituitary level. The high TSH released from the thyrotrophs continuously stimulates growth of the thyroid gland.[6]

Natural Goitrogens

Natural goitrogens (**Table 1**) may be considered significant determinants of the prevalence of goiter, either in iodine-deficient areas or in localities where iodine intake is abundant, as in the coal-rich Appalachian area of eastern Kentucky.[15] Goitrogenic effects may be related to the consumption of certain foodstuffs (cassava, millet, babassu coconut, piñon, vegetables from the genus *Brassica*, and soybean).[16–27] The goitrogenic factor in cassava is related to the hydrocyanic acid liberated from the cyanogenetic glucoside (linamarin) and converted endogenously to thiocyanate. These compounds, competitively, inhibit trapping and promote the efflux of intrathyroidal iodine.[16] Pearl millet is one of the most important food crops in the semiarid tropics (large portions of Africa and Asia). Millet porridge is rich in *C*-glucosylflavones and also contains thiocyanate. Both are additive in their antithyroid effects. Babassu coconut is largely consumed in northern Brazil, and studies have shown the presence of flavonoids in the edible part of the nut.[17] Studies of soy isoflavones in experimental animals suggest possible adverse effects like enhancement of reproductive organs, modulation of endocrine function, and antithyroid effects. Antithyroid effects may also be extended by increasing the loss of T_4 from the blood via bile into the gut, and may cause goiter when iodine intake is limited.[18,19]

Table 1
Natural goitrogens associated with goiter prevalence

Goitrogens	Agent	Action
Millet, soy	Flavonoids	Impairs thyroperoxidase activity
Cassava, sweet potato, sorghum	Cyanogenic glucosides metabolized to thiocyanates	Inhibits iodine thyroidal uptake
Babassu coconut, mandioca	Flavonoids	Inhibits thyroperoxidase
Cruciferous vegetables: cabbage, cauliflower, broccoli, turnips	Glucosinolates	Impairs iodine thyroidal uptake
Seaweed (kelp)	Iodine excess	Inhibits release of thyroidal hormones
Malnutrition	Vitamin A deficiency Iron deficiency	Increases TSH stimulation Reduces heme-dependent thyroperoxidase thyroidal activity
Selenium	Selenium deficiency	Accumulates peroxides and causes deiodinase deficiency; impairs thyroid hormone synthesis

Adapted and modified from Medeiros-Neto G, Knobel M. Iodine deficiency disorders. In: Jameson JL, De Groot LJ, editors. Endocrinology. 6th edition. Philadelphia: WB Saunders Co; 2010; with permission.

Excess of Nutritional Iodine

Excess consumption of iodine-rich kelp (dry seaweed, 80–200 mg iodine per day) has caused sporadic and even endemic goiter in humans. In these cases, goiter is common in some families and more frequent in girls at puberty, which suggests the influence of additional genetic and hormonal factors. The organification of iodine and, consequently, the synthesis of T_4 and triiodothyronine (T_3) were lower than normal, and iodine-rich colloid goiter was observed in patients from the goiter-endemic coast of Hokkaido, Japan.[20]

Generalized malnutrition (protein-caloric deprivation) has been recognized as an additive factor in the prevalence of goiter in populations with mild iodine deficiency.[21–27] Epidemiologic data recorded in 5-year-old to 14-year-old South African children showed that vitamin A supplements are effective in treating goiter in areas of mild iodine deficiency. It has also an additional benefit: through suppression of the pituitary *TSHβ* gene, vitamin A supplements can decrease TSH secretion and the subsequent over-stimulation of the thyroid. These events reduce the risk of goiter.[21,22] Iron, selenium, and zinc are essential for normal thyroid hormone metabolism. Iron deficiency impairs thyroid hormone synthesis by reducing activity of heme-dependent thyroid peroxidase. Iron-deficiency anemia blunts and iron supplementation improves the efficacy of iodine supplementation.[23]

Natural goitrogenesis, protein-caloric malnutrition, iron, selenium, and zinc as well as environmental disruptors have a limited if any effect in a normal iodine environment. In clinical practice, these factors are of minor pathologic action in patients with SDG or MNG.

Oxidative stress has been previously evaluated[10] and considered an important factor in goitrogenesis. Certain drugs may induce damage to the follicular cells, with a possible induction of goiter.

Heterogeneity of Thyroid Cells

Cells of the thyroid gland are often polyclonal rather than monoclonal in origin.[14] From a functional aspect, it seems that through developmental processes the thyroid epithelial cells forming a follicle are functionally polyclonal and possess widely different qualities regarding biochemical steps leading to growth and to thyroid hormone synthesis.[6] As a consequence, there is marked heterogeneity of growth and function within the thyroid and even within a single follicle.[14]

An example of genetic qualities acquisition is the identification in the last few years of constitutively activating somatic mutations not only in solitary toxic adenoma but also in hyperfunctioning nodules of MNGs.[13]

Environmental Disruptors Affecting Thyroid Function

In addition to the natural goitrogens mentioned earlier, exposure to environmental chemicals may have deleterious effects on the thyroid system in humans during development, especially in the nervous system.[28] Disruptors may also adversely affect thyroid hormone metabolism.[29,30] However, these agents have not proved to be goitrogenic.

Smoking

Tobacco smoking is a major source of thiocyanate in humans, which inhibits the function of the iodide transporter in the lactating mammary gland. Smoking during the period of breastfeeding dose-dependently reduces breast-milk iodine content to about half and, consequently, exposes the infant to increased risk of iodine deficiency.[31]

GENES ASSOCIATED WITH MNG

In contrast to sporadic goiters, caused by recessive genomic variation, most cases of familial goiter present an autosomal-dominant pattern of inheritance, indicating predominant genetic defects. Gene-gene interactions of various polygenic mechanisms (ie, synergistic effects of several variants or polymorphisms) could increase the complexity of the pathogenesis of nontoxic MNG and offer an explanation for its genetic heterogeneity.[32–40] A strong genetic predisposition is indicated by family and twin studies.[33] Thus, children from parents with goiter have a significantly higher risk of developing goiter compared with children from nongoitrous parents. The high incidence in females and the higher concordance rate in monozygotic instead of dizygotic twins have also suggested a genetic predisposition. Moreover, there is preliminary evidence of a positive family history for thyroid diseases in those who have postoperative relapse of goiter, which can occur from months to years after surgery.

A genome-wide linkage analysis has identified a candidate locus, MNG1 on chromosome 14q31, in a large Canadian family with 18 affected individuals.[32]

This focus was confirmed in a German family with recurrent euthyroid goiters.[34] A dominant pattern of inheritance with high penetrance was assumed in both investigations. Moreover, a region on 14q31 between MNG1 and the TSH-R gene was identified as a potential positional candidate region for nontoxic goiter. Furthermore, an X-linked autosomal-dominant pattern and linkage to a second locus MNG2 (Xp22) was identified in an Italian pedigree with nontoxic familial goiter.[35] A study in Japan identified 2 independent multigenerational families with MNG with euthyroidism.[37] An autosomal-dominant pattern of inheritance has been suggested in both families. Linkage analysis mapped a single locus on 3q26.1-q263. These findings indicate that the MNG phenotype observed in the pedigree was not caused by impairment of genes directly involved in thyroid hormonogenesis. An unknown protein may be involved in the biochemical pathway of thyroid hormone synthesis.

Genome-wide Linkage Analysis

To identify further candidate regions, the first extended genome-wide linkage analysis was performed to detect susceptibility loci in 18 Danish, German, and Slovakian families.[38] Assuming genetic heterogeneity and a dominant pattern of inheritance, 4 novel candidate loci on chromosomes 3p, 2q, 7q, and 8p were identified. An individual contribution was attributable to 4 families for the 3p locus and to 1 family for each of the other loci, respectively. From the candidate regions identified earlier and the established environmental factors, nontoxic goiter can consequently be defined as a complex disease. However, a more prevalent putative locus, present in 20% of the investigated families, has been identified.[38]

Moreover, the sum of several weak genetic variations in different genomic regions could lead to goiter predisposition. Therefore, the widely accepted risk factors such as iodine deficiency, smoking, old age, and female gender are likely to interact with or trigger the genetic susceptibility.[36]

Thyroglobulin gene mutations have been implicated in the genesis of nontoxic goiter.[41–44] Two studies from Spain have indicated monoallelic mutations in the TG gene causing euthyroid diffuse goiter.[41,42] In 1 patient a homozygous mutation in exon 43 induced the synthesis of an abnormal TG protein that was mostly retained in the endoplasmic reticulum.[44] Thus, the defective TG protein that reached the colloidal space was rapidly hydrolyzed and thyroid hormone released into the circulation. However, serum TSH level was mildly increased and a large diffuse goiter was present (**Fig. 3**). The high iodine intake had a positive role for generation of barely normal serum T_3 and T_4 levels.

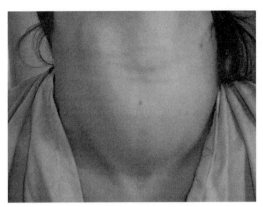

Fig. 3. A large diffuse goiter in a 39-year-old woman with serum TSH 4.19 mIU/mL, free T_4 = 0.63 ng/dL, low serum Tg (4.2 ng/mL) not responsive to stimulation by rhTSH. Iodine nutrition was normal, as confirmed by a urinary iodine of 239 μg/L. A thyroglobulin gene mutation in exon 43 (Ala 2215 Asp) led to an expressive retention of TG-mutated protein in the endoplasmic reticulum. Hormone synthesis and release were only mildly affected, possibly by the high iodine ingestion. Goiter was probably caused by excessive and persistent TSH stimulation. (*Data from* Pardo V, Vono-Toniolo J, Rubio IG, et al. The p.A2215D thyroglobulin gene mutation leads to deficient synthesis and secretion of the mutated protein and congenital hypothyroidism with wide phenotype variation. J Clin Endocrinol Metab 2009;94: 2938–44.)

CLINICAL EVALUATION

Most patients with SDG and MNG have few or no symptoms except for those with large MNG. Many patients are referred to hospital for cosmetic reasons or, more frequently, for compression of cervical structures causing tracheal deviation. Rarely dyspnea, cough, and dysphasia are present. Often patients have a family history of goiter and nodules removed by surgery in their relatives. SDG commonly develops slowly in school-age children during adolescence. Goiter asymmetry is common. In older people, MNG is the most frequently diagnosed entity. Aside from cosmetic complaints, a sudden transient pain with enlargement of a side of the MNG secondary to hemorrhage is the major complaint by patients. Compression symptoms are more often seen when there is an intrathoraxic extension of the MNG (**Fig. 4**). Such goiters develop insidiously in elderly individuals when there is a substantial growth into the thorax (anterior mediastinum); they may lead to compression of the subclavia arterial/venous flow with the surge of collateral circulation in the upper thoracic region. Intrathoraxic localization may cause respiratory distress in 30% to 85% of patients referred for surgery.[5,6] Tracheal compression results in dyspnea, stridor, cough, and a sensation of shock. Intrathoraxic MNG symptoms of respiratory distress are amplified in a recumbent position (**Fig. 5**). Several patients with MNG may present signs and symptoms related to subclinical hyperthyroidism/clinical hyperthyroidism. These symptoms are probably caused by autonomous nodules inside the MNG[13] or, more frequently, by an excess of nutritional iodine or iodinated drugs, or radiological contrasts containing iodine.[6]

LABORATORY INVESTIGATION AND IMAGING PROCEDURES

TSH assays are sensitive in detecting thyroid dysfunction and are therefore preferred as a first approach by more than half of clinicians.[45,46] Depending on the geographic localization of the attending physician (North and South America, Europe,

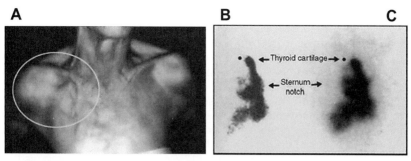

Fig. 4. An elderly woman with a large and long-standing MNG that migrated to the upper mediastinal region with subsequent compression of the subclavian system. Note the subcutaneous enlarged venous circulation (*A*). Scintillographic studies after a tracer dose of ^{131}I (*B*) before and (*C*) after simulation by 0.45 mg of rhTSH. (*From* Silva MN, Rubió IG, Romão R, et al. Administration of a single dose of recombinant human thyrotrophin enhances the efficacy of radioiodine treatment of large compressive multinodular goitres. Clin Endocrinol (Oxf) 2004;60:302; with permission.)

and Asia/Oceania), thyroidologists frequently also ask for thyroid hormone determination (free T_4, free T_3, total T_4, total T_3) in the initial evaluation of the patient. Antithyroid peroxidase (anti-TPO) antibodies are measured by half of clinicians. The information provided by a positive anti-TPO test is relevant for future treatment with radioiodine (as a risk factor for thyroiditis and hypothyroidism). Serum thyroglobulin (Tg) is an important marker for the rare condition of a mutation in the TG gene leading to a paradoxic low Tg serum level in a large MNG (see **Fig. 3**).

Imaging Procedures

Sonography of the thyroid
It is widely accepted that neck palpation is imprecise both for assessment of thyroid morphology and size (weight) determination. Therefore, sonography has been

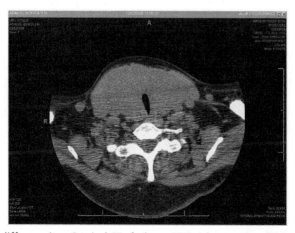

Fig. 5. Familial diffuse goiter. Cervical CT of a large SDG. A large goiter (230 mL) in a 42-year-old woman from an iodine-sufficient area. The thyroid volume apparently started to grow after her third pregnancy. Her mother and 2 sisters also have goiters. The patient complained of dyspnea, compression symptoms, and stridor. Serum TSH level was 6.0 mIU/mL, free T_4 1.1 ng/dL, and anti-TPO was negative. Serum TG level was increased (186 ng/mL). Note the tracheal compression with a reduced area (8 × 18 mm).

introduced, with a dramatic effect on clinical practice. Sonographic portable machines are available at a reasonable price, and in many countries the endocrinologist (after training) may perform echography of the neck in their patients, to image the thyroid gland. Sonography also provides an accurate estimate of the goiter/nodule volume, identifies thyroid nodules/cysts, detects microcalcifications, and specifies the degree of echogenicity of the nodule(s).

In the presence of an SDG, echographic measurements produce reliable information about the effect of treatment on goiter volume in relation to time. Moreover, serial echographic studies may detect the emergence of cysts, hemorrhages, and nodular structures in follow-up of the patient. For MNG, the ellipsoid method for volume estimation may underestimate the goiter size by 17% compared with magnetic resonance imaging (MRI). An important feature of the sonographic methodology for imaging is the use of a Doppler technique to evaluate the flow of the vascular (arterial) bed in nodules. Moreover, the new three-dimensional sonographic machines may improve volume estimation and possibly avoid the use of other methods (MRI, computed tomography [CT]).

Scintillography

Scintillography of thyroid isotope imaging has little place in the evaluation of SDG or MNG. However, isotope uptake by the MNG may be measured before and after stimulation by recombinant human TSH (rhTSH) (see **Fig. 4**). It has been clearly shown that after rhTSH stimulation, the uptake of the nodules (within the MNG) increases dramatically. This finding indicates a therapeutic choice for a dose of radioiodine preceded by rhTSH.

CT and MRI

CT and MRI provide high-resolution three-dimensional visualization of the thyroid gland and are specially useful for an MNG that extends to the upper mediastinum. Another advantage of CT and MRI is the possibility for planimetric volume estimations, especially in large MNG before and after a radioiodine therapeutic dose. Moreover, both imaging methods provide an accurate view of the degree of tracheal compression (see **Fig. 5**). As the MNG progressively shrinks in volume, the trachea lumen expands to its normal size. This expansion can be accurately measured in serial MRI.

Fine-needle aspiration and cytology

Fine-needle aspiration biopsy (FNAB) should be performed in MNG before surgery or a radioiodine therapeutic dose. Usually, a dominant nodule and 1 or 2 other nodules are aspirated under sonographic imaging. The risk of malignancy in a long-standing MNG has been considered as small both in surgical and in autopsy specimens. Thus, the FNAB is usually conducted to enable the surgeon/nuclear medical group to search for suspicious lymph nodes before a surgical or medical intervention. If a nodule within an MNG has a cytologic diagnosis of papillary cancer, surgery should be performed.

TREATMENT

There is no ideal therapeutic option for SDG.[47] As discussed earlier, SDG results from a combination of genetic factors and environmental conditions. Frequently a mild iodine deficiency is present.[4] Therefore, iodine supplementation seems to be an adequate approach (400 μg iodine for 8–12 months). A significant reduction was observed in SDG. However, in patients with MNG, iodine therapy may induce autoimmune thyroiditis and also the risk of iodine-induced hyperthyroidism (Jod-Basedow phenomenon). Therefore aside from a few European countries, iodine is no longer used for treatment of goiter (SDG, MNG).

This situation leaves 3 therapeutic options (**Table 2**):

a. surgery
b. L-T$_4$–suppressive therapy
c. radioiodine (^{131}I) alone/preceded by rhTSH.

Surgery

In the United States (and possibly in most other countries), surgery is the preferred treatment for patients with euthyroid, large obstructive, and substernal MNG.[45,46] This preference was clearly shown in questionnaires sent to members of the American Thyroid Association and the European Thyroid Association. Small MNGs were preferentially treated with suppressive L-T$_4$ therapy by more than half of the responders to the questionnaire. By contrast, European thyroidologists tended to treat MNG with radioiodine (^{131}I) alone or preceded by rhTSH as an alternative to surgery. In countries

Table 2
Treatment of nontoxic MNGs

Therapeutic Options	Data Favoring	Data Against	Comments
Surgery	Rapid goiter reduction and cervical decompression obtained Pathologic examination	Higher cost ($$$) Hospitalization Postoperative complications (2%–5%) Hypothyroidism/ recurrence Higher risk in intrathoracic goiters	Standard therapy when high-volume thyroid surgeons are available Not all patients may be eligible Elderly patients may be high risk
L-T$_4$ and L-T$_4$ plus iodine	Outpatient treatment Low cost Prevent new nodule formation Association with iodine may be more effective	Goiter reduction in only 30% Treatment is for life TSH suppressed Possible subclinical hyperthyroidism Effects in bone and heart Compliance may be low	Currently indicated in small MNG Association with iodine may result in higher efficacy May be recommended as first option
Radioiodine (preceded by rhTSH)	Goiter volume reduced (50%) after 1 y Few side effects Low cost for the public health system, specially in emergent countries	Reduction of goiter sizes gradual Larger goiters may have a lower reduction Transient thyroiditis Increased levels of T$_4$ and T$_3$ hypothyroidism (30%)	Has replaced surgery in European and emergent countries Best option for those who decline or are not fit for surgery

Adapted and modified from Hegedus, L, Paschke R, Krohn K, et al. Multinodular goiter. In: Jameson LJ, De Groot LJ, editors. Endocrinology. 6th edition. Philadelphia: Saunders-Elsevier; 2010. p. 1636–49; with permission.

with a past history of chronic iodine deficiency, MNG is common in elderly patients, many of whom are considered to have a higher risk for surgery because of the presence of other chronic disorders, hence the need for an alternative therapeutic procedure to replace the obvious surgical intervention. In most patients with large MNG, near total or total thyroidectomy is the procedure of choice.[48–59] Complications of surgery such as injury to the recurrent laryngeal nerve tracheal lesions, nonintentional removal of the parathyroid glands resulting in permanent hypoparathyroidism with lifelong need for continuous treatment are, apparently, more common in large and substernal goiters rather than those undergoing surgery for cervical goiters.[55–57] To minimize the risks of complications, those patients with substernal goiters should be referred to an experienced thyroid surgeon.[11] However, in many settings, thyroid surgeons may not be easily available and general surgeons are indicated for MNG surgery. Frequently a subtotal thyroidectomy is performed, and the recurrence risk of MNG may reach 60% of patients within many years of the surgical procedure.[51,58] Another point of controversy is the use of L-T_4 after a subtotal thyroidectomy. Total removal of the thyroid (MNG) leads to hypothyroidism and treatment with L-T_4 is mandatory. Patients who are left with a substantial residual thyroid tissue may be treated with L-T_4.[51] The use of routine L-T_4 therapy is questioned by others.[52] Because of the high long-term recurrence rate after subtotal thyroidectomy for MNG, most clinicians treat these patients with L-T_4.[45,46]

A reoperation for the recurrent MNG accounts for approximately 10% to 15% of thyroidectomies (mostly subtotal surgery), resulting in a 3-fold to 10-fold increase in risk of surgical complications, as indicated earlier.[5] An alternative is the use of radioiodine preceded by rhTSH stimulation, as discussed in the last section of the therapeutic approaches to MNG.

L-T_4–suppressive Therapy for MNG

L-T_4–suppressive therapy is used extensively in Europe, the United States, and Latin America, according to their respective surveys.[45,46] A beneficial effect of L-T_4 has been shown in diffuse goiters in many controlled trials.[60–66] A goiter reduction of 20% to 40% can be expected in 6 to 12 months of therapy, the goiter returning to the pretreatment size after L-T_4 withdrawal. The efficacy of L-T_4 depends on the degree of TSH suppression. For nontoxic MNG, there are controlled studies in which sonography was used for objective size monitoring. A randomized, double-blind trial showed that the goiter volume was reduced by 15% (9 months of L-T_4 therapy). In the placebo group, the goiter continued to increase in size by more than 20% in the 9-month period.[60] The goiter volume returned to baseline values after discontinuation of the therapy. Others[61] studied 62 patients with nodular goiter. Thirty per cent of patients were regarded as responders (reduction >50% of the initial volume). In the control group, 87% showed no change or an increase in goiter size. Another randomized trial[62] compared L-T_4 with ^{131}I therapy. The median reduction of goiter volume in the radioiodine-treated group was 38% to 44%, whereas only 7% of the L-T_4–treated patients had a significant goiter reduction.

An Italian group[63] treated 83 goitrous patients (nodular goiter) with suppressive doses of L-T_4, comparing the results with a control group. The L-T_4 therapy was extended for 5 years. There was a decrease in nodular size in the L-T_4–treated group and a mean volume increase in the control group. After 5 years, sonograms detected 28.5% new nodules in the control group but only 7.5% in the L-T_4–treated group. Long-term TSH suppression by L-T_4 induced volume reduction in a subgroup of thyroid nodules but effectively prevented the appearance of new nodules. Another recently controlled study from Italy[67] studied patients with MNG treated with L-T_4

compared with a control group for 1 year. These investigators concluded that L-T$_4$ reduced significantly the goiter volume, compared with the control group. Thyroid volume was evaluated by sonography.

A study conducted in Brazil[65] evaluated 42 women with a nodular goiter. Twenty-one patients were treated with 2.7 µg/kg of L-T$_4$ for 1 year. Six of the 21 treated patients had a greater than 50% reduction of the goiter. Nodule volume has been evaluated by sonography. Nodule volume reduction has been observed in only 2 (of 24 patients) who received a placebo. These investigators concluded that L-T$_4$ therapy is associated with 17% of reduction of a single colloid nodule and may inhibit growth in other patients. They also conducted a meta-analysis of 6 prospective controlled trials and concluded that 4 of 7 studies favor treatment with L-T$_4$. More recently, a study conducted in Germany[66] in a large cohort (1024 patients), in a multicenter setting evaluated L-T$_4$ alone, L-T$_4$ plus iodine, iodine alone, and placebo in thyroid nodules. Nodular volume was reduced by 17.3% in the group receiving L-T$_4$ and iodine compared with 7.3% in the group treated with L-T$_4$ alone. Both treatments were more effective in goiter (nodule) reduction compared with placebo. These investigators concluded that in a region with sufficient iodine the combination of L-T$_4$ plus iodine is more effective than another component alone or placebo. The treatment of single nodules or MNG with L-T$_4$ is an open issue, because the reduction of the nodule/MNG is obtained in only about one-third of patients. The possible unwanted effects of L-T$_4$ therapy have also to be considered.[5,6]

Radioiodine in the Treatment of MNG

Radioiodine treatment of nontoxic MNGs was introduced in some European countries about 25 years ago.[68,69] Patients were selected for ablation with radioiodine when they had comorbidities that increased the risk for a surgical procedure (total thyroidectomy) or when they refused surgery. In these earlier studies, radioiodine therapy induced a mean goiter reduction of about 40% in 1 year of therapy.[68] The individual response to the ablative dose was variable mostly because of low iodine uptake by the MNG. Moreover, for large MNG, a high radioiodine dose was needed to have an adequate ^{131}I accumulation in the distinct nodular areas of the MNG. With the approval of rhTSH for diagnostic use in thyroid disease and later extended for ablation of remnant thyroid tissue after surgery for thyroid cancer, it was suggested that rhTSH might be used before radioiodine to increase the uptake of the radioiodine in the various nodules of the MNG. Therefore several groups in Europe (Denmark, the Netherlands, Germany, Italy), Israel, United States, and Brazil started the use of rhTSH before ablation by radioiodine.[67,69-83] Iodine uptake after a single dose of rhTSH was markedly increased within the various nodular areas of the MNG (see **Fig. 4**). This finding reduces the total ^{131}I dose administered, also reducing the radiation to the whole body. Depending on the regulations of each country, the radioiodine can be administered on an outpatient basis, thus saving the costs of hospitalization.[72]

Acute adverse effects

Acute adverse effects are caused by the surge of thyroid hormone in blood and the goiter increase in volume (in the first 48 hours of radioiodine therapy), which may cause local tenderness, tracheal compression, and, frequently, cardiac symptoms. These conditions may be minimized by the use of corticoids and β-blockers.[74]

Several recent articles[77-83] have indicated that these adverse effects are probably dose dependent and are negligible with lower rhTSH doses.

In the case of patients with MNG with subclinical/clinical hyperthyroidism, it is recommended to precede the ablation with 60 days of a high dose of methimazole and a low-iodine diet. Both precautions reduce the amount of thyroid hormone within the MNG and prevent the possible complications of a surge of thyroid hormone after ablation.[75]

Long-term adverse effects of combined rhTSH plus [131]I

Hypothyroidism is the result of a total thyroidectomy. Similarly, the combined use of rhTSH and radioiodine therapy induces permanent hypothyroidism in about one-third of patients. In 3 reported randomized controlled studies, permanent hypothyroidism at 1 year was reported in 21%, 63%, and 65% of rhTSH-treated patients compared with 7%, 11%, and 21%, respectively, in the control groups.[67,70,71]

Radioiodine treatment may induce the surge of autoantibodies against thyroid antigens independently from rhTSH, and a few and rare cases of Graves disease have been reported.

rhTSH use as an adjuvant of radioiodine therapy for MNG is still off-label, but the evidence gathered indicates that it potentiates a ^{131}I cytolytic effect in treating large MNG with improvement of goiter volume reduction, and this is sufficient to reduce compression and eliminate areas of thyroid autonomy.[78] Moreover, it is easier to perform in an outpatient mode, with reduced costs to the public health system, particularly in countries with limited resources and lack of high-volume thyroid surgeons.

SUMMARY

SDG and MNG affect millions of people worldwide. The main causes are mild iodine deficiency, natural goitrogens, smoking, and other environmental agents. Clinical evaluation is based on TSH, free T_4, and anti-TPO determinations followed by ultrasonographic imaging. Large goiters with substernal invasion may require CT or MRI. More recently, it has been accepted that there is a strong genetic influence in some familial goiters, and it is suggested that goiters are derived from a combination of genetic and environmental factors. Goiters are frequently treated by L-T_4–suppressive therapy (small goiters), subtotal thyroidectomy, followed by L-T_4 therapy. Radioiodine alone or preceded by rhTSH is widely used in Europe and other countries. Each of these therapeutic options has advantages and disadvantages, with acute and long-term side effects.

REFERENCES

1. Merke F. History and iconography of endemic goiter and endemic cretinism. Stuttgart and Wien: Verlag Hans Huber; 1974 [in German].
2. Medeiros-Neto G, Sawin CT. Francisco Freire-Alemão (1797–1874) and the early study of endemic goiter in Brazil. Endocrinologist 1996;6:353–5.
3. Zimmermann MB, Jooste PL, Pandav CS. Iodine deficiency disorders. Lancet 2008;372:1251–62.
4. Delange F, Benker G, Caron P, et al. Thyroid volume and urinary iodine in European schoolchildren; standardization values for assessment of iodine deficiency. Eur J Endocrinol 1997;136:180–7.
5. Hegedus L, Bonnema SJ, Bennedbaek FN. Management of simple nodular goiter: current status and future perspectives. Endocr Rev 2003;24:102–32.
6. Medeiros-Neto G, Henneman G: Multimodular goiter. Available at: http://www.thyroidmanager.org. 2010. Accessed November 7, 2011.
7. Turbridge WM, Evered DC, Hall R, et al. The spectrum of thyroid disease in a community: the Wickham survey. Clin Endocrinol 1977;7:481–93.

8. Vander JB, Gastón EA, Dawber TR. Significance of solitary nontoxic nodules. preliminary report. N Engl J Med 1954;251:970–6.
9. Berghout A, Wiersinga WM, Smits NJ, et al. Interrelationships between age, thyroid volume, thyroid nodularity and thyroid function in patients with sporadic non-toxic goiters. Am J Med 1995;89:602–8.
10. Hegedus L, Paschke R, Krohn K, et al. Multinodular goiter. In: Jamenson JL, Degroot LJ, editors. Endocrinology. 6th edition. Philadelphia: Saunders-Elsevier; 2010. p. 1636–49.
11. Bahn RS, Castro MR. Approach to the patient with non-toxic multinodular goiter. J Clin Endocrinol Metab 2011;96:1202–12.
12. Hegedus L, Brix TH, Paschke R. Etiology of simple goiter. Thyroid 2009;19: 209–11.
13. Krohn K, Wohlgenuth S, Gerber H, et al. Hot microscopic areas of iodine deficient thyroid goiters contain constitutively TSH-receptor mutations. J Pathol 2000;192: 37–42.
14. Studer H, Peter HJ, Gerber H. Natural heterogeneity of thyroid cells: the basis for understanding thyroid function and nodular growth. Endocr Rev 1989;10: 125–34.
15. Gaitan E, Cooksey RC, Legan J, et al. Antithyroid and goitrogenic effects of coal-water extracts from iodine-sufficient goiter areas. Thyroid 1993;3:49–53.
16. Ngudi DD, Kuo YH, Lambein F. Cassava cyanogens and free amino acids in raw and cooked leaves. Food Chem Toxicol 2003;41:1193–7.
17. Gaitan E, Cooksey RC, Legan J, et al. Antithyroid effects in vivo and in vitro of babassu and mandioca: a staple food in goiter areas of Brazil. Eur J Endocrinol 1994;131:138–44.
18. Schröder-van der Elst JP, Smit JW, Romijn HA, et al. Dietary flavonoids and iodine metabolism. Biofactors 2003;19:171–6.
19. Doerge DR, Chang HC. Inactivation of thyroid peroxidase by soy isoflavones, in vitro and in vivo. J Chromatogr B Analyt Technol Biomed Life Sci 2002;777: 269–79.
20. Suzuki H, Higuchi T, Sawa K, et al. Endemic coast goitre in Hokkaido, Japan. Acta Endocrinol 1965;50:161–76.
21. Zimmermann MB, Jooste PL, Mabapa NS, et al. Vitamin A supplementation in iodine-deficient African children decreases thyrotropin stimulation of the thyroid and reduces the goiter rate. Am J Clin Nutr 2007;86:1040–4.
22. Ingenbleek Y. Vitamin A deficiency impairs the normal mannosylation, conformation and iodination of the thyroglobulin: a new etiological approach to endemic goiter. Experientia Suppl 1983;44:264–97.
23. Zimmermann MB. The influence of iron status on iodine utilization and thyroid function. Annu Rev Nutr 2006;26:367–89.
24. Brauer VF, Schweizer U, Köhrle J, et al. Selenium and goiter prevalence in border-line iodine sufficiency. Eur J Endocrinol 2006;155:807–12.
25. Kralik A, Eder K, Kirchgessner M. Influence of zinc and selenium deficiency on parameters relating to thyroid hormone metabolism. Horm Metab Res 1996;28:223–6.
26. Ruz M, Codoceo J, Galgani J, et al. Single and multiple selenium-zinc-iodine deficiencies affect rat thyroid metabolism and ultrastructure. J Nutr 1999;129:174–80.
27. Wada L, King JC. Effect of low zinc intakes on basal metabolic rate, thyroid hormones and protein utilization in adult men. J Nutr 1986;116:1045–53.
28. Brucker-Davis F. Environmental disrupters of thyroid hormone action. In: Henry HL, Norman AN, editors. Encyclopedia of hormones. New York: Elsevier-Academic Press; 2003. p. 535–7.

29. Lindsay RH, Hill JB, Gaitan E, et al. Antithyroid effects of coal-derived pollutants. J Toxicol Environ Health 1992;37:467–81.

30. Braverman LE. Clinical studies of exposure to perchlorate in the United States. Thyroid 2007;17:819–22.

31. Laurberg P, Nøhr SB, Pedersen KM, et al. Iodine nutrition in breast-fed infants is impaired by maternal smoking. J Clin Endocrinol Metab 2004;89:181–7.

32. Bignell GR, Canzian F, Shayeghi M, et al. Familial nontoxic multi-nodular thyroid goiter locus maps to chromosome 14q but does not account for familial nonmedullary thyroid cancer. Am J Hum Genet 1997;61(5):1123–30.

33. Brix TH, Kyvik KO, Hegedüs L. Major role of genes in the etiology of simple goiter in females: a population-based twin study. J Clin Endocrinol Metab 1999;84(9):3071–5.

34. Neumann S, Willgerodt H, Ackermann F, et al. Linkage of familial euthyroid goiter to the multinodular goiter-1 locus and exclusion of the candidate genes thyroglobulin, thyroperoxidase, and Na+/I- symporter. J Clin Endocrinol Metab 1999;84:3750–6.

35. Capon F, Tacconelli A, Giardina E, et al. Mapping a dominant form of multinodular goiter to chromosome Xp22. Am J Hum Genet 2000;67:1004–7.

36. Brix TH, Hegedüs L. Genetic and environmental factors in the aetiology of simple goitre. Ann Med 2000;32:153–6.

37. Takahashi T, Nozaki J, Komatsu M, et al. A new locus for a dominant form of multinodular goiter on 3q26.1-q26.3. Biochem Biophys Res Commun 2001;284:650–4.

38. Bayer Y, Neumann S, Meyer B, et al. Genome-wide linkage analysis reveals evidence for four new susceptibility loci for familial euthyroid goiter. J Clin Endocrinol Metab 2004;89:4044–52.

39. Krohn K, Führer D, Bayer Y, et al. Molecular pathogenesis of euthyroid and toxic multinodular goiter. Endocr Rev 2005;26:504–24.

40. Ngan ES, Lang BH, Liu T, et al. A germline mutation (A339V) in thyroid transcription factor-1 (TITF-1/NKX2.1) in patients with multinodular goiter and papillary thyroid carcinoma. J Natl Cancer Inst 2009;101:162–75.

41. Corral M, Perez R, Sanchez I, et al. Thyroglobulin gene point mutation associated with non-endemic simple goiter. Lancet 1993;341:462–4.

42. González-Sarmiento R, Corral J, Mories MT, et al. Monoallelic deletion in the 5' region of the thyroglobulin gene as a cause of sporadic nonendemic simple goiter. Thyroid 2001;11:789–93.

43. Rubio IG, Medeiros-Neto G. Mutations in the thyroglobulin gene and its relevance to thyroid disorders. Curr Opin Endocrinol Diabetes Obes 2009;16:373–8.

44. Pardo V, Vono-Toniolo J, Rubio IG, et al. The p.A2215D thyroglobulin gene mutation leads to deficient synthesis and secretion of the mutated protein and congenital hypothyroidism with wide phenotype variation. J Clin Endocrinol Metab 2009; 94:2938–44.

45. Bonnema SJ, Bennedbaek FN, Ladenson PW, et al. Management of the nontoxic multinodular goiter: a North American survey. J Clin Endocrinol Metab 2002;87: 112–7.

46. Bonnema SJ, Bennedbaek FN, Wiersinga WM, et al. Management of the nontoxic multinodular goitre: a European questionnaire study. Clin Endocrinol (Oxf) 2000; 53(1):5–12.

47. Samuels MH. Evaluation and treatment of sporadic nontoxic goiter–some answers and more questions [editorial]. J Clin Endocrinol Metab 2001;86:994–7.

48. Abdel Rahim AA, Ahmed ME, Hassan MA. Respiratory complications after thyroidectomy and the need for tracheostomy in patients with a large goitre. Br J Surg 1999;86:88–90.

49. Torre G, Borgonovo G, Amato A, et al. Surgical management of substernal goiter: analysis of 237 patients. Am Surg 1995;61:826–31.
50. Vadasz P, Kotsis L. Surgical aspects of 175 mediastinal goiters. Eur J Cardiothorac Surg 1998;14:393–7.
51. Röjdmark J, Järhult J. High long term recurrence rate after subtotal thyroidectomy for nodular goitre. Eur J Surg 1995;161:725–7.
52. Hegedüs L, Nygaard B, Hansen JM. Is routine thyroxine treatment to hinder postoperative recurrence of nontoxic goiter justified? J Clin Endocrinol Metab 1999; 84:756–60.
53. Berghout A, Wiersinga WM, Drexhage HA, et al. The long-term outcome of thyroidectomy for sporadic non-toxic goitre. Clin Endocrinol (Oxf) 1989;31:193–9.
54. Miccoli P, Antonelli A, Iacconi P, et al. Prospective, randomized, double-blind study about effectiveness of levothyroxine suppressive therapy in prevention of recurrence after operation: result at the third year of follow-up. Surgery 1993; 114:1097–101 [discussion: 1101–2].
55. Hussain M, Hisham AN. Total thyroidectomy: the procedure of choice for toxic goitre. Asian J Surg 2008;31:59–62.
56. Riju R, Jadhav S, Kanthaswamy R, et al. Is total thyroidectomy justified in multinodular goitre. J Indian Med Assoc 2009;107(4):223–5.
57. Cannon CR, Lee R, Didlake R. Management of the substernal goiter: a team approach. J Miss State Med Assoc 2010;51(7):179–82.
58. Albayral Y, Demiryilmaz I, Kaya Z, et al. Comparison of total thyroidectomy, bilateral subtotal thyroidectomy and Dunhill operations in the treatment of benign thyroid disorders. Minerva Chir 2011;66(3):189–95.
59. Dogan L, Karaman N, Yilmaz KB, et al. Total thyroidectomy for the surgical treatment of multinodular goiter. Surg Today 2011;41(3):323–7.
60. Güllü S, Gürses MA, Başkal N, et al. Suppressive therapy with levothyroxine for euthyroid diffuse and nodular goiter. Endocr J 1999;46(1):221–6.
61. Lima N, Knobel M, Cavaliere H, et al. Levothyroxine suppressive therapy is partially effective in treating patients with benign, solid thyroid nodules and multinodular goiters. Thyroid 1997;7:691–7.
62. Wesche MF, Tiel-V Buul MM, Lips P, et al. A randomized trial comparing levothyroxine with radioactive iodine in the treatment of sporadic nontoxic goiter. J Clin Endocrinol Metab 2001;86:998–1005.
63. Papini E, Petrucci L, Guglielmi R, et al. Long-term changes in nodular goiter: a 5-year prospective randomized trial of levothyroxine suppressive therapy for benign cold thyroid nodules. J Clin Endocrinol Metab 1998;83:780–3.
64. Cesareo R, Iozzino M, Isgrò MA, et al. Short term effects of levothyroxine treatment in thyroid multinodular disease. Endocr J 2010;57(9):803–9.
65. Zelmanovitz F, Genro S, Gross JL. Suppressive therapy with levothyroxine for solitary thyroid nodules: a double-blind controlled clinical study and cumulative meta-analyses. J Clin Endocrinol Metab 1998;83:3881–5.
66. Grussendorf M, Reiners C, Paschke R, et al. Reduction of thyroid nodule volume by levothyroxine and iodine alone and in combination: a randomized, placebo-controlled trial. J Clin Endocrinol Metab 2011;96:2786–95.
67. Nielsen VE, Bonnema SJ, Boel-Jørgensen H, et al. Stimulation with 0.3-mg recombinant human thyrotropin prior to iodine 131 therapy to improve the size reduction of benign nontoxic nodular goiter: a prospective randomized double-blind trial. Arch Intern Med 2006;166(14):1476–82.
68. Hegedüs L, Hansen BM, Knudsen N, et al. Reduction of size of thyroid with radioactive iodine in multinodular non-toxic goitre. BMJ 1988;297:661–2.

69. Bonnema SJ, Hegedüs L. A 30-year perspective on radioiodine therapy of benign nontoxic multinodular goiter. Curr Opin Endocrinol Diabetes Obes 2009;16: 379–84.

70. Silva MN, Rubió IG, Romão R, et al. Administration of a single dose of recombinant human thyrotrophin enhances the efficacy of radioiodine treatment of large compressive multinodular goitres. Clin Endocrinol (Oxf) 2004;60:300–8.

71. Bonnema SJ, Nielsen VE, Boel-Jørgensen H, et al. Improvement of goiter volume reduction after 0.3 mg recombinant human thyrotropin-stimulated radioiodine therapy in patients with a very large goiter: a double-blinded, randomized trial. J Clin Endocrinol Metab 2007;92(9):3424–8.

72. Medeiros-Neto G, Marui S, Knobel M. An outline concerning the potential use of recombinant human thyrotropin for improving radioiodine therapy of multinodular goiter. Endocrine 2008;33:109–17.

73. Fast S, Nielsen VE, Grupe P, et al. Optimizing 131I uptake after rhTSH stimulation in patients with nontoxic multinodular goiter: evidence from a prospective, randomized, double-blind study. J Nucl Med 2009;50:732–7.

74. Fast S, Nielsen VE, Bonnema SJ, et al. Time to reconsider nonsurgical therapy of benign non-toxic multinodular goitre: focus on recombinant human TSH augmented radioiodine therapy. Eur J Endocrinol 2009;160:517–28.

75. Hegedüs L. Therapy: a new nonsurgical therapy option for benign thyroid nodules? Nat Rev Endocrinol 2009;5:476–8.

76. Romão R, Rubio IG, Tomimori EK, et al. High prevalence of side effects after recombinant human thyrotropin-stimulated radioiodine treatment with 30 mCi in patients with multinodular goiter and subclinical/clinical hyperthyroidism. Thyroid 2009;19:945–51.

77. Cubas ER, Paz-Filho GJ, Olandoski M, et al. Recombinant human TSH increases the efficacy of a fixed activity of radioiodine for treatment of multinodular goitre. Int J Clin Pract 2009;63:583–90.

78. Ceccarelli C, Brozzi F, Bianchi F, et al. Role of the recombinant human TSH in the management of large euthyroid multinodular goiter: a new therapeutic option? Pros and cons. Minerva Endocrinol 2010;35(3):161–71.

79. Fast S, Nielsen VE, Bonnema SJ, et al. Recombinant human TSH (rh TSH) augmented radioiodine treatment of benign multinodular goitre. Available at: http://www.hotthyroidology.com/. 2010. Accessed November 7, 2011.

80. Fast S, Nielsen VE, Bonnema SJ, et al. Dose-dependent acute effects of recombinant human TSH (rhTSH) on thyroid size and function: comparison of 0.1, 0.3 and 0.9 mg of rhTSH. Clin Endocrinol (Oxf) 2010;72:411–6.

81. Ceccarelli C, Antonangeli L, Brozzi F, et al. Radioiodine 131I treatment for large nodular goiter: recombinant human thyrotropin allows the reduction of radioiodine 131I activity to be administered in patients with low uptake. Thyroid 2011;21:759–64.

82. Graf H, Fast S, Pacini F, et al. Modified-release recombinant human TSH (MRrhTSH) augments the effect of (131)I therapy in benign multinodular goiter: results from a multicenter international, randomized, placebo-controlled study. J Clin Endocrinol Metab 2011;96:1368–76.

83. Fast S, Bonnema SJ, Hegedüs L. Radioiodine therapy of benign non-toxic goitre: potential role of recombinant human TSH. Ann Endocrinol (Paris) 2011;72(2): 129–35.

Approach to and Treatment of Differentiated Thyroid Carcinoma

Furio Pacini, MD*, Maria Grazia Castagna, MD

KEYWORDS

- Thyroglobulin • rhTSH • ^{131}I whole-body scan
- Radioiodine therapy

Thyroid cancer is the most common endocrine malignancy, although representing fewer than 1% of all human tumors. Differentiated thyroid carcinoma (DTC) includes the papillary and follicular histotypes and their variants, accounting for more than 90% of all thyroid cancers. The incidence of thyroid cancer has been increasing in many countries over the last 30 years (from 3.6 per 100,000 in 1973 to 8.7 per 100,000 in 2002), while mortality has been slowly decreasing.[1] This phenomenon is mainly attributable to an increase in the incidence of small papillary (<2 cm) tumors while there has been no significant change in incidence of the less common histologic categories: follicular, medullary, and anaplastic cancers. The increase is attributable to the better detection of small papillary carcinomas as a result of improved diagnostic accuracy (neck ultrasonography [US] and fine-needle aspiration cytology [FNAC]). Given the changing presentation of DTC in the last years, the aim of thyroid cancer management is to ensure the most effective but least invasive treatment, and adequate follow-up for a disease that nowadays is mostly cured just with surgery and is rarely fatal. This review addresses the multiple steps of current management, based on previous assumptions.

EPIDEMIOLOGY OF DTC

Nearly 60% to 80% of thyroid carcinomas detected nowadays in thyroid cancer referral centers are micropapillary thyroid carcinomas (<1 cm in size) carrying an excellent long-term prognosis,[2] and the features of the disease have changed dramatically in comparison with the previous decades.[3] Papillary thyroid carcinoma (PTC)

Section of Endocrinology and Metabolism, Department of Internal Medicine, Endocrinology & Metabolism and Biochemistry, University of Siena, Policlinico Santa Maria alle Scotte, Viale Bracci 1, 53100 Siena, Italy
* Corresponding author.
E-mail address: pacini8@unisi.it

Med Clin N Am 96 (2012) 369–383
doi:10.1016/j.mcna.2012.01.002
0025-7125/12/$ – see front matter © 2012 Elsevier Inc. All rights reserved.

affects women more often than men, and in 2006 it was predicted to be one of the top 7 leading causes of new cases of cancer in women, representing 3% of all cancers in women, about 1% in men, and about 1.4% of all cancers in children.[4] The onset of PTC occurs between the ages of 30 and 50 years. The incidence of PTC in the United States is 5.7 per 100,000 person-years, with a rate of 8.8 per 100,000 woman-years and 2.7 per 100,000 man-years.[5] Among women, PTC was higher among whites (10.39 per 100,000 woman-years) and lower among blacks (4.9 per 100,000 woman-years). Among men, PTC was higher among whites (3.58 per 100,000 woman-years) and lower among blacks (1.56 per 100,000 woman-years).[5] Follicular thyroid cancer (FTC) tends to occur in patients who are older (>40 years of age) than patients who have papillary cancer. The incidence of FTC in the United States is 0.82 per 100,000 person-years, with a rate of 1.06 per 100,000 woman-years and 0.59 per 100,000 man-years. The incidence of follicular cancer did not vary substantially by race/ethnicity,[5] although it is well known that its frequency is affected by iodine intake.[6] The incidence of anaplastic thyroid cancer in the United States is 0.21 per 100,000 person-years, without substantial difference by race/ethnicity and sex.

Despite the increasing incidence, the mortality from thyroid cancer has declined over the last 3 decades. In the European Union from 1992 to 2002, the mortality for thyroid cancer declined in both men and women (−23% and −28%, respectively).[7] It is unclear how much of the decline in mortality is due to early diagnosis rather than improved treatment of the disease. The age-adjusted death rate was 0.5 per 100,000 men and women per year, increasing from 0.1% in those younger than 20 years to 30% in their seventh and eighth decades.[8]

PATHOGENESIS OF DTC

The process of oncogenesis is characterized by a series of genetic events associated with hypothetical environmental factors. In the past several years, the genetic alterations responsible for thyroid cancer have been extensively studied and partially defined. Mutations in genes coding for elements of the mitogen-activated protein kinase pathway are often responsible for the transformation of thyroid follicular cells. The most frequent genetic alterations are represented by somatic activating mutations of proto-oncogenes, including BRAF and RAS or rearrangements of RET and TRK, or inactivating mutations of tumor suppressor genes, such as p53 and PPAR-γ. Mutations in the BRAF gene are the most frequent alterations of papillary carcinoma, with a prevalence of 49%.[9] In the case of RET and TRK, the genetic alteration is represented by the rearrangement of these genes with various ubiquitous genes (rearranged RET/PTC and TRK rearrangements).[10,11] Unlike BRAF and RET/PTC, which are papillary carcinoma–specific, mutations of RAS are found in a small proportion of papillary carcinomas, follicular adenomas, and follicular carcinomas.[12,13] The PAX8–PPAR-γ rearrangement is found in 35% to 45% of follicular carcinomas, 4% to 33% in follicular adenomas, and rarely in oncocytic carcinomas.[14,15] Aberrant activation (*PIK3CA* amplification and *ras* mutations) of the phosphatidylinositol-3 kinase (PI3K)/Akt pathway plays a fundamental role in thyroid tumorigenesis, particularly in FTC and aggressive thyroid cancer, such as anaplastic thyroid cancer (ATC), and less frequently in PTC. Epigenetic silencing of the *PTEN* gene, a negative regulator of the PI3K/AKT pathway, also occurs in thyroid tumors, but its relationship with genetic alterations in this pathway is unclear.[16] PTC and FTC tumors may progress to poorly differentiated or anaplastic phenotype by inactivating mutations of p53 proto-oncogene that deprive the cell of a major thyroid tumor suppressor gene.[17,18]

Familial predisposition in DTC is reported in 3% to 10% of the cases,[19,20] in the absence of recognized predisposing syndromes (Cowden syndrome, Werner syndrome, Carney complex, familial adenomatous polyposis), and the risk of developing the same tumor in first-degree relatives of subjects with DTC is significantly higher than in the general population.[21,22] No specific genetic alterations have been demonstrated in the blood of patients with familial nonmedullary thyroid carcinoma (FNMTC), apart from susceptibility loci found in a few pedigrees with FNMTC.[23] Among molecular mechanisms possibly underlying the familial predisposition to FNMTC, alteration in the telomere-telomerase complex has been recently reported.[24,25]

Although genetic factors have been well defined in recent decades, the role of environmental factors is still controversial. The only established environmental risk factor for thyroid carcinoma is exposure to ionizing radiation, and the risk, particularly of papillary carcinoma, is greater in subjects of younger age at exposure. This finding is supported by epidemiologic studies in the survivors of the atomic bomb attacks and following the explosion of the Chernobyl nuclear reactor in 1986, when a dramatic increase in the incidence of malignant thyroid tumors (80 times more) was observed in subjects who were children at the time of the accident and who were living in an extensive area surrounding the reactor.[26–31] In addition, studies in patients who received external radiation on the neck for the treatment of several diseases demonstrated a causative role of irradiation in the development of thyroid cancer.[32–34]

PRESENTATION AND DIAGNOSIS

Thyroid cancer presents as a thyroid nodule detected by palpation or, more frequently, by the fortuitous discovery at neck US. Although thyroid nodules are frequent (4%–50% depending on the diagnostic procedures and patients' age),[35] thyroid cancer is rare (approximately 5% of all thyroid nodules). The US features associated with malignancy are hypoechogenicity, microcalcifications, absence of peripheral halo, irregular borders, solid aspect, intranodular blood flow, and shape (taller than wide). All these patterns taken individually are poorly predictive of malignancy, but when multiple patterns suggestive of malignancy are simultaneously present, the specificity of US increases.[36] However, despite the overall utility of US, the gold standard for the differential diagnosis of thyroid nodules is still based on FNAC. According to the available guidelines,[37,38] FNAC should be performed in any thyroid nodule larger than 1 cm and in those smaller than 1 cm if there is any clinical (history of head and neck irradiation, family history of thyroid cancer, suspicious features at palpation, presence of cervical adenopathy) or US suspicion of malignancy. The results of FNAC are very sensitive for the differential diagnosis of benign and malignant nodules, although there are limitations: inadequate samples and follicular neoplasia. In the event of inadequate samples FNAC should be repeated, whereas in the case of follicular neoplasia with normal thyrotropin (TSH), surgery should be considered.[37,38] Among various methods proposed to increase the diagnostic accuracy of FNAC, mutation status of the tumor (presence or absence of oncogene mutations) is gaining increasing attention after reports demonstrating that the integration of traditional cytology with mutations analysis significantly increases sensitivity and specificity.[39,40] Thyroid function test and thyroglobulin (Tg) measurement are of little help in the diagnosis of thyroid cancer. However, measurement of serum calcitonin is a reliable tool for the diagnosis of the few cases of medullary thyroid cancer (5%–7% of all thyroid cancers), and has higher sensitivity compared with FNAC. Hence measurement of calcitonin should be an integral part of the diagnostic evaluation of thyroid nodules.[41] In the case of undifferentiated thyroid carcinoma, the diagnosis is usually based on typical clinical aspects: large, hard mass invading the neck and causing compressive symptoms (dyspnea, cough, vocal cord paralysis, dysphagia, and hoarseness). Cervical metastases are palpable on examination in 40% of patients.

TREATMENT OF DTC
Surgery

The initial treatment of DTC is total or near-total thyroidectomy whenever the diagnosis is made before surgery. Less extensive surgical procedures may be accepted in the case of unifocal DTC diagnosed at final histology after surgery performed for benign thyroid disorders, provided that the tumor is small, intrathyroidal, and of favorable histologic type (classic papillary or follicular variant of papillary or minimally invasive follicular). The initial treatment of DTC should always be preceded by careful exploration of the neck by US to assess the status of lymph node chains. Clinically evident lymph node metastases are present in approximately one-third of patients with PTC at presentation. Microscopic metastases are present in one-half. The most common site of lymph node involvement is the central compartment (level 6). The lateral lymph node chains (levels 2–4) are the next most common sites of cervical node involvement. Lymph nodes in the posterior triangle of the neck (level 5) may also develop metastases. Unlike papillary carcinoma, cervical metastases from follicular carcinomas are uncommon. The benefit of prophylactic central node dissection in the absence of evidence of nodal disease is controversial. There is no evidence that in PTC prophylactic central node dissection may improve the recurrence or mortality rate, but it does allow accurate staging of the disease that may guide subsequent treatment and follow-up.[37,38] Compartment-oriented dissection of lymph nodes should be performed in cases of preoperatively suspected and/or intraoperatively proven lymph node metastases. Prophylactic lymph node dissection is not indicated in FTC. In expert hands, surgical complications such as laryngeal nerve palsy and hypoparathyroidism are extremely rare (<1%–2%).[37,38]

Staging and Risk Assessment

Both papillary- and follicular-differentiated thyroid cancer have usually a good prognosis, with an overall mortality of less than 10%.[42] This favorable prognosis results from the combination of the biological properties of most thyroid carcinomas and effective primary therapy. In the last several years, an increased emphasis has been placed on using individual estimates of risk to guide postablative remnant ablation and follow-up in patients with DTC. Several different risk stratification systems have been published, the most popular being the American Joint Committee on Cancer/Union Internationale Contre le Cancer system.[43] All of the systems have been developed to predict the risk of death but not of recurrence and, being based on clinical pathologic factors available soon after diagnosis and initial surgical therapy, do not change over time. To overcome this limitation, both the American Thyroid Association (ATA) and the European Thyroid Association (ETA) have recently published practical guidelines[37,38] in which they grade the risk of recurrence in 3 categories of increasing risk based on tumor-related parameters (pTNM and histologic variant) integrated with other clinical features, including the result of the postablative whole-body scan (WBS) and serum Tg measurement (**Table 1**).

Table 1
Risk stratification according to the ATA and ETA guidelines

ATA Risk Stratification		
Low Risk	**Intermediate Risk**	**High Risk**
No local or distant metastases	Microscopic invasion of tumor into the perithyroidal soft tissues at initial surgery	Macroscopic tumor invasion
All macroscopic tumors have been resected		Incomplete tumor resection
No tumor invasion of locoregional tissues or structures	Cervical lymph node metastases or	Distant metastases
	^{131}I uptake outside the thyroid bed on the posttherapeutic WBS	Thyroglobulinemia out of proportion to what is seen on the postablative WBS scan
No aggressive histology or vascular invasion		
If ^{131}I was given, no ^{131}I uptake outside the thyroid bed on the posttherapeutic WBS	Tumor with aggressive histology or vascular invasion	

ETA Risk Stratification		
Very Low Risk	**Low Risk**	**High Risk**
Complete surgery	No local or distant metastases	Less than total thyroidectomy
Patients with unifocal microcarcinoma (<1 cm) with no extension beyond the thyroid capsule and without lymph node metastases	No tumor invasion of locoregional tissues or structures	Tumor invasion of locoregional tissues or structures
	No aggressive histology or vascular invasion	Cervical lymph node metastases
		Distant metastases
		Aggressive histology or vascular invasion

Data from Pacini F, Schlumberger M, Dralle H, et al. European Thyroid Cancer Taskforce. European consensus for the management of patients with differentiated thyroid carcinoma of the follicular epithelium. Eur J Endocrinol 2006;154:787–803; and Cooper DS, Doherty GM, Haugen BR, et al. Revised American Thyroid Association management guidelines for patients with thyroid nodules and differentiated thyroid cancer. Thyroid 2009;19:1167–214.

Recent reports have developed the new concept of Ongoing Risk Stratification or Delayed Risk Stratification (DRS), which better defines the patient risk based on the results of the initial treatment.[44,45] This concept is based on the continuous integration of the initial risk stratification (at the time of diagnosis) with the clinical, radiologic, and laboratory data becoming available during follow-up. Although the risk stratification guidelines proposed by ATA[38] and ETA[37] are a good starting point for initial decision-making, they are less accurate in predicting the long-term outcome in patients with DTC. Indeed, both systems have a very low positive predictive value (PPV), due to a large number of patients (about 60%) who are classified at intermediate/high risk being in complete remission at the end of follow-up.[45] This drawback is probably due to the lack of consideration of the effects of the initial therapy. When patients are restratified according to the results of the 8- to 12-month control after initial treatment, a significant number of patients who were initially considered (misleadingly) as high risk were reclassified as low risk and, most interestingly, almost all of these patients continued to be in apparent remission up to the end of follow-up.[45] This DRS allows improved modulation of the subsequent follow-up excluding a significant number of intermediate-/high-risk patients from unnecessary intensive workup.

Radioiodine Ablative Therapy

Surgery is usually followed by the administration of radioiodine (^{131}I) aimed at ablating any remnant thyroid tissue and potential microscopic residual tumor. This procedure does not seem to have an influence on mortality rate, but in most series seems to reduce the risk of regional recurrence and facilitates the long-term surveillance based on serum Tg measurement and diagnostic ^{131}I WBS. In addition, the high activity of ^{131}I allows obtaining a highly sensitive posttherapeutic WBS. According to several guidelines,[37,38] the recommendations for remnant thyroid ablation are modulated on the basis of risk factors. ^{131}I ablation is indicated in high-risk patients but not in low-risk patients. In patients at intermediate risk, ^{131}I remnant ablation may be indicated, but the decision must be individualized (**Table 2**).[37,38]

Effective thyroid ablation requires adequate stimulation by TSH. This may be achieved by thyroid hormone withdrawal (THW) or after the administration of recombinant human TSH (rhTSH). The latter procedure is considered the method of choice based on several reports[46–48] demonstrating equal efficacy compared with THW but better acceptance from the patients. In addition, in recent years successful thyroid ablation has been achieved using low activities of ^{131}I (1110–1850 MBq).[47,48]

Recent studies show that rhTSH-assisted ^{131}I ablative therapy is associated with similar rates of persistent disease and clinically evident recurrence than those observed after traditional THW preparation, at least in the short-term follow-up.[49,50] Based on these data, the use of rhTSH for postthyroidectomy ^{131}I ablation represents a safe and effective option for the postoperative management of patients with thyroid cancer. In addition, preparation with either rhTSH or THW seems to have similar effects of adjuvant therapy on small-volume ^{131}I-avid disease identified outside the thyroid bed at the time of initial ^{131}I remnant ablation.[47,51] ^{131}I-avid metastatic disease discovered at the time of rhTSH-stimulated remnant ablation was successfully treated in approximately 70% of locoregional lymph nodes[47,51] and in approximately 70% of pulmonary micrometastases.[51]

Table 2 Indications for remnant ablative therapy	
RAI is Recommended	**RAI is Not Recommended**
All Patients with: • Known distant metastases • Documented lymph node metastases • Gross extrathyroidal extension of the tumor regardless of tumor size • Primary tumor size >2 cm even in the absence of other higher-risk features[a] For Selected Patients with 1–2-cm Thyroid Cancers Confined to the Thyroid, with • Documented lymph node metastases, or • Other higher-risk features[a]	Patients with unifocal cancer <1 cm without other higher-risk features[a] Patients with multifocal cancer when all foci are <1 cm in the absence of other higher-risk features[a]

Abbreviation: RAI, radioiodine (^{131}I).

[a] Higher-risk features: histologic subtypes (tall cell, columnar, insular and solid variant as well as poorly DTC, follicular and Hurthle cell cancer), intrathyroidal vascular invasion, gross or microscopic multifocal disease.

Levothyroxine Therapy

Thyroid hormone suppression therapy is an important part of the treatment of thyroid cancer. Immediately after surgery, thyroid hormone therapy is initiated with a dual aim: to replace thyroid hormone and to suppress the potential growth stimulus of TSH on tumor cells (TSH-suppressive therapy). The drug of choice is levothyroxine (LT$_4$) and the suppressive dose varies according to age and body mass index.[52] TSH-suppressive treatment with LT$_4$ is of benefit in high-risk patients with thyroid cancer in whom the treatment may decrease the progression of metastatic disease, thus reducing cancer-related mortality. No significant benefits are demonstrated in low-risk patients.[53,54] The results of these studies suggest that more aggressive TSH suppression with LT$_4$ is important in patients with high-risk disease or recurrent tumor, whereas less aggressive TSH suppression is reasonable in low-risk patients.[53,54] This provides a rationale to target TSH levels to the lower part of the normal range in low-risk patients with DTC, as recommended by the ATA[38] and the ETA.[37] In particular, in the presence of persistent or metastatic disease an undetectable serum TSH (<0.1 mU/L) should be maintained during follow-up. In patients free of disease, regardless of their initial risk class, LT$_4$ therapy may be shifted from suppressive to replacement.

FOLLOW-UP
Short-Term Follow-Up

The aim of follow-up is the early discovery and treatment of persistent or recurrent locoregional or distant disease. Most recurrences develop and are detected in the first 5 years after diagnosis, whereas local or distant recurrence may develop in late follow-up, even 20 years after the initial treatment in a few cases.

After 2 to 3 months of initial treatment thyroid function tests (FT$_3$, FT$_4$, TSH) should be obtained to check the adequacy of LT$_4$ suppressive therapy. At 6 to 12 months, the follow-up is aimed to ascertain whether the patient is free of disease and is based on physical examination, neck US, and basal and rhTSH-stimulated serum Tg measurement, with or without diagnostic WBS.[37,38] At this time most (nearly 80%) of the patients will belong to the low-risk category, and will disclose normal results in neck US and undetectable (<1.0 ng/mL) basal and stimulated serum Tg values in the absence of serum Tg antibodies. Diagnostic WBS does not add any clinical information in this setting, and may be omitted.[55,56]

Recently, new methods for serum Tg measurement with functional sensitivity less than 0.1 ng/mL became available. Using these assays some investigators reported that an undetectable basal serum Tg value (<0.1 ng/mL) may give the same information as a stimulated serum Tg value, thus avoiding the need for Tg stimulation.[57–64] However, the higher negative predictive value (NPV) of these tests is at the expense of a very low specificity and PPV (**Table 3**), and there is a risk of exposing large numbers of patients, probably free of disease, to extensive testing and/or unnecessary treatment. In clinical practice, when the basal serum Tg level is up to 0.1 ng/mL and the neck US result is unremarkable, patients may be considered free of disease (NPV = 100%) and can avoid an rhTSH stimulation. On the contrary, when basal serum Tg is greater than 0.1 ng/mL but less than 1.0 ng/mL, it is not possible to distinguish between absence or presence of disease. In these cases, an rhTSH stimulation test may still be informative because it may detect those patients in whom serum Tg level increases to more than 1 ng/mL. In these patients a more intensive follow-up may be useful.[63]

Table 3
Diagnostic accuracy of basal serum thyroglobulin using sensitive assays

References	Criterion	N	Tg FS	Sens (%)	Spec (%)	PPV (%)	NPV (%)	FP (%)	FN (%)
Schlumberger et al,[59] 2007	Clinical status	944	0.11	78	63	NA	NA	37	22
Smallridge et al,[57] 2007	rhTSH-Tg (>2.0 ng/mL)	194	0.11	91.6	73.5	44	97.5	26.4	8.4
Iervasi et al,[58] 2007	rhTSH-Tg (>2.0 ng/mL)	160	0.11	100	90.1	34.7	100	10	0
Rosario and Purisch,[60] 2008	THW-Tg (<1.0 ng/mL)	178	0.11	80	81.6	41.6	96.1	18.4	20
Spencer et al,[62] 2010	rhTSH-Tg (>2.0 ng/mL)	1029	0.05	99.3	66.5	53.8	99.5	33.4	1.1
Castagna et al,[45,63] 2011	Clinical status	215	0.11	83.3	85.5	58.3	95.4	14.4	16.6
Malandrino et al,[64] 2011	rhTSH-Tg (>2.0 ng/mL)	425	0.11	91.6	84.3	35.1	99.0	15.7	8.4

Abbreviations: FN, false negative; FP, false positive; FS, functional sensitivity; NPV, negative predictive value; PPV, positive predictive value; Sens, sensitivity; Spec, specificity.

Long-Term Follow-Up

The subsequent follow-up of patients considered free of disease at the time of their first follow-up will consist of physical examination, basal serum Tg measurement on LT_4 therapy, and neck US once a year. No other biochemical or morphologic tests are indicated unless some new suspicion arises during evaluation. The question of whether a second rhTSH-stimulated Tg test should be performed in patients free of disease is a matter of debate. Recent studies reported that this procedure has little clinical utility in patients who had no biochemical (undetectable serum Tg) or clinical (imaging) evidence of disease at the time of their first control after initial therapy. In this group, the second test confirmed complete remission in almost all patients (**Table 4**).[55,56,65–68]

At the time of the first control after initial therapy, about 20% of patients may have detectable basal or stimulated serum Tg levels. If serum Tg level is detectable in the basal condition, the chance of a visible disease in the patient is very high, hence

Table 4
Prevalence of recurrences in patients free of disease at the first control after initial therapy, based on stimulated serum Tg measurement, neck ultrasonography, and diagnostic WBS

References	N	Stimulus	Follow-up (y)	Recurrence (%)
Pacini et al,[55] 2002	315	Hypothyroidism	12	0.6
Cailleux et al,[56] 2000	256	Hypothyroidism	5.0	0.9
Kloos and Mazzaferri,[65] 2005	68	rhTSH	3.3	1.4
Castagna et al,[66] 2008	68	rhTSH	3.0	1.5
Crocetti et al,[67] 2008	89	rhTSH	3.0	1.1
Brassard et al,[68] 2011	715	Hypothyroidism/rhTSH	7.0	1.1

imaging techniques must be applied. If serum Tg level is detectable in the low range after rhTSH stimulation, the chance of serum Tg to convert from detectable to undetectable level during follow-up is about 50%,[69] therefore observation is all that is required. On the contrary, the trend of serum Tg level to increase over time is a hallmark of possible disease to be localized by imaging techniques including therapeutic doses of ^{131}I.[37,38] During the evaluation of metastatic patients, positron emission tomography with fludeoxyglucose F 18 (^{18}F FDG-PET) scanning is gaining more attention as a diagnostic and prognostic tool.[70] The sensitivity of ^{18}F FDG-PET is not superior to that of traditional techniques, such as computed tomography and magnetic resonance imaging, therefore the main indication for ^{18}F FDG-PET is in patients with metastasis who have lost ^{131}I uptake. Patients who have negative results on ^{131}I WBS and positive results on ^{18}F FDG-PET show a group of tumors with more aggressive and less differentiated phenotype carrying a worse prognosis compared with patients who have positive results on ^{131}I WBS and negative results on ^{18}F FDG-PET.[70]

TREATMENT OF METASTATIC DISEASE

Treatment of persistent or recurrent locoregional disease during follow-up is based on surgical procedures whenever possible. Radioiodine therapy may be an option in the case of lesions not amenable to surgery with proven ^{131}I avidity. External beam radiotherapy may be indicated when complete surgical excision is not possible or when there is no significant ^{131}I uptake in the tumor.[37,38]

Approximately 20% of patients with DTC have distant metastases at diagnosis or during follow-up. Distant metastases are more successfully cured if they take up ^{131}I, are of small size, and are located in the lungs (not visible on radiographs). Lung

Table 5
Results of clinical trials with tyrosine kinase inhibitors in DTC

References	Phase	Drug	N	Partial Response (%)	Stable Disease >6 Months (%)	Median PFS (mo)
Gupta-Abramson et al,[75] 2008	II	Sorafenib	30	23	53	20
Kloos et al,[74] 2009	II	Sorafenib	41	15	56	15
Hoftijzer et al,[80] 2009	II	Sorafenib	32	25	34	13.5
Ahmed et al,[76] 2011	II	Sorafenib	19	18	82	<24
Sherman et al,[81] 2008	II	Motesanib	93	14	35	9
Cohen et al,[73] 2008	II	Axitinib	45	31	46	18.1
Carr et al,[77] 2010	II	Sunitinib	28	29	50	12.8
Bible et al,[78] 2010	II	Pazopanib	39	49	NR	11.7
Sherman et al,[79] 2011	II	Lenvatinib	58	45	46	13.3

Abbreviation: NR, not reported.

macronodules may benefit from ^{131}I therapy, but the definitive cure rate is very low.[71] Bone metastases have the worst prognosis even when aggressively treated by a combination of ^{131}I therapy and external beam radiotherapy.[37,38] Brain metastases are rare and usually carry a poor prognosis. Surgical resection and external beam radiotherapy represent the only therapeutic options.

TREATMENT OF METASTATIC DISEASE REFRACTORY TO CONVENTIONAL THERAPY

Treatment of distant metastases with ^{131}I therapy provides complete remission in only one-third of patients with distant metastases. The other patients have ^{131}I refractory disease defined as no ^{131}I-avid lesions or ^{131}I-avid lesions that do not benefit from repeated treatment courses of [131]I. These patients are candidates for systemic therapies. The selection is based on clinical prognostic indicators, including age, performance status, histology, extent and location of disease, and progression rate. Usually patients who are treated are those with significant progressive disease and with low life expectancy. In these patients, chemotherapy has limited effectiveness, with a response rate typically less than 20% and short lasting.[72]

Recently, molecules that block kinase activity at distal steps in the mitogen-activated protein kinase pathway have been identified as logical candidate drugs for refractory thyroid cancer. Tyrosine kinase inhibitors being tested against DTC in phase I and II trials include axitinib, lenvatinib, motesanib, pazopanib, sorafenib, sunitinib, and vandetanib. None of these are specific for 1 oncogene protein, but they target several tyrosine kinase receptors and proangiogenic growth factors. The results of phase I and II clinical trials have clearly confirmed the clinical benefits of these compounds. No compound has yet achieved the regulatory approval of Food and Drug Administration and European Medicines Agency for the therapy of advanced and progressive DTC, but some treatment guidelines recommend the use of available agents for selected patients with progressive metastatic disease based on the phase II results.[38] The results of phase I and II clinical trials conducted so far are promising, with a partial response ranging from 14% to 49% and stable disease ranging from 34% to 82% (**Table 5**).[73–81]

REFERENCES

1. Davies L, Welch HG. Increasing incidence of thyroid cancer in the United States, 1973-2002. JAMA 2006;295:2164–7.
2. Leenhardt L, Bernier MO, Boin-Pineau MH, et al. Advances in diagnostic practices affect thyroid cancer incidence in France. Eur J Endocrinol 2004;150:133–9.
3. Elisei R, Molinaro E, Agate L, et al. Are the clinical and pathological features of differentiated thyroid carcinoma really changed over the last 35 years? Study on 4187 patients from a single Italian institution to answer this question. J Clin Endocrinol Metab 2010;95:1516–27.
4. Jemal A, Siegel R, Ward E. Cancer statistics 2006. CA Cancer J Clin 2006;56: 106–30.
5. Aschebrook-Kilfoy B, Ward MH, Sabra MM, et al. Thyroid cancer incidence patterns in the United States by histologic type, 1992-2006. Thyroid 2011;21: 125–34.
6. Belfiore A, La Rosa GL, La Porta GA, et al. Cancer risk in patients with cold thyroid nodules: relevance of iodine intake, sex, age, and multinodularity. Am J Med 1992;93:363–9.

7. Bosetti C, Bertuccio P, Levi F, et al. Cancer mortality in the European Union, 1970-2003, with a joinpoint analysis. Ann Oncol 2008;19:631–40.

8. Howlader N, Noone AM, Krapcho M, et al, editors. SEER Cancer Statistics Review, 1975-2008. Bethesda (MD): National Cancer Institute; 2011. Available at. http://seer.cancer.gov/csr/1975_2008/. based on November 2010 SEER data submission, posted to the SEER web site.

9. Xing M. BRAF mutation in thyroid cancer. Endocr Relat Cancer 2005;12:245–62.

10. Fugazzola L, Pilotti S, Pinchera A, et al. Oncogenic rearrangements of the RET proto-oncogene in papillary thyroid carcinomas from children exposed to the Chernobyl nuclear accident. Cancer Res 1995;55:5617–20.

11. Ito T, Seyama T, Iwamoto KS, et al. Activated RET oncogene in thyroid cancers of children from areas contaminated by Chernobyl accident. Lancet 1994; 344(8917):259.

12. Karga H, Lee JK, Vickery AL Jr, et al. Ras oncogene mutations in benign and malignant thyroid neoplasms. J Clin Endocrinol Metab 1991;73:832–6.

13. Vasko V, Ferrand M, Di Cristofaro J, et al. Specific pattern of RAS oncogene mutations in follicular thyroid tumors. J Clin Endocrinol Metab 2003;88: 2745–52.

14. Marques AR, Espadinha C, Catarino AL, et al. Expression of PAX8-PPAR gamma 1 rearrangements in both follicular thyroid carcinomas and adenomas. J Clin Endocrinol Metab 2002;87:3947–52.

15. Nikiforova MN, Biddinger PW, Caudill CM, et al. PAX8-PPARgamma rearrangement in thyroid tumors: RT-PCR and immunohistochemical analyses. Am J Surg Pathol 2002;26:1016–23.

16. Xing M. Genetic alterations in the phosphatidylinositol-3 kinase/Akt pathway in thyroid cancer. Thyroid 2010;20:697–706.

17. Pollina L, Pacini F, Fontanini G, et al. bcl-2, p53 and proliferating cell nuclear antigen expression is related to the degree of differentiation in thyroid carcinomas. Br J Cancer 1996;73:139–43.

18. Nikiforova MN, Kimura ET, Gandhi M, et al. BRAF mutations in thyroid tumors are restricted to papillary carcinomas and anaplastic or poorly differentiated carcinomas arising from papillary carcinomas. J Clin Endocrinol Metab 2003;88: 5399–404.

19. Loh KC. Familial nonmedullary thyroid carcinoma: a meta-review of case series. Thyroid 1997;7:107–13.

20. Goldgar DE, Easton DF, Cannon-Albright LA, et al. Systematic population-based assessment of cancer risk in first-degree relatives of cancer probands. J Natl Cancer Inst 1994;86:1600–8.

21. Hemminki K, Eng C, Chen B. Familial risks for nonmedullary thyroid cancer. J Clin Endocrinol Metab 2005;90:5747–53.

22. Canzian F, Amati P, Harach HR, et al. A gene predisposing to familial thyroid tumors with cell oxyphilia maps to chromosome 19p13.2. Am J Hum Genet 1998;63:1743–8.

23. Malchoff CD, Sarfarazi M, Tendler B, et al. Papillary thyroid carcinoma associated with papillary renal neoplasia: genetic linkage analysis of a distinct heritable tumor syndrome. J Clin Endocrinol Metab 2000;85:1758–64.

24. Capezzone M, Marchisotta S, Cantara S, et al. Familial non-medullary thyroid carcinoma displays the features of clinical anticipation suggestive of a distinct biological entity. Endocr Relat Cancer 2008;15:1075–81.

25. Capezzone M, Cantara S, Marchisotta S, et al. Short telomeres, telomerase reverse transcriptase gene amplification, and increased telomerase activity in

the blood of familial papillary thyroid cancer patients. J Clin Endocrinol Metab 2008;93:3950–7.

26. Nagataki S, Aashizawa K, Yamashita S. Cause of childhood thyroid cancer after the Chernobyl accident. Thyroid 1998;8:115–7.

27. Mettler FA Jr, Williamson MR, Royal HD, et al. Thyroid nodules in the population living around Chernobyl. JAMA 1992;5(268):616–9.

28. Anspaugh LR, Catlin RJ, Goldman M. The global impact of the Chernobyl reactor accident. Science 1988;16(242):1513–9.

29. Pacini F, Vorontsova T, Molinaro E, et al. Thyroid consequences of the Chernobyl nuclear accident. Acta Paediatr Suppl 1999;88:23–7.

30. Tronko MD, Bogdanova TI, Komissarenko IV, et al. Thyroid carcinoma in children and adolescents in Ukraine after the Chernobyl nuclear accident: statistical data and clinicomorphologic characteristics. Cancer 1999;86:149–56.

31. Jacob P, Bogdanova TI, Buglova E, et al. Thyroid cancer among Ukrainians and Belarusians who were children or adolescents at the time of the Chernobyl accident. J Radiol Prot 2006;26:51–67.

32. Sarne D, Schneider AB. External radiation and thyroid neoplasia. Endocrinol Metab Clin North Am 1996;25:181–96.

33. Ron E, Kleinerman RA, Boice JD Jr, et al. A population-based case-control study of thyroid cancer. J Natl Cancer Inst 1987;79:1–12.

34. Ron E, Lubin JH, Shore RE, et al. Thyroid cancer after exposure to external radiation: a pooled analysis of seven studies. Radiat Res 1995;141:259–77.

35. Dean DS, Gharib H. Epidemiology of thyroid nodules. Best Pract Res Clin Endocrinol Metab 2008;22:901–11.

36. Rago T, Vitti P. Role of thyroid ultrasound in the diagnostic evaluation of thyroid nodules. Best Pract Res Clin Endocrinol Metab 2008;226:913–28.

37. Pacini F, Schlumberger M, Dralle H, et al. European Thyroid Cancer Taskforce. European consensus for the management of patients with differentiated thyroid carcinoma of the follicular epithelium. Eur J Endocrinol 2006;154:787–803.

38. Cooper DS, Doherty GM, Haugen BR, et al. Revised American Thyroid Association management guidelines for patients with thyroid nodules and differentiated thyroid cancer. Thyroid 2009;19:1167–214.

39. Nikiforov YE, Steward DL, Robinson-Smith TM, et al. Molecular testing for mutations in improving the fine-needle aspiration diagnosis of thyroid nodules. J Clin Endocrinol Metab 2009;94:2092–8.

40. Cantara S, Capezzone M, Marchisotta S, et al. Impact of proto-oncogene mutation detection in cytological specimens from thyroid nodules improves the diagnostic accuracy of cytology. J Clin Endocrinol Metab 2010;95:1365–9.

41. Elisei R, Bottici V, Luchetti F, et al. Impact of routine measurement of serum calcitonin on the diagnosis and outcome of medullary thyroid cancer: experience in 10,864 patients with nodular thyroid disorders. J Clin Endocrinol Metab 2004; 89:163–8.

42. Mazzaferri EL, Kloos RT. Clinical review 128: current approaches to primary therapy for papillary and follicular thyroid cancer. J Clin Endocrinol Metab 2001;86:1447–63.

43. American Joint Committee on Cancer: AJCC. Cancer staging manual. 7th edition. New York: Springer; 2010.

44. Tuttle RM, Tala H, Shah J, et al. Estimating risk of recurrence in differentiated thyroid cancer after total thyroidectomy and radioactive iodine remnant ablation: using response to therapy variables to modify the initial risk estimates predicted by the DRS American Thyroid Association staging system. Thyroid 2010;20:1341–9.

45. Castagna MG, Maino F, Cipri C, et al. Delayed risk stratification, to include the response to initial treatment (surgery and radioiodine ablation), has better outcome predictivity in differentiated thyroid cancer patients. Eur J Endocrinol 2011;165(3):441–6.

46. Pacini F, Ladenson PW, Schlumberger M, et al. Radioiodine ablation of thyroid remnants after preparation with recombinant human thyrotropin in differentiated thyroid carcinoma: results of an international, randomized, controlled study. J Clin Endocrinol Metab 2006;91:926–32.

47. Pilli T, Brianzoni E, Capoccetti F, et al. A comparison of 1850 (50 mCi) and 3700 MBq (100 mCi) 131-iodine administered doses for recombinant thyrotropin-stimulated postoperative thyroid remnant ablation in differentiated thyroid cancer. J Clin Endocrinol Metab 2007;92:3542–6.

48. Chianelli M, Todino V, Graziano FM, et al. Low-activity (2.0 GBq; 54 mCi) radioiodine post-surgical remnant ablation in thyroid cancer: comparison between hormone withdrawal and use of rhTSH in low-risk patients. Eur J Endocrinol 2009;160:431–6.

49. Elisei R, Schlumberger M, Driedger A, et al. Follow-up of low-risk differentiated thyroid cancer patients who underwent radioiodine ablation of postsurgical thyroid remnants after either recombinant human thyrotropin or thyroid hormone withdrawal. J Clin Endocrinol Metab 2009;94:4171–9.

50. Tuttle RM, Brokhin M, Omry G, et al. Recombinant human TSH-assisted radioactive iodine remnant ablation achieves short-term clinical recurrence rates similar to those of traditional thyroid hormone withdrawal. J Nucl Med 2008;49:764–70.

51. Tuttle RM, Lopez N, Leboeuf R, et al. 8. Radioactive iodine administered for thyroid remnant ablation following recombinant human thyroid stimulating hormone preparation also has an important adjuvant therapy function. Thyroid 2010;20:257–63.

52. Santini F, Pinchera A, Marsili A, et al. Lean body mass is a major determinant of levothyroxine dosage in the treatment of thyroid diseases. J Clin Endocrinol Metab 2005 Jan;90(1):124–7.

53. Jonklaas J, Sarlis NJ, Litofsky D, et al. Outcomes of patients with differentiated thyroid carcinoma following initial therapy. Thyroid 2006;16:1229–42.

54. Hovens GC, Stokkel MP, Kievit J, et al. Associations of serum thyrotropin concentrations with recurrence and death in differentiated thyroid cancer. J Clin Endocrinol Metab 2007;92:2610–5.

55. Pacini F, Capezzone M, Elisei R, et al. Diagnostic 131-iodine whole-body scan may be avoided in thyroid cancer patients who have undetectable stimulated serum Tg levels after initial treatment. J Clin Endocrinol Metab 2002;87:1499–501.

56. Cailleux AF, Baudin E, Travagli JP, et al. Is diagnostic iodine-131 scanning useful after total thyroid ablation for differentiated thyroid cancer? J Clin Endocrinol Metab 2000;85:175–8.

57. Smallridge RC, Meek SE, Morgan MA, et al. Monitoring thyroglobulin in a sensitive immunoassay has comparable sensitivity to recombinant human TSH-stimulated thyroglobulin in follow-up of thyroid cancer patients. J Clin Endocrinol Metab 2007;92:82–7.

58. Iervasi A, Iervasi G, Ferdeghini M, et al. Clinical relevance of highly sensitive Tg assay in monitoring patients treated for differentiated thyroid cancer. Clin Endocrinol 2007;67:434–41.

59. Schlumberger M, Hitzel A, Toubert ME, et al. Comparison of seven serum thyroglobulin assays in the follow-up of papillary and follicular thyroid cancer patients. J Clin Endocrinol Metab 2007;92:2487–95.

60. Rosario PW, Purisch S. Does a highly sensitive thyroglobulin (Tg) assay change the clinical management of low-risk patients with thyroid cancer with Tg on T4 <1 ng/ml determined by traditional assays? Clin Endocrinol 2008;68:338–42.

61. Giovanella L, Maffioli M, Ceriani L, et al. Unstimulated high sensitive thyroglobulin measurement predicts outcome of differentiated thyroid carcinoma. Clin Chem Lab Med 2009;47:1001–4.

62. Spencer C, Fatemi S, Singer P, et al. Serum basal thyroglobulin measured by a second-generation assay correlates with the recombinant human thyrotropin-stimulated thyroglobulin response in patients treated for differentiated thyroid cancer. Thyroid 2010;20:587–95.

63. Castagna MG, Tala Jury HP, Cipri C, et al. The use of ultrasensitive thyroglobulin assays reduces but does not abolish the need for TSH stimulation in patients with differentiated thyroid carcinoma. J Endocrinol Invest 2011;34:219–23.

64. Malandrino P, Latina A, Marescalco S, et al. Risk-adapted management of differentiated thyroid cancer assessed by a sensitive measurement of basal serum thyroglobulin. J Clin Endocrinol Metab 2011;96:1703–9.

65. Kloos RT, Mazzaferri EL. A single recombinant human thyrotropin-stimulated serum thyroglobulin measurement predicts differentiated thyroid carcinoma metastases three to five years later. J Clin Endocrinol Metab 2005;90:5047–57.

66. Castagna MG, Brilli L, Pilli T, et al. Limited value of repeat recombinant human thyrotropin (rhTSH)-stimulated thyroglobulin testing in differentiated thyroid carcinoma patients with previous negative rhTSH-stimulated thyroglobulin and undetectable basal serum thyroglobulin levels. J Clin Endocrinol Metab 2008;93:76–81.

67. Crocetti U, Durante C, Attard M, et al. Predictive value of recombinant human TSH stimulation and neck ultrasonography in differentiated thyroid cancer patients. Thyroid 2008;18:1049–53.

68. Brassard M, Borget I, Edet-Sanson A, et al. THYRDIAG Working Group. Long-term follow-up of patients with papillary and follicular thyroid cancer: a prospective study on 715 patients. J Clin Endocrinol Metab 2011;96:1352–9.

69. Kloos RT. Thyroid cancer recurrence in patients clinically free of disease with undetectable or very low serum thyroglobulin values. J Clin Endocrinol Metab 2010;95:5241–8.

70. Robbins RJ, Wan Q, Grewal RK, et al. Real-time prognosis for metastatic thyroid carcinoma based on 2-[^{18}F]fluoro-2-deoxy-D-glucose-positron emission tomography scanning. J Clin Endocrinol Metab 2006;91:498–505.

71. Durante C, Haddy N, Baudin E, et al. Long-term outcome of 444 patients with distant metastases from papillary and follicular thyroid carcinoma: benefits and limits of radioiodine therapy. J Clin Endocrinol Metab 2006;91:2892–9.

72. Haugen BR. Management of the patient with progressive radioiodine non-responsive disease. Semin Surg Oncol 1999;16:34–41.

73. Cohen EE, Rosen LS, Vokes EE, et al. Axitinib is an active treatment for all histologic subtypes of advanced thyroid cancer: results from a phase II study. J Clin Oncol 2008;26:4708–13.

74. Kloos RT, Ringel MD, Knopp MV, et al. Phase II trial of sorafenib in metastatic thyroid cancer. J Clin Oncol 2009;27:1675–84.

75. Gupta-Abramson V, Troxel AB, Nellore A, et al. Phase II trial of sorafenib in advanced thyroid cancer. J Clin Oncol 2008;26:4714–9.

76. Ahmed M, Barbachano Y, Riddell A, et al. Analysis of the efficacy and toxicity of sorafenib in thyroid cancer: a phase II study in a UK based population. Eur J Endocrinol 2011;165:315–22.

77. Carr LL, Mankoff DA, Goulart BH, et al. Phase II study of daily sunitinib in FDG-PET-positive, iodine-refractory differentiated thyroid cancer and metastatic medullary carcinoma of the thyroid with functional imaging correlation. Clin Cancer Res 2010;16:5260–8.
78. Bible KC, Suman VJ, Molina JR, et al. Endocrine Malignancies Disease Oriented Group; Mayo Clinic Cancer Center; Mayo Phase 2 Consortium. Efficacy of pazopanib in progressive, radioiodine-refractory, metastatic differentiated thyroid cancers: results of a phase 2 consortium study. Lancet Oncol 2010;11:962–72.
79. Sherman SI, Jarzab B, Cabanillas ME, et al. A phase II trial of the multitargeted kinase inhibitor E7080 in advanced radioiodine (RAI)-refractory differentiated thyroid cancer (DTC) [abstract]. J Clin Oncol 2011;29:a5503.
80. Hoftijzer H, Heemstra KA, Morreau H, et al. Beneficial effects of sorafenib on tumor progression, but not on radioiodine uptake in patients with differentiated thyroid cancer. Eur J Endocrinol 2009;161:923–31.
81. Sherman SI, Wirth LJ, Droz JP, et al. Motesanib Thyroid Cancer Study Group. Motesanib diphosphate in progressive differentiated thyroid cancer. N Engl J Med 2008;3(359):31–42.

Thyroid Emergencies

Joanna Klubo-Gwiezdzinska, MD, PhD[a,b],
Leonard Wartofsky, MD, MPH, MACP[c],*

KEYWORDS

- Myxedema coma • Thyrotoxic storm • Diagnosis
- Management

Thyroid emergencies are rare, life-threatening conditions resulting from either severe deficiency of thyroid hormones (myxedema coma) or, by contrast, decompensated thyrotoxicosis with the increased action of thyroxine (T4) and triiodothyronine (T3) exceeding metabolic demands of the organism (thyrotoxic storm). The understanding of the pathogenesis of these conditions, appropriate recognition of the clinical signs and symptoms, and their prompt and accurate diagnosis and treatment are crucial in optimizing survival.

MYXEDEMA COMA
Epidemiology and Precipitating Events

Myxedema coma is the extreme expression of severe hypothyroidism and fortunately is rare, with an incidence rate of 0.22 per million per year.[1] The most common presentation of the syndrome is in hospitalized elderly women with long-standing hypothyroidism, with 80% of cases occurring in women older than 60 years. However, myxedema coma occurs in younger patients as well, with 36 documented cases of pregnant women.[2,3]

The syndrome will typically present in patients who develop a systemic illness such as pulmonary or urinary infections, congestive heart failure, or cerebrovascular accident (**Table 1**), superimposed on previously undiagnosed hypothyroidism. Sometimes a history of antecedent thyroid disease, thyroidectomy, treatment with radioactive iodine, or T4 replacement therapy discontinued for no apparent reason can be elicited. A pituitary or hypothalamic basis for hypothyroidism is encountered in about 5% or, according to some studies, in up to 10% to 15% of patients.[4]

The authors have nothing to disclose.

[a] Division of Endocrinology, Department of Medicine, Washington Hospital Center, 110 Irving Street Northwest, Washington, DC 20010-2910, USA
[b] Department of Endocrinology and Diabetology, Collegium Medicum in Bydgoszcz, Nicolaus Copernicus University in Torun, ul. M. Sklodowskiej-Curie 9, 85-094 Bydgoszcz, Poland
[c] Department of Medicine, Washington Hospital Center, 110 Irving Street Northwest, Washington, DC 20010-2910, USA
* Corresponding author.
E-mail address: leonard.wartofsky@medstar.net

Med Clin N Am 96 (2012) 385–403
doi:10.1016/j.mcna.2012.01.015
0025-7125/12/$ – see front matter © 2012 Elsevier Inc. All rights reserved.

Table 1	
Factors precipitating thyroid emergencies: myxedema coma and thyrotoxic storm	
Precipitating Factors	
Myxedema Coma	**Thyrotoxic Storm**
Drugs	Drugs
Withdrawal of L-thyroxine	Withdrawal of antithyroid drug treatment
Anesthetics	Radioactive iodine treatment
Sedatives	Thyroxine/triiodothyronine overdosage
Tranquilizers	Cytotoxic chemotherapy
Narcotics	Aspirin overdosage
Amiodarone	Iodinated contrast dyes
Lithium carbonate	Organophosphates
Infections, sepsis	Sepsis, infection
Cerebrovascular accidents	Seizure disorder
Congestive heart failure	Pulmonary thromboembolism
Low temperatures	Burn injury
Trauma	Surgery, trauma, vigorous palpation of thyroid
Metabolic disturbances	Metabolic disturbances
Acidosis	Diabetic ketoacidosis
Hypoglycemia	Hypoglycemia
Hyponatremia	
Hypercapnia	
Other	Other
Gastrointestinal bleeding	Parturition
Ingestion of raw bok choy	Emotional stress

Patients with myxedema coma generally present in the winter months, suggesting that external cold may be an aggravating factor.[5] Some abnormalities such as hypoglycemia, hypercalcemia, hyponatremia, hypercapnia, and hypoxemia, may be either precipitating factors or secondary consequences of myxedema coma. Moreover, the comatose state is associated with the risk of aspiration pneumonia and sepsis. In hospitalized patients, drugs such as anesthetics, narcotics, sedatives, antidepressants, and tranquilizers may depress respiratory drive and thereby either cause or compound the deterioration of the hypothyroid patient into coma.[6,7] The effect of these drugs should be taken into consideration as a potential causative mechanism. In fact, Church and Callen[8] described a 41-year-old male patient without any history of thyroid disease who developed myxedema coma after being administered combined therapy with aripiprazole and sertraline.

There is also a report of myxedema coma induced by chronic ingestion of large amounts of raw bok choy. This Chinese white cabbage contains glucosinolates, which break down products such as thiocyanates, nitriles, and oxazolidines, and inhibit iodine uptake and production of thyroid hormones by the thyroid gland. When eaten raw, digestion of the vegetable releases the enzyme myrosinase, which accelerates production of the aforementioned thyroid disruptors.[9]

Clinical Signs and Symptoms

Hypothermia (often profound to 80°F [26.7°C]) and unconsciousness constitute 2 of the cardinal features of myxedema coma.[10] Of importance is that coincident infection may be masked by hypothyroidism, with a patient presenting as afebrile despite an underlying severe infection. In view of the latter and the fact that undiagnosed infection might lead inexorably to vascular collapse and death, some authorities have advocated the routine use of antibiotics in patients with myxedema coma. Underlying hypoglycemia may further compound the decrement in body temperature.

Although coma is the predominant clinical presentation, a history of disorientation, depression, paranoia, or hallucinations (myxedema madness) may often be elicited. The neurologic findings may also include cerebellar signs (poorly coordinated purposeful movements of the hands and feet, ataxia, adiadochokinesia), poor memory and recall, or even frank amnesia, and abnormal findings on electroencephalography (low amplitude and a decreased rate of α-wave activity). Status epilepticus has been also described[11] and up to 25% of patients may experience seizures possibly related to hyponatremia, hypoglycemia, or hypoxemia.

Respiratory System

The mechanism for hypoventilation in profound myxedema is a combination of a depressed hypoxic respiratory drive and a depressed ventilatory response to hypercapnia.[12,13] Partial obstruction of the upper airway caused by edema of the tongue or vocal cords may also play a role. Hypothyroid patients may be predisposed to increased airway hyperresponsiveness and chronic inflammation.[14] Tidal volume may be additionally reduced by other factors such as pleural effusion or ascites. to achieve appropriately effective pulmonary function in myxedema coma, prolonged mechanically assisted ventilation is usually required.

Cardiovascular Manifestations

Patients diagnosed with myxedema coma are at increased risk for shock and potentially fatal arrhythmias. Typical electrocardiographic (ECG) findings include bradycardia, varying degrees of block, low voltage, flattened or inverted T waves, and prolonged Q-T interval, which can result in torsades de pointes ventricular tachycardia.[15] Myocardial infarction should also be ruled out by the usual diagnostic procedures, because aggressive or injudicious T4 replacement may increase the risk of myocardial infarction. Moreover, cardiac contractility is impaired, leading to reduced stroke volume and cardiac output. Reduced stroke volume in severe cases may also be due to the cardiac tamponade caused by the accumulation of fluid rich in mucopolysaccharides within the pericardial sac.

Electrolyte Disturbances and Renal Manifestations

Hyponatremia is a common finding observed in patients with myxedema coma. The mechanism accounting for the hyponatremia is associated with increased serum antidiuretic hormone[16] and impaired water diuresis caused by reduced delivery of water to the distal nephron.[17] Depending on its duration and severity, hyponatremia will add to altered mental status, and when severe may be largely responsible for precipitating the comatose state. Alterations in renal function observed in myxedema coma include decreases in glomerular filtration rate and renal plasma flow, and increases in total body water. Atony of the urinary bladder with retention of large residual urine volumes is commonly seen. Renal failure may occur as a result of underlying rhabdomyolysis with extremely high levels of creatine kinase.[18–21]

Gastrointestinal Manifestations

The gastrointestinal tract in myxedema may be marked by mucopolysaccharide infiltration and edema of the muscularis, as well as neuropathic changes leading to gastric atony, impaired peristalsis, and even paralytic ileus. Ascites may occur, and has been documented in one report of 51 cases.[22] Another potential complication is gastrointestinal bleeding secondary to an associated coagulopathy.[23] It is important to recognize the underlying mechanisms of these acute gastrointestinal complications so as to avoid unnecessary surgery for an apparent acute abdomen.[24]

Hematological Manifestations

In contrast to the tendency to thrombosis seen in mild hypothyroidism, severe hypothyroidism is associated with a higher risk of bleeding caused by coagulopathy related to an acquired von Willebrand syndrome (type 1) and decreases in factors V, VII, VIII, IX, and X.[25] The von Willebrand syndrome is reversible with T4 therapy.[26] Another cause of bleeding may be disseminated intravascular coagulation associated with sepsis. Patients with myxedema coma have increased preponderance to severe infections, including sepsis, because of granulocytopenia and a decreased cell-mediated immunologic response. Such patients may also present with a microcytic anemia secondary to hemorrhage, or a macrocytic anemia caused by vitamin B_{12} deficiency, which may also worsen the neurologic state.

Diagnosis

To summarize the aforementioned clinical manifestations, the typical patient presenting with myxedema coma is a woman in the later decades of life who may have a history of thyroid disease and who is admitted to hospital, typically in winter, with pneumonia. Physical findings could include bradycardia, macroglossia, hoarseness, delayed reflexes, dry skin, general cachexia, hypoventilation, and hypothermia, commonly without shivering. Laboratory evaluation may indicate hypoxemia, hypercapnia, anemia, hyponatremia, hypercholesterolemia, and increased serum lactate dehydrogenase and creatine kinase. On lumbar puncture there is increased pressure and the cerebrospinal fluid has high protein content.

Although an elevated serum thyrotropin (TSH) concentration is the most important laboratory evidence for the diagnosis, the presence of severe complicating systemic illness or treatment with drugs such as dopamine, dobutamine, or corticosteroids may serve to reduce the elevation in TSH levels.[27,28] There may also be a pituitary cause for the hypothyroidism, in which case an increased TSH would not be found.

Treatment

Myxedema coma as a true medical emergency requires a multifaceted approach to treatment in a critical care setting.

Airways and ventilation

The patient's comatose state is perpetuated by hypoventilation, with CO_2 retention and respiratory acidosis. The maintenance of an adequate airway is the single most important supportive measure, because of the high mortality rate associated with the inexorable respiratory failure. Mechanical ventilation is usually required during the first 36 to 48 hours, but in some patients it may be necessary to continue assisted ventilation for as long as 2 to 3 weeks. The hypercapnia may be rapidly relieved with mechanical ventilation, but the hypoxia tends to persist, possibly because of shunting in nonaerated lung areas.[29] It is advisable, therefore, not to extubate the patients prematurely and to wait until full consciousness is attained.

Thyroid hormone therapy

One of the most controversial aspects of the management of myxedema coma is which thyroid hormone preparation to give and how to give it (dose, frequency, and route of administration). The optimum treatment remains uncertain, because of the scarcity of clinical studies and obvious difficulties with performing controlled trials. There is a necessity to balance the need for quickly attaining physiologically effective thyroid hormone levels against the risk of precipitating a fatal tachyarrhythmia or myocardial infarction. All patients should have continuous ECG monitoring, with reduction in thyroid hormone dosage should arrhythmias or ischemic changes be detected.

Parenteral preparations of either T4 or T3 are available for intravenous administration. Although oral forms of either T3 or T4 can be given by nasogastric tube in the comatose patient, this route is fraught with risks of aspiration and uncertain absorption, particularly in the presence of gastric atony or ileus. The single intravenous bolus of T4 was popularized by reports[30] suggesting that replacement of the entire estimated pool of extrathyroidal T4 (usually 300–600 μg) was desirable to restore near-normal hormonal status. This initial loading dose is followed by the maintenance dose of 50 to 100 μg given daily (either intravenously or by mouth if the patient is adequately alert). Larger doses of T4 probably have no advantage and may, in fact, be more dangerous.[31] There is also evidence showing improved outcomes with lower doses of thyroid hormone.[32] Rodriguez and colleagues[1] performed a prospective trial in which patients were randomized to receive either a 500-μg loading dose of T4 followed by a 100-μg daily maintenance dose, or only the maintenance dose. The overall mortality rate was 36.4%, with a lower mortality rate in the high-dose group (17%) than in the low-dose group (60%). Although suggestive, the difference was not statistically significant.

The rate of conversion of T4 to T3 is reduced in many systemic illnesses (the euthyroid sick or low T3 syndrome),[28] hence T3 generation may be reduced in myxedema coma as a consequence of any associated illness (hypothyroid sick syndrome). As a consequence, some clinicians suggest that small supplements of T3 should be given along with T4 during the initial few days of treatment, especially if obvious associated illness is present. When therapy is approached with T3 alone, it may be given as a 10- to 20-μg bolus followed by 10 μg every 4 hours for the first 24 hours, dropping to 10 μg every 6 hours for days 2 to 3, by which time oral administration should be feasible.[6] T3 has a much quicker onset of action than T4, and increases in body temperature and oxygen consumption may occur 2 to 3 hours after intravenous T3, compared with 8 to 14 hours after intravenous T4. The other advantage of T3 is that it crosses the blood-brain barrier more rapidly than T4, which may be particularly important in patients with profound neuropsychological symptoms.[33] One clinical example of the possible benefit of T3 is a case report of a patient with myxedema coma and cardiogenic shock who responded to T3 therapy but not to T4 therapy.[34] On the other hand, treatment with T3 alone is associated with large and unpredictable fluctuations in serum T3 levels, and high serum T3 levels during treatment have been associated with fatal outcomes.[35] A more conservative but seemingly rational approach is to provide combined therapy with both T4 and T3.[36] Rather than administer 300 to 500 μg T4 intravenously initially, a dose of 4 μg/kg lean body weight (or about 200–300 μg) is given, and an additional 100 μg is given 24 hours later. By the third day, the dose is reduced to a daily maintenance dose of 50 μg, which can be given by mouth as soon as the patient is conscious.[36] Simultaneously with the initial dose of T4, a bolus of 10 μg T3 is given and intravenous T3 is continued at a dosage of 10 μg every 8 to 12 hours until the patient is conscious and taking maintenance T4. Clinical improvement has been seen with even a single dose of only 2.5 μg of T3.[37]

Hypothermia
Treatment with T4 and/or T3 enables restoration of body temperature to normal. Simultaneously, blankets or increasing the room temperature can be used as additional interventions to keep the patient warm until the thyroid hormone effect is

achieved. Too aggressive warming may cause peripheral vasodilatation, which may then lead to hypotension or shock.

Hypotension

Hypotension should also be correctable by treatment with T4 and/or T3. However, a hypotensive patient may require additional volume-repletion therapy. Fluids may be administered cautiously as 5% to 10% glucose in 0.5 N sodium chloride if hypoglycemia is present, or as isotonic normal saline if hyponatremia is present. An agent such as dopamine might be used to maintain coronary blood flow, but patients should be weaned off the vasopressor as soon as possible because of the risk of a pressor-induced ischemic event.

Because of the risk of relative adrenal insufficiency, it is wise to administer hydrocortisone until the hypotension is corrected. The typical dosage of hydrocortisone is 50 to 100 mg every 6 to 8 hours during the first 7 to 10 days, with tapering of the dosage thereafter based on clinical response and any plans for further diagnostic evaluation. Decreased adrenal reserve has been found in 5% to 10% of patients, based on either hypopituitarism or primary adrenal failure accompanying Hashimoto disease (Schmidt syndrome). The other rationale for the treatment with corticosteroids is the potential risk of precipitating acute adrenal insufficiency caused by the accelerated metabolism of cortisol that follows T4 therapy. The clinicians should be aware of signs and symptoms signaling coexisting adrenal insufficiency such as hypotension, hypothermia, hypoglycemia, hyperkalemia, and hyponatremia.

Hyponatremia

Low serum sodium may cause a semicomatose state or seizures even in euthyroid patients, and the severe hyponatremia (105–120 mmol/L) in profound myxedema is likely to contribute substantially to the coma in these patients. Mortality rates in critically ill patients with symptomatic hyponatremia have been reported to be 60-fold higher than in patients without hyponatremia.[38] The appropriate management of severe hyponatremia often requires administration of a small amount of hypertonic saline (50–100 mL 3% sodium chloride), enough to increase sodium concentration by about 2 mmol/L early in the course of treatment, followed by an intravenous bolus dose of 40 to 120 mg furosemide to promote a water diuresis.[39] A small, quick increase in the serum sodium concentration (2–4 mmol/L) is effective in acute hyponatremia because even a slight reduction in brain swelling results in a substantial decrease in intracerebral pressure.[40] On the other hand, too rapid correction of hyponatremia can cause a dangerous complication, the osmotic demyelination syndrome. In patients with chronic hyponatremia, this complication is avoided by limiting the sodium correction to less than 10 to 12 mmol/L in 24 hours and less than 18 mmol/L in 48 h. After achieving a sodium level of more than 120 mmol/L, restriction of fluids may be all that is necessary to correct hyponatremia. It must be emphasized that fluid or saline therapy requires careful monitoring of volume status based on clinical parameters and measurements of central venous pressure, especially in patients with significant cardiovascular decompensation.

The other therapeutic option is treatment with an intravenous vasopressin antagonist, conivaptan. Conivaptan has been approved by the US Food and Drug Administration for the treatment of hospitalized patients with euvolemic and hypervolemic hyponatremia in a setting of the syndrome of inappropriate secretion of antidiuretic hormone, hypothyroidism, adrenal insufficiency, or pulmonary disorders.[41] The rationale for application of conivaptan in this clinical setting is based on the high vasopressin levels observed in myxedema coma. Current dosing recommendations are for a 20-mg loading dose to be infused over 30 minutes followed by 20 mg/d continuous infusion for up to 4 days. Unfortunately, no data are available on the use of conivaptan in severe hyponatremia (<115 mEq/L) in hypothyroid patients.[42,43]

General supportive measures

In addition to the specific therapies outlined, other treatments will be indicated as in the management of any other elderly patient with multisystem problems. Management might include the treatment of underlying problems such as infection, congestive heart failure, diabetes, or hypertension. The dosage of specific medications (eg, digoxin for congestive heart failure) may need to be modified based on their altered distribution and slowed metabolism in myxedema.

Prognosis

Even with this vigorous therapy, the prognosis for myxedema coma remains grim, and patients with severe hypothermia and hypotension seem to do the worst. In the past the mortality rate was as high as 60% to 70%, but this has now been reduced to 20%–25% with the advances in intensive care management.[44] Several prognostic factors may be associated with a fatal outcome,[1,5,32,35,45] and include older age, persistent hypothermia or bradycardia, lower degree of consciousness by Glasgow Coma Scale, multiorgan impairment indicated by an APACHE II score (Acute Physiology and Chronic Health Evaluation) of more than 20, or SOFA score (Sequential Organ Failure Assessment) of more than 6. The most common causes of death are respiratory failure, sepsis, and gastrointestinal bleeding. Early diagnosis and prompt treatment, with meticulous attention to the details of management during the first 48 hours, remain critical for effective therapy.

THYROTOXIC STORM

Thyroid crisis or thyrotoxic storm is characterized by severely exaggerated manifestations of thyrotoxicosis. The underlying cause of thyrotoxicosis is commonly Graves disease or toxic multinodular goiter. Rarely, thyrotoxic storm may occur with subacute thyroiditis or factitious thyrotoxicosis caused by intentional thyroxine overdose.[46,47]

Epidemiology and Precipitating Events

An accurate estimation of the incidence of thyroid storm is impossible to determine because of the considerable variability in the criteria for its diagnosis. The syndrome does appear to be less common today than in the past, perhaps because of earlier diagnosis and treatment of thyrotoxicosis, thereby precluding its progression to the stage of crisis. Nevertheless, it may occur in 1% to 2% of hospital admissions for thyrotoxicosis.[48] Thyrotoxic storm is rarely seen after thyroid surgery, because of the routine preparation of patients for elective thyroidectomy by treatment with antithyroid drugs. However, several types of nonthyroidal surgeries or other traumas have precipitated surgical thyrotoxic storm in patients with previously undiagnosed thyrotoxicosis. The crisis may be related to perioperative events, such as anesthesia, stress, and volume depletion, because these conditions are associated with increases in the concentration of free thyroid hormone. Thyroid storm has been seen in pregnancy, during labor, and in complicated deliveries such as those with placenta previa.[49] An acute discharge of hormones in the appropriate clinical setting may trigger a crisis, and cases have been reported following vigorous palpation of the thyroid, radioactive iodine therapy,[50] withdrawal of propylthiouracil therapy, or after administration of lithium, stable iodine, or iodinated contrast dyes. The other conditions known to be associated with increased free fraction of T4 and T3 include stress, infections, burns, cytotoxic chemotherapy for acute leukemia, aspirin overdose, ketoacidosis, or organophosphate intoxication (see **Table 1**).[45,51–55] Amiodarone, an antiarrhythmic and antianginal drug that is also rich in iodine, may cause either an iodine-induced thyrotoxicosis (type 1) or a destructive thyroiditis (type 2); the latter has been reported as a cause of thyroid storm refractory to the usual treatment.[56] There is also a case report of thyrotoxic storm precipitated by food poisoning with marine neurotoxin after ingestion of seafood.[57] Notwithstanding the multiplicity of precipitating factors, in hospitalized patients the most common event associated with thyrotoxic storm is some type of infection.

Clinical Signs and Symptoms

The clinical diagnosis is based on the identification of signs and symptoms that suggest decompensation of several organ systems. Some of these cardinal manifestations include fever out of proportion to an apparent infection and dramatic diaphoresis. Hyperthermia in thyroid crisis can represent defective thermoregulation by the hypothalamus and/or increased basal metabolic rate, increased oxidation of lipids being responsible for more than 60% of the resting energy expenditure.[58] The other key components of thyrotoxic storm include tachycardia out of proportion to the fever, and gastrointestinal dysfunction, which can include nausea, vomiting, diarrhea and, in severe cases, jaundice. As the storm progresses, symptoms of central nervous system dysfunction simulating an encephalopathic picture will appear, which may include increasing agitation and emotional lability, confusion, paranoia, psychosis, and coma.[59] Patients have been reported who presented with thyroid storm associated with status epilepticus and stroke and with bilateral basal ganglia infarction.[60] In patients with neurologic symptoms, a high index of suspicion for cerebral sinus thrombosis should be considered, because of the higher prevalence of this condition in severe hyperthyroidism.[61] Paralysis observed in thyroid crisis might be due to not only the cerebrovascular accident but also thyrotoxic periodic paralysis with hypokalemia, as frequently may present in Asian men.[62] In older patients, the thyrotoxic storm may present as so-called masked or apathetic thyrotoxicosis.[63]

Cardiovascular Manifestations

The most common cardiovascular manifestations are rhythm disturbances such as sinus tachycardia, atrial fibrillation, or other supraventricular tachyarrhythmias, and rarely, ventricular tachyarrhythmias, which can be observed even in patients without previous heart disease.[64] Congestive heart failure or a reversible dilated cardiomyopathy[65] also may be present even in young or middle-aged patients without known antecedent cardiac disease. A high-output state is present, attributable to the increased preload secondary to activation of the renin-angiotensin-aldosterone axis and to decreased afterload secondary to a direct relaxing effect of thyroid hormones on vascular muscle cells. Therefore, most patients present with systolic hypertension with widened pulse pressure. The hyperthyroid heart is characterized by higher than usual oxygen demands and hence myocardial infarction can be observed, even in young patients.[66,67] A relatively rare complication of severe hyperthyroidism is pulmonary hypertension, which is presumed to be on an autoimmune basis when associated with Graves disease, but which also may be secondary to an augmented blood volume, cardiac output, and sympathetic tone, leading to pulmonary vasoconstriction and increased pulmonary arterial pressure. This condition is usually reversible after treatment with antithyroid drugs. The other possible reason for pulmonary hypertension is pulmonary embolism caused by the thrombotic or hypercoagulable state that has been observed in severe hyperthyroidism.

Respiratory Manifestations

The main pulmonary symptom is dyspnea and tachypnea related to an increased oxygen demand. The excessive work of the respiratory muscles may eventually lead to diaphragmatic dysfunction.[68] Respiratory failure may result from the hyperdynamic cardiomyopathy but also from preexistent underlying pulmonary disease.[69,70]

Gastrointestinal Manifestations

The most common symptoms are diarrhea and vomiting, which can aggravate volume depletion, postural hypotension, and shock with vascular collapse. The diffuse abdominal pain, possibly caused by impaired neurohormonal regulation of gastric myoelectrical activity with delayed gastric emptying,[71] may even lead to a presentation such as acute abdomen[72] or intestinal obstruction.[73] The liver function abnormalities and presence of jaundice warrant immediate and vigorous therapy. Although most presentations of an acute abdomen in thyrotoxicosis are medical in nature, surgical conditions may also occur.[74]

Electrolyte Disturbances and Renal Manifestations

Increased serum calcium levels, caused by both hemoconcentration and known effects of thyroid hormone on bone resorption, may be seen. The sodium, potassium, and chloride levels are usually normal. Because of the augmented lipolysis and ketogenesis, and the basal metabolic demands that exceed oxygen delivery, ketoacidosis and lactic acidosis are observed.

Hyperthyroidism is often associated with an accelerated glomerular filtration rate, which may progress to glomerulosclerosis and excessive proteinuria. There are case reports of renal failure caused by rhabdomyolysis,[75] urinary retention associated with dyssynergy of the detrusor muscle and bladder dysfunction,[76] and an autoimmune complex–mediated nephritis concomitant with Graves disease.[77]

Hematological Manifestations

A moderate leukocytosis with a mild shift to the left is a common finding, even in the absence of infection. Hyperthyroidism may be associated with hypercoagulability caused by increased concentrations of fibrinogen, factors VIII and IX, tissue plasminogen activator inhibitor 1, von Willebrand factor, increase in red blood cell mass secondary to erythropoietin upregulation, and a tendency to augmented platelet plug formation.[78] Major thromboembolic complications are responsible for 18% of deaths caused by thyrotoxicosis.[79–83]

Diagnosis

Diagnosis can be established predominantly on the basis of clinical presentation, because the laboratory findings may not be much different than those observed in uncomplicated hyperthyroidism. Indeed, serum total T3 levels may be even within normal limits, as these patients may have some underlying precipitating illness that reduces T4 to T3 conversion as is seen in the euthyroid sick syndrome.[84] Therefore, a semiquantitative scale (**Table 2**) assessing the presence and severity of the most common signs and symptoms has been developed to aid in the diagnosis.[85]

Other laboratory abnormalities may include a modest hyperglycemia in the absence of diabetes mellitus, probably as a result of augmented glycogenolysis and catecholamine-mediated inhibition of insulin release, as well as increased insulin

Table 2
Semiquantitative scale assessing the presence and severity of the most common signs and symptoms

Criteria	Score
Thermoregulatory Dysfunction	
Temperature 99°–99.9°F (37.2°–37.7°C)	5
Temperature 100°–100.9°F (37.8°–38.2°C)	10
Temperature 101°–101.9°F (38.3°–38.8°C)	15
Temperature 102°–102.9°F (38.9°–39.3°C)	20
Temperature 103°–103.9°F (39.4°–39.9°C)	25
Temperature ≥104°F (40°C) or higher	30
Central Nervous System Effects	
Absent	0
Mild agitation	10
Delirium, psychosis, lethargy	20
Seizure or coma	30
Gastrointestinal Dysfunction	
Absent	0
Diarrhea, nausea, vomiting, abdominal pain	10
Unexplained jaundice	20
Cardiovascular Dysfunction (beats/min)	
90–109	5
110–119	10
120–129	15
130–139	20
≥140	25
Congestive Heart Failure	
Absent	0
Mild (edema)	5
Moderate (bibasilar rales)	10
Severe (pulmonary edema)	15
Atrial Fibrillation	
Absent	0
Present	10
History of Precipitating Event	
Absent	0
Present	10

Based on the total score, the likelihood of the diagnosis of thyrotoxic storm is: unlikely, <25; impending, 25–44; highly likely, >45.

Data from Burch HB, Wartofsky L. Life-threatening thyrotoxicosis. Thyroid storm. Endocrinol Metab Clin North Am 1993;22:263–77.

clearance and insulin resistance. When thyrotoxicosis is prolonged, leading to the depletion of glycogen deposits, hypoglycemia may occur, particularly in older people when aggravated by malnutrition secondary to emesis or abdominal pain.[86] Hepatic dysfunction in thyroid storm results in elevated levels of serum lactate dehydrogenase, aspartate aminotransferase, and bilirubin. Increased levels of serum alkaline phosphatase are also observed, predominantly because of increased osteoblastic bone activity in response to the augmentation of bone resorption.

Of importance, adrenal reserve may be exceeded in thyrotoxic crisis because of the inability of the adrenal gland to meet the metabolic demands and accelerated turnover of glucocorticoids. Moreover, there is known coincidence of adrenal insufficiency with Graves disease. This diagnosis should be considered when there is hypotension and suggestive electrolyte abnormalities.

Treatment

To avoid a disastrous outcome, a complex approach to management is recommended.[87] First, specific antithyroid drugs must be used to reduce the increased thyroid production and release of T4 and T3. The second approach comprises treatment intended to block the effects of the remaining but excessive circulating concentrations of free T4 and T3 in blood. The third arm involves treatment of any systemic decompensation, for example, congestive heart failure, and shock. The final component addresses any underlying precipitating illness such as infection or ketoacidosis.

Therapy directed to the thyroid gland

Inhibition of new synthesis of the thyroid hormones is achieved by administration of thionamide antithyroid drugs, such as carbimazole, methimazole (Tapazole), and propylthiouracil. These drugs in the comatose or uncooperative patient are given by nasogastric tube or per rectum as enemas or suppositories.[88-91] There are no available intravenous preparations of these compounds in the United States, but they are successfully used in some European countries such as the United Kingdom, Germany, and Poland.[92-94] According to the recently published guidelines by the American Thyroid Association and the Association of Clinical Endocrinologists, propylthiouracil can be started with a loading dose of 500 to 1000 mg followed by 250 mg every 4 hours, and methimazole should be administered at daily dose of 60 to 80 mg.[87] It is thought that propylthiouracil will provide more rapid clinical improvement because it has the additional advantage of inhibiting conversion of T4 to T3, a property not shared by methimazole. Because thionamides reduce new hormone synthesis but not thyroidal secretion of preformed glandular stores of hormone, separate treatment must be administered to inhibit proteolysis of colloid and the continuing release of T4 and T3 into the blood. Either inorganic iodine or lithium carbonate may be used for this purpose. Iodides may be given either orally as Lugol solution or as a saturated solution of potassium iodide (3–5 drops every 6 hours). An earlier mainstay of treatment, the use of an intravenous infusion of sodium iodide (0.5–1 g every 12 hours), has not been feasible recently because sterile sodium iodide has not been available for intravenous use.

It is important that iodine should be administered no sooner than 1 hour after prior thionamide dosage. Otherwise iodine will enhance thyroid hormone synthesis, enrich hormone stores within the gland, and thereby permit further exaggeration of thyrotoxicosis. When iodine is administered in conjunction with full doses of antithyroid drugs, dramatic rapid decreases in serum T4 are seen, with values approaching the normal range within 4 or 5 days.[95] Other agents that theoretically could be used in this manner are the radiographic contrast dyes ipodate (Oragrafin) and iopanoic acid (Telepaque), which act not only by decreasing thyroid hormone release but also by slowing the peripheral conversion of T4 to T3, as well as possibly blocking binding of both T3 and T4 to their cellular receptors. Unfortunately, these agents are no longer available in the United States.

In patients who may be allergic to iodine, lithium carbonate may be used as an alternative agent to inhibit hormonal release.[96,97] Lithium should be administered initially as 300 mg every 6 hours, with subsequent adjustment of dosage as necessary to maintain serum lithium levels at about 0.8 to 1.2 mEq/L.

Therapy directed at the continuing effects of thyroid hormone in the periphery
Given the presence and likelihood of high levels of circulating T4 and T3 in a large vascular pool and tissue distribution space, in severe cases treatment with antithyroid drugs alone is not sufficient. Plasmapheresis and therapeutic plasma exchange are effective alternative therapies, which can reduce T4 and T3 levels within 36 hours. Plasma or albumin solution given during therapeutic plasma exchange provides new binding sites to reduce circulating levels of free thyroid hormones.[98–100] However, this effect is transient and lasts only about 24 to 48 hours, and thus should be followed by a more definitive therapy. Early thyroidectomy has been reported to reduce the mortality rate from 20% to 40% under standard treatment to less than 10%.[101]

Peritoneal dialysis or experimental hemoperfusion through a resin bed[102] or charcoal columns[103] has also been used. Another therapeutic adjunct is the oral administration of cholestyramine resin, resulting in removal of T4 and T3 by binding thyroid hormone entering the gut via enterohepatic recirculation, with the subsequent excretion of the resin-hormone complex.[104]

Hughes[105] was the first to treat a patient with thyrotoxic storm with a β-adrenergic blocker to ameliorate the manifestations of thyroid hormone excess. Propranolol is the most commonly used agent in the United States. The oral dosage of 60 to 80 mg every 4 hours or intravenous doses of 0.5 to 1 mg followed by subsequent doses of 2 to 3 mg given intravenously over 10 to 15 min every several hours are recommended, alongside constant cardiac rhythm monitoring.[87,106,107] There may be a theoretical benefit derived from the inhibitory effect of propranolol on the conversion of T4 to T3,[108] but a significant effect is seen only with oral doses higher than 160 mg/d. Usage of β-blockers not only corrects the heart rate and diminishes the oxygen demand of the cardiac muscle, but also improves agitation, convulsions, psychotic behavior, tremor, diarrhea, fever, and diaphoresis. In some patients, there may be a relative risks or contraindications to the use of these agents. In patients with a history of bronchospasm or asthma and treatment with either selective β1-blockers or reserpine, guanethidine should be considered instead. A short-acting β-adrenergic blocker, esmolol, has also been used successfully in the management of thyroid storm. An initial loading dose of 0.25 to 0.5 mg/kg is followed by continuous infusion of 0.05 to 0.1 mg/kg per minute.[109,110]

The other important medications characterized by a high therapeutic potency and modest ability to inhibit peripheral conversion of T4 to T3 are steroids. An initial dose of 300 mg hydrocortisone followed by 100 mg every 8 hours during the first 24 to 36 hours should be adequate. Thyroid storm has been reported to recur when steroids had been discontinued after initial clinical improvement.[111] The additional rationale behind the routine use of steroids is perhaps theoretical and unproven, but relates to possible relative adrenal insufficiency secondary to increased metabolic demands and more rapid turnover of cortisol.

Some authorities have suggested that the supplemental administration of 1α(OH) vitamin D_3 might accelerate the reduction of serum T4 and T3.[112] In a recent study, the administration of 2 g/d L-carnitine in thyrotoxic storm facilitated a dose reduction of methimazole. The mechanism appears to be related to an inhibition by L-carnitine of T3 and T4 entry into cell nuclei.[113,114] Although these preliminary findings are of interest, the utility of this adjunct to therapy requires confirmation.

Therapy directed at systemic decompensation
Fluid depletion caused by hyperpyrexia and diaphoresis, as well as by vomiting or diarrhea, must be vigorously replaced to avoid vascular collapse. Appropriate fluid therapy will usually correct hypercalcemia, if present. Judicious replacement of fluids

is necessary in elderly patients with congestive heart failure or other cardiac compromise. Intravenous fluids containing 10% dextrose in addition to electrolytes will better restore depleted hepatic glycogen. Vitamin supplements may be added to the intravenous fluids to replace probable coexistent deficiency. Hypotension not readily reversed by adequate hydration may temporarily require pressor and/or glucocorticoid therapy.

For fever, acetaminophen rather than salicylates is the preferred antipyretic, because salicylates inhibit thyroid hormone binding and could increase free T4 and T3, thereby transiently worsening the thyrotoxic crisis. Hyperthermia also responds well to external cooling with alcohol sponging, cooling blankets, and ice packs. Some investigators advocate the use of the skeletal muscle relaxant dantrolene,[115] but significant risk associated with its use precludes routine recommendation. When present, congestive heart failure should be treated routinely. Although less commonly used today, when digoxin is used, larger than usual doses may be required because of its increased turnover in the thyrotoxic state.

Therapy directed at the precipitating illness

The therapy is not complete unless a diagnosis of the possible precipitating event is made and early treatment as indicated for that underlying illness is implemented. This is not a problem in obvious cases, when trauma, surgery, labor, or premature withdrawal of antithyroid drugs are known to have been the precipitants of thyrotoxic crisis, and which may require no additional management. However, when none of the latter precipitating factors is apparent, a diligent search for some focus of infection must be performed. Routine cultures of urine, blood, and sputum should be obtained in the febrile thyrotoxic patient, and cultures of other sites may be warranted on clinical grounds. Broad-spectrum antibiotic coverage on an empiric basis may be required initially while awaiting results of cultures.

Conditions such as ketoacidosis, pulmonary thromboembolism, or stroke may underlie thyrotoxic crisis, particularly in the obtunded or psychotic patient, and require the same vigorous management as routinely indicated.

Prognosis

Even with early diagnosis, death can occur, and reported mortality rates have ranged from 10% to 75% in hospitalized patients.[85,116,117] In most patients who survive thyrotoxic crisis, clinical improvement is dramatic and demonstrable within the first 24 hours. During the recovery period of the next few days, supportive therapy such as corticosteroids, antipyretics, and intravenous fluids may be tapered and gradually withdrawn, based on patient status, oral intake of calories and fluids, vasomotor stability, and continuing improvement. After the crisis has been resolved, attention may be turned to consideration of the definitive treatment of thyrotoxicosis. Should thyroidectomy be considered, thyrotoxicosis will need to have been adequately treated preoperatively, to obviate any likelihood of another episode of crisis during the surgery. Total thyroidectomy is the procedure of choice, in view of reports of recurrent severe thyrotoxicosis and thyroid crisis after less than total thyroidectomy.[118]

Radioactive iodine as definitive treatment is often precluded by the recent use of inorganic iodine in virtually all cases of storm, but it could be considered at a later date, in which case antithyroid thionamide therapy is continued to restore and maintain euthyroidism until such a time as ablative therapy can be administered. Continuing treatment with antithyroid drugs alone, in the hope of the patient's sustaining a spontaneous remission, is also possible.

SUMMARY

The life-threatening thyroid emergencies of myxedema coma and thyrotoxic crisis require a high index of suspicion in the appropriate clinical setting, followed by prompt and accurate diagnosis and urgent multifaceted therapy to reduce the risk of fatal outcome.

REFERENCES

1. Rodriguez I, Fluiters E, Perez-Mendez LF, et al. Factors associated with mortality of patients with myxedema coma: prospective study in 11 cases treated in a single institution. J Endocrinol 2004;80:347–50.
2. Blignault EJ. Advanced pregnancy in severely myxedematous patient. A case report and review of the literature. S Afr Med J 1980;57:1050–1.
3. Patel S, Robinson S, Bidgood RJ, et al. A pre-eclamptic-like syndrome associated with hypothyroidism during pregnancy. Q J Med 1991;79:435–41.
4. Mathew V, Misgar RA, Ghosh S, et al. Myxedema coma: a new look into an old crisis. J Thyroid Res 2011;2011:493462.
5. Dutta P, Bhansali A, Masoodi SR, et al. Predictors of outcome in myxedema coma: a study from a tertiary care centre. Crit Care 2008;12:1–8.
6. Klubo-Gwiezdzinska J, Wartofsky L. Myxedema coma. In: Oxford textbook of endocrinology and Diabetes. 2nd edition. Oxford: Oxford Univ. Press; 2011. p. 537–43.
7. Kwaku MP, Burman KD. Myxedema coma. J Intensive Care Med 2007;22: 224–31.
8. Church CO, Callen EC. Myxedema coma associated with combination aripiprazole and sertraline therapy. Ann Pharmacother 2009;43:2113–6.
9. Chu M, Seltzer TF. Myxedema coma induced by ingestion of raw bok choy. N Engl J Med 2010;20(362):1945–6.
10. Reinhardt W, Mann K. Incidence, clinical picture and treatment of hypothyroid coma. Results of a survey. Med Klin 1997;92:521–4.
11. Jansen HJ, Doebe SR, Louwerse ES, et al. Status epilepticus caused by a myxedema coma. Neth J Med 2006;64:202–5.
12. Zwillich CW, Pierson DJ, Hofeldt FD, et al. Ventilatory control in myxedema and hypothyroidism. N Engl J Med 1975;292:662–5.
13. Ladenson PW, Goldenheim PD, Ridgway EC. Prediction of reversal of blunted respiratory responsiveness in patients with hypothyroidism. Am J Med 1988; 84:877–83.
14. Birring SS, Patel RB, Parker D, et al. Airway function and markers of airway inflammation in patients with treated hypothyroidism. Thorax 2005;60:249–53.
15. Schenck JB, Rizvi AA, Lin T. Severe primary hypothyroidism manifesting with torsades de pointes. Am J Med Sci 2006;331:154–6.
16. Skowsky RW, Kikuchi TA. The role of vasopressin in the impaired water excretion of myxedema. Am J Med 1978;64:613–21.
17. DeRubertis FR Jr, Michelis MF, Bloom ME, et al. Impaired water excretion in myxedema. Am J Med 1971;51:41–53.
18. Ardalan MR, Ghabili K, Mirnour R, et al. Hypothyroidism-induced rhabdomyolysis and renal failure. Ren Fail 2011;33:553–4.
19. Nikolaidou C, Gouridou E, Ilonidis G, et al. Acute renal dysfunction in a patient presenting with rhabdomyolysis due to hypothyroidism attributed to Hashimoto's disease. Hippokratia 2010;4:281–3.
20. Kar PM, Hirani A, Allen MJ. Acute renal failure in a hypothyroid patient with rhabdomyolysis. Clin Nephrol 2003;60:428–9.

21. Birewar S, Oppenheimer M, Zawada ET Jr. Hypothyroid acute renal failure. S D J Med 2004;57:109–10.
22. Ji JS, Chae HS, Cho YS, et al. Myxedema ascites: case report and literature review. J Korean Med Sci 2006;21:761–4.
23. Fukunaga K. Refractory gastrointestinal bleeding treated with thyroid hormone replacement. J Clin Gastroenterol 2001;33:145–7.
24. Bergeron E, Mitchell A, Heyen F, et al. Acute colonic surgery and unrecognized hypothyroidism: a warning. Report of six cases. Dis Colon Rectum 1997;40: 859–61.
25. Manfredi E, van Zaane B, Gerdes VE, et al. Hypothyroidism and acquired von Willebrand's syndrome: a systematic review. Haemophilia 2008;14:423–33.
26. Michiels JJ, Schroyens W, Berneman Z, et al. Acquired von Willebrand syndrome type 1 in hypothyroidism: reversal after treatment with thyroxine. Clin Appl Thromb Hemost 2001;7:113–5.
27. Hooper MJ. Diminished TSH secretion during acute non-thyroidal illness in untreated primary hypothyroidism. Lancet 1976;1:48–9.
28. Wartofsky L, Burman KD. Alterations in thyroid function in patients with systemic illness: the 'euthyroid sick syndrome'. Endocr Rev 1982;3:164–217.
29. Nicoloff JT. Thyroid storm and myxedema coma. Med Clin North Am 1985;69: 1005–17.
30. Holvey DN, Goodner CJ, Nicoloff JT, et al. Treatment of myxedema coma with intravenous thyroxine. Arch Intern Med 1964;113:139–46.
31. Ridgway EC, McCammon JA, Benotti J, et al. Acute metabolic responses in myxedema to large doses of intravenous l-thyroxine. Ann Intern Med 1972;77: 549–55.
32. Yamamoto T, Fukuyama J, Fujiyoshi A. Factors associated with mortality of myxedema coma: report of eight cases and literature survey. Thyroid 1999;9:1167–74.
33. Chernow B, Burman KD, Johnson DL, et al. T3 may be a better agent than T4 in the critically ill hypothyroid patient: evaluation of transport across the blood-brain barrier in a primate model. Crit Care Med 1983;11:99–104.
34. McKerrow SD, Osborn LA, Levy H, et al. Myxedema-associated cardiogenic shock treated with triiodothyronine. Ann Intern Med 1992;117:1014–5.
35. Hylander B, Rosenqvist U. Treatment of myxedema coma: factors associated with fatal outcome. Acta Endocrinol (Copenh) 1985;108:65–71.
36. Wartofsky L. Myxedema coma. Endocrinol Metab Clin North Am 2006;35: 687–98.
37. McCulloch W, Price P, Hinds CJ, et al. Effects of low dose oral triiodothyronine in myxedema coma. Intensive Care Med 1985;11:259–62.
38. Vachharajani TJ, Zaman F, Abreo KD. Hyponatremia in critically ill patients. J Intensive Care Med 2003;18:3–8.
39. Pereira VG, Haron ES, Lima-Neto N, et al. Management of myxedema coma: report on three successfully treated cases with nasogastric or intravenous administration of triiodothyronine. J Endocrinol Invest 1982;5:331–4.
40. Verbalis JG, Goldsmith SR, Greenberg A, et al. Hyponatremia treatment guidelines 2007: expert panel recommendations. Am J Med 2007;120:1–21.
41. Vaprisol (conivaptan HCl injection) [package insert]. Deerfield (IL): Astellas Tokai Co; 2006.
42. Hline SS, Pham PT, Pham PT, et al. Conivaptan: a step forward in the treatment of hyponatremia. Ther Clin Risk Manag 2008;4:315–26.
43. Li-Ng M, Verbalis JG. Conivaptan: evidence supporting its therapeutic use in hyponatremia. Core Evid 2010;4:83–92.

44. Devdhar M, Ousman YH, Burman KD. Hypothyroidism. Endocrinol Metab Clin North Am 2007;36:595–615.

45. Jordan RM. Myxedema coma. Pathophysiology, therapy, and factors affecting prognosis. Med Clin North Am 1995;79:185–94.

46. Swinburne JL, Kreisman SH. A rare case of subacute thyroiditis causing thyroid storm. Thyroid 2007;17:73–6.

47. Yoon SJ, Choi SR, Kim DM, et al. A case of thyroid storm due to thyrotoxicosis factitia. Yonsei Med J 2003;44:351–4.

48. Klubo-Gwiezdzinska J, Wartofsky L. Thyrotoxic storm. In: Oxford textbook of endocrinology and diabetes. 2nd edition. Oxford: Oxford Univ. Press; 2011. p. 454–61.

49. Tewari K, Balderston KD, Carpenter SE, et al. Papillary thyroid carcinoma manifesting as thyroid storm of pregnancy: case report. Am J Obstet Gynecol 1998; 179:818–9.

50. McDermott MT, Kidd GS, Dodson LE, et al. Radioiodine-induced thyroid storm. Am J Med 1983;75:353–9.

51. Naito Y, Sone T, Kataoka K, et al. Thyroid storm due to functioning metastatic thyroid carcinoma in a burn patient. Anesthesiology 1997;87:433–5.

52. Al-Anazi KA, Inam S, Jeha MT, et al. Thyrotoxic crisis induced by cytotoxic chemotherapy. Support Care Cancer 2005;13:196–8.

53. Sebe A, Satar S, Sari A. Thyroid storm induced by aspirin intoxication and the effect of hemodialysis: a case report. Adv Ther 2004;21:173–7.

54. Hirvonen EA, Niskanen LK, Niskanen MM. Thyroid storm prior to induction of anaesthesia. Anaesthesia 2004;59:1020–2.

55. Yuan YD, Seak CJ, Lin CC, et al. Thyroid storm precipitated by organophosphate intoxication. Am J Emerg Med 2007;25:861.

56. Samaras K, Marel GM. Failure of plasmapheresis, corticosteroids and thionamides to ameliorate a case of protracted amiodarone-induced thyroiditis. Clin Endocrinol 1996;45:365–8.

57. Noh KW, Seon CS, Choi JW, et al. Thyroid storm and reversible thyrotoxic cardiomyopathy after ingestion of seafood stew thought to contain marine neurotoxin. Thyroid 2011;21:679–82.

58. Riis AL, Gravholt CH, Djurhuus CB, et al. Elevated regional lipolysis in hyperthyroidism. J Clin Endocrinol Metab 2002;87:4747–53.

59. Aiello DP, DuPlessis AJ, Pattishall EG III, et al. Thyroid storm presenting with coma and seizures. Clin Pediatr (Phila) 1989;28:571–4.

60. Lee TG, Ha CK, Lim BH. Thyroid storm presenting as status epilepticus and stroke. Postgrad Med J 1997;73:61.

61. Dai A, Wasay M, Dubey N, et al. Superior sagittal sinus thrombosis secondary to hyperthyroidism. J Stroke Cerebrovasc Dis 2000;9:89–90.

62. Lu KC, Hsu YJ, Chiu JS, et al. Effects of potassium supplementation on the recovery of thyrotoxic periodic paralysis. Am J Emerg Med 2004;22:544–7.

63. Feroza M, May H. Apathetic thyrotoxicosis. Int J Clin Pract 1997;51:332–3.

64. Jao YT, Chen Y, Lee WH, et al. Thyroid storm and ventricular tachycardia. South Med J 2004;976:604–7.

65. Daly MJ, Wilson CM, Dolan SJ, et al. Reversible dilated cardiomyopathy associated with post-partum thyrotoxic storm. QJM 2009;102:217–9.

66. Opdahl H, Eritsland J, Sovik E. Acute myocardial infarction and thyrotoxic storm— a difficult and dangerous combination. Acta Anaesthesiol Scand 2005;49: 707–11.

67. Lee SM, Jung TS, Hahm JR, et al. Thyrotoxicosis with coronary spasm that required coronary artery bypass surgery. Intern Med 2007;46:1915–8.

68. Liu YC, Tsai WS, Chau T, et al. Acute hypercapnic respiratory failure due to thyrotoxic periodic paralysis. Am J Med Sci 2004;327:264–7.
69. Mezosi E, Szabo J, Nagy EV, et al. Nongenomic effect of thyroid hormone on free-radical production in human polymorphonuclear leukocytes. J Endocrinol 2005;185:121–9.
70. Luong KV, Nguyen LT. Hyperthyroidism and asthma. J Asthma 2000;37:125–30.
71. Barczynski M, Thor P. Reversible autonomic dysfunction in hyperthyroid patients affects gastric myoelectrical activity and emptying. Clin Auton Res 2001;114: 243–9.
72. Bhattacharyya A, Wiles PG. Thyrotoxic crisis presenting as acute abdomen. J R Soc Med 1997;90:681–2.
73. Cansler CL, Latham JA, Brown PM Jr, et al. Duodenal obstruction in thyroid storm. South Med J 1997;90:1143–6.
74. Leow MK, Chew DE, Zhu M, et al. Thyrotoxicosis and acute abdomen: still as defying and misunderstood today? Brief observations over the recent decade. QJM 2008;101:943–7.
75. van Hoek I, Daminet S. Interactions between thyroid and kidney function in pathological conditions of these organ systems: a review. Gen Comp Endocrinol 2008;160:205–15.
76. Goswami R, Seth A, Goswami AK, et al. Prevalence of enuresis and other bladder symptoms in patients with active Graves' disease. Br J Urol 1997; 804:563–6.
77. Kahara T, Yoshizawa M, Nakaya I, et al. Thyroid crisis following interstitial nephritis. Intern Med 2008;47:1237–40.
78. Homonick M, Gessl A, Ferlitsch A, et al. Altered platelet plug formation in hyperthyroidism and hypothyroidism. J Clin Endocrinol Metab 2007;92:3006–12.
79. Romualdi E, Squizzato A, Ageno W. Venous thrombosis: a possible complication of overt hyperthyroidism. Eur J Intern Med 2008;19:386–7.
80. Pekdemir M, Yilmaz S, Ersel M, et al. A rare cause of headache; cerebral venous sinus thrombosis due to hyperthyroidism. Am J Emerg Med 2008;26:383.
81. Osman F, Gamma MD, Sheppard MC, et al. Clinical review 142: cardiac dysrhythmias and thyroid dysfunction: the hidden menace? J Clin Endocrinol Metab 2002;87:963–7.
82. Squizzato A, Gerdes VE. Thyroid disease and haemostasis: a relationship with clinical implications? Thromb Haemost 2008;100:727–8.
83. Lippi G, Franchini M, Targher G, et al. Hyperthyroidism is associated with shortened APTT and increased fibrinogen values in a general population of unselected outpatients. J Thromb Thrombolysis 2008;28:362–5.
84. Wartofsky L. The low T3 or 'sick euthyroid syndrome': update 1994. In: Braverman LE, Refetoff S, editors. Endocrine Reviews monographs. 3. Clinical and molecular aspects of diseases of the thyroid. Bethesda (MD): The Endocrine Society; 1994. p. 248–51.
85. Burch HB, Wartofsky L. Life-threatening thyrotoxicosis. Thyroid storm. Endocrinol Metab Clin North Am 1993;22:263–77.
86. Kobayashi C, Sasaki H, Kosuge K, et al. Severe starvation hypoglycemia and congestive heart failure induced by thyroid crisis, with accidentally induced severe liver dysfunction and disseminated intravascular coagulation. Intern Med 2005;44:234–9.
87. Bahn Chair RS, Burch HB, Cooper DS, et al. American Thyroid Association; American Association of Clinical Endocrinologists. Hyperthyroidism and other causes of thyrotoxicosis: management guidelines of the American Thyroid

Association and American Association of Clinical Endocrinologists. Thyroid 2011;21:593–646.

88. Nareem N, Miner DJ, Amatruda JM. Methimazole: an alternative route of administration. J Clin Endocrinol Metab 1982;54:180–1.

89. Yeung SC, Go R, Balasubramanyam A. Rectal administration of iodide and propylthiouracil in the treatment of thyroid storm. Thyroid 1995;5:403–5.

90. Zweig SB, Schlosser JR, Thomas SA, et al. Rectal administration of propylthiouracil in suppository form in patients with thyrotoxicosis and critical illness: case report and review of literature. Endocr Pract 2006;12:43–7.

91. Ogiso S, Inamoto S, Hata H, et al. Successful treatment of gastric perforation with thyrotoxic crisis. Am J Emerg Med 2008;26:3–4.

92. Thomas DJ, Hardy J, Sarwar R, et al. Thyroid storm treated with intravenous methimazole in patients with gastrointestinal dysfunction. Br J Hosp Med (Lond) 2006;67:492–3.

93. Weissel M. Withdrawal of the parenterally applicable form of thyrostatic drugs in Austria. Thyroid 2005;15:1203.

94. Sowiński J, Junik R, Gembicki M. Effectiveness of intravenous administration of methimazole in patients with thyroid crisis. Endokrynol Pol 1988;39:67–73.

95. Wartofsky L, Ransil BJ, Ingbar SH. Inhibition by iodine of the release of thyroxine from the thyroid glands of patients with thyrotoxicosis. J Clin Invest 1970;49:78–86.

96. Boehm TM, Burman KD, Barnes S, et al. Lithium and iodine combination therapy for thyrotoxicosis. Acta Endocrinol (Copenh) 1980;94:174–83.

97. Reed J, Bradley EL III. Postoperative thyroid storm after lithium preparation. Surgery 1985;98:983–6.

98. Vyas AA, Vyas P, Fillipon NL, et al. Successful treatment of thyroid storm with plasmapheresis in a patient with methimazole-induced agranulocytosis. Endocr Pract 2010;16:673–6.

99. Ozbey N, Kalayoglu-Besisik S, Gul N, et al. Therapeutic plasmapheresis in patients with severe hyperthyroidism in whom antithyroid drugs are contraindicated. Int J Clin Pract 2004;58:554–8.

100. Ezer A, Caliskan K, Parlakgumus A, et al. Preoperative therapeutic plasma exchange in patients with thyrotoxicosis. J Clin Apher 2009;24:111–4.

101. Enghofer M, Badenhoop K, Zeuzem S, et al. Fulminant hepatitis A in a patient with severe hyperthyroidism; rapid recovery from hepatic coma after plasmapheresis and total thyroidectomy. J Clin Endocrinol Metab 2000;85:1765–9.

102. Burman KD, Yeager HC, Briggs WA, et al. Resin hemoperfusion: a method of removing circulating thyroid hormones. J Clin Endocrinol Metab 1976;42:70–8.

103. Candrina R, DiStefano O, Spandrio S, et al. Treatment of thyrotoxic storm by charcoal plasmaperfusion. J Endocrinol Invest 1989;12:133–4.

104. Solomon BL, Wartofsky L, Burman KD. Adjunctive cholestyramine therapy for thyrotoxicosis. Clin Endocrinol (Oxf) 1993;38:39–43.

105. Hughes G. Management of thyrotoxic crisis with a beta-adrenergic blocking agent (pronethalol). Br J Clin Pract 1966;20:579–81.

106. Feely J, Forrest A, Gunn A, et al. Propranolol dosage in thyrotoxicosis. J Clin Endocrinol Metab 1980;51:658–61.

107. Rubenfeld S, Silverman VE, Welch KM, et al. Variable plasma propranolol levels in thyrotoxicosis. N Engl J Med 1979;300:353–4.

108. Wiersinga WM. Propranolol and thyroid hormone metabolism. Thyroid 1991;1:273–7.

109. Brunette DD, Rothong C. Emergency department management of thyrotoxic crisis with esmolol. Am J Emerg Med 1991;9:232–4.

110. Knighton JD, Crosse MM. Anaesthetic management of childhood thyrotoxicosis and the use of esmolol. Anaesthesia 1997;52:67–70.

111. Kidess AJ, Caplan RH, Reynertson MD, et al. Recurrence of ^{131}I induced thyroid storm after discontinuing glucocorticoid therapy. Wis Med J 1991;90:463–5.

112. Kawakami-Tani T, Fukawa E, Tanaka H, et al. Effect of alpha hydroxyvitamin D3 on serum levels of thyroid hormones in hyperthyroid patients with untreated Graves' disease. Metabolism 1997;46:1184–8.

113. Benvenga S, Lapa D, Cannavo S, et al. Successive thyroid storms treated with l-carnitine and low doses of methimazole. Am J Med 2003;115:417–8.

114. Benvenga S, Ruggeri RM, Russo A, et al. Usefulness of l-carnitine, a naturally occurring peripheral antagonist of thyroid hormone action, in iatrogenic hyperthyroidism: a randomized, double-blind, placebo-controlled clinical trial. J Clin Endocrinol Metab 2001;86:3579–94.

115. Bennett MH, Wainwright A. Acute thyroid crisis on induction of anesthesia. Anaesthesia 1989;44:28–30.

116. Dillman WH. Thyroid storm. Curr Ther Endocrinol Metab 1997;6:81–5.

117. Tietgens ST, Leinung MC. Thyroid storm. Med Clin North Am 1995;79:169–84.

118. Leow MK, Loh KC. Fatal thyroid crisis years after two thyroidectomies for Graves' disease: is thyroid tissue auto transplantation for postthyroidectomy hypothyroidism worthwhile? J Am Coll Surg 2002;195:434–5.

Index

Note: Page numbers of article titles are in **boldface** type.

A

Abscess, thyroid, 188–189
Acetaminophen, for thyrotoxic storm, 397
Adenomas
 pituitary, TSH-secreting, 185
 thyroid, 181–182
Adipose tissue, in Graves ophthalmopathy, 312
Adrenal failure, in myxedema coma, 390
Airway resuscitation, for myxedema coma, 388
Albumin, as hormone carrier, 170
Alemtuzumab, thyroid function effects of, 289
Allopurinol, for Graves ophthalmopathy, 318–319
Aluminum hydroxide, interfering with levothyroxine absorption, 291
American Thyroid System, cancer risk stratification guidelines of, 372–373
Amiodarone
 hyperthyroidism due to, 286–287
 hypothyroidism due to, 206, 263–264, 286
 thyrotoxicosis due to, 191–193, 264
Anaplastic thyroid cancer, 303
Ankle-jerk reflex, in hypothyroidism, 207
Antioxidant therapy, for Graves ophthalmopathy, 318–319
Antithyroid drugs
 for Graves disease, 180–182, 242–243
 hyperthyroidism due to, 286–287
Arrhythmias
 in myxedema coma, 387
 in thyrotoxic storm, 392
Artificial tears, for Graves ophthalmopathy, 318
Atrial fibrillation, in hyperthyroidism, 262–263, 299
Autoimmune thyroiditis, 204–206

B

Basal metabolism, in hypothyroidism, 207
Beta blockers
 for Graves disease, 243
 for hyperthyroidism, 300
 for subacute thyroiditis, 226
 for thyrotoxic storm, 396
Bethesda System for Reporting Thyroid Cytopathology, 338
Bexarotene, in TSH suppression, 284–285

doi:10.1016/S0025-7125(12)00056-9
0025-7125/12/$ – see front matter © 2012 Elsevier Inc. All rights reserved.